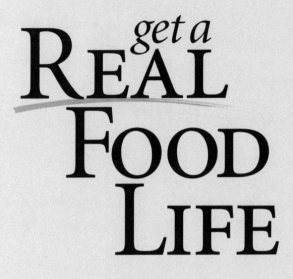

Get a Slimmer Body, Increased Energy, a Better Mood,
and Good Health for Life

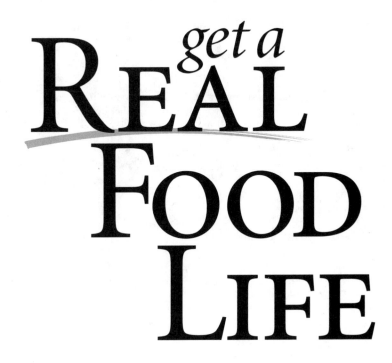

get a
REAL
FOOD
LIFE

Janine Whiteson, M.Sc.,
with Marion Rosenfeld

Medical Advisor: Lisa Hark, R.D., Ph.D., director of the nutrition
education and prevention program at the University of Pennsylvania
Medical Center in Philadelphia

RODALE

© 2002 by Janine Whiteson
Cover photograph by Lisa Koenig

Printed in the United States of America
Rodale Inc. makes every effort to use acid-free ∞, recycled paper ♻.

Interior Design by Joanna Williams
Cover Design by Christina Gaugler

Library of Congress Cataloging-in-Publication Data

Whiteson, Janine.
    Get a real food life : get a slimmer body, increased energy, a better mood, and good health for life / Janine Whiteson with Marion Rosenfeld.
        p.   cm.
    Includes index.
    ISBN 1–57954–485–1   hardcover
    1. Nutrition.   I. Rosenfeld, Marion.   II. Title.
RA784 .W595 2001
613.2—dc21   2001005874

Distributed to the book trade by St. Martin's Press

2   4   6   8   10   9   7   5   3   hardcover

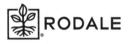

RODALE

WE **INSPIRE** AND **ENABLE** PEOPLE TO IMPROVE
THEIR LIVES AND THE WORLD AROUND THEM

FOR MORE OF OUR PRODUCTS
WWW.RODALESTORE.COM
(800) 848-4735

This book is dedicated to my husband, Jonathan,

for without you there would be no book,

and to my son, Harris,

the source of my inspiration.

Contents

Part Four: The Real Food Life Recipes

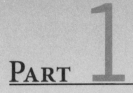

PART **1**

The Good
FOOD
LIFE

1 LET'S GET REAL

Satisfaction. Pleasure. Comfort. Food can make us feel all of these things. But it can also make us feel guilty, gluttonous, and overwhelmed.

Okay, maybe food *itself* doesn't have the power to make us feel these things—but ever since we were children, we were fed values about food along with our daily breakfasts, lunches, and dinners.

Maybe we were told it was a sin to waste food. Or perhaps we were scolded for eating certain foods we craved. Maybe our friends assigned positive or negative traits to a certain food based on what they thought it could do to their bodies, and we blindly followed along. So we shunned chocolate because we were sure it would cause our faces to break out. Or the athletes among us overloaded on protein be-cause we thought it would make us bulk up.

And then, of course, there was all the food for special occasions. The birthday cake, the Halloween candy, the summer picnic hamburgers and macaroni salad, the Thanksgiving dinner with its huge turkey and 10 different side dishes.

Even now that we're adults, food is entwined in our social and professional lives. On dates, we splurge on popcorn and sodas at the movies. A candlelit dinner for two usually ends with a deca-dent dessert. Many of us feed our ambi-tion at our workplaces with a steady diet of coffee or caffeinated sodas and whatever chips or candy bars are avail-able in the company vending machines. And if we have jobs that allow us to travel and have our own expense ac-counts, we often find ourselves dining on rich meals that leave our clients impressed but our tummies bloated. Then there are all those other things that affect our relationships with food: children, worries about bills, stress.

Whether you're a man or a woman, a high school student or a person nearing retirement age, a stay-at-home parent or a corporate executive, food affects you every day. And, no doubt, you spend an inordinate amount of time thinking about it.

What you need is a Real Food Life.

What Does It Mean to Have a Real Food Life?

Simply put, a Real Food Life is a life where you enjoy food and make conscious decisions about the best food to put in your body so that it works at an optimum level. It means not being obsessed by food, and not feeling guilty when you eat something you crave. A Real Food Life means enjoying all the food you eat because you know it is nutritious, delicious, and satisfying to your physical and emotional being.

It shouldn't be confused with having a "perfect" food life. Indeed, I believe that the reason so many of us have a mixed-up relationship with food is because we've bought into the myth of a "perfect" diet. We think that if we can just eat "perfectly"—never splurging or giving in to cravings—all of our problems

will dissolve. But nothing and no one is perfect—not me, not you. Having a Real Food Life means eating when you are actually hungry, not because you are tired, stressed, lonely, or angry. It means being in control of your food, not the other way around. When you're in control, even an "indulgence" will be a conscious choice because you know where the treat fits into the rest of your food plan.

In this chapter, I'll explain how I came to develop an approach to food that eliminates the guilt and obsessiveness and gets back to using food for what it is—fuel to make our bodies and minds run efficiently and effectively. I'll also introduce you to some strategies you can start using *right now* to overcome everyday food obstacles.

In the chapters that follow, you'll get all the information you need to revamp your food life. You'll identify the obstacles that are hindering you and hone in on what you want out of your new food life. Perhaps you want to lose weight—and keep it off for good. Or maybe you're finding yourself in a "food fog" after certain meals and want to learn how to use food for optimum performance. Perhaps you crash every afternoon and need to find some new, interesting lunches that will keep you humming along all afternoon and evening. Maybe, like many of us, your diet includes far too many food "crutches" to get you through the day—caffeinated sodas, coffee, sweets, or junk food—and you've fi-

Kitchen CURES

Simple Steps to Boost Your Brainpower

With our fast-paced lifestyles, there's rarely a time when we *don't* need to be at our mental best. If you're having trouble focusing and staying mentally sharp, try out these all-natural strategies.

- Carbohydrates are the main source of brain fuel. So smarten up with a variety of vegetables and fruits. Also try whole grain bread, crackers, and cereal with some protein, such as hummus, low-fat cheese, or turkey breast.
- There's a reason why fish has a reputation for being brain food. It's rich in B vitamins, which fortify cognitive skills and memory. Plus, it's an excellent source of protein and omega-3 fatty acids. Be sure to serve up fish a few times a week.
- If you're getting too little of any of the B vitamins, you can become mildly depressed and have lowered mental functions. Eggs, brown rice, whole grains, seafood, dairy, and nuts all have a good variety of B vitamins.
- Make sure you're eating a healthful breakfast. It really is the most important meal of the day, and it keeps your brain ticking all day long.
- Exercise increases mental function and improves memory and concentration. Be smart and exercise several times a week. It's a good workout for your body and your mind.

nally decided that you need to start feeding your body more nutritious fare. Whatever your motive, this book will give you the tools you need to get real with your food.

In order to understand how to best modify your diet, you'll need to learn a little bit about nutrition. In part 2 of this book, I'll introduce you to some basics. You'll learn the difference between simple and complex carbohydrates—and what each does for your body. Why certain kinds of fat are actually good for you. Why drinking lots of water—at least eight 8-ounce glasses each day—will not only keep your body running smoothly but actually give you energy. Armed with information such as this, you'll be ready to start the 8-Week Food Life Makeover Plan.

Through the 8-week makeover plan, I'll

guide you every step of the way as you work toward getting a Real Food Life. No matter what your ultimate goal—having more energy, eating more healthfully, losing weight—I'll help you to customize the plan to reach it. By keeping a journal of everything you eat, you'll be able to analyze your eating patterns and identify previously unrecognized roadblocks. You'll also gain insight into how your body uses and reacts to various types of food, such as proteins, carbohydrates, and so on.

Together, we'll make over your kitchen so that you can't *help* but succeed. I'll also give you pointers so that as you grocery shop you choose foods with a new awareness of what works best for your body. I'll even provide menu suggestions, tips for dining out, recipes, exercise hints, and much, much more.

How do I know all this works? Personal experience.

How I Developed the Real Food Life Program

I am Janine Whiteson and I'm a nutritionist. My clients call me their Food Life Coach, but I don't wear a whistle and I've never made anyone run wind sprints. I received a masters of science degree in nutrition and weight-loss programs from Kings College in London.

For more than 11 years, I've helped thousands of people to get a better food life. I've worked with nationally known TV personali-

ties and shy high school students, with busy executives and new mothers, with the skinny, the obese, the healthy, the sick, the young and the old, the exercise fiends and the sedentary homebodies. The one thing they all had in common was a need to get a better food life.

I'm not into fad diets. They're usually unhealthy and have no positive long-term effects. Plus, because we all have different needs and different lifestyles, the fact that these diets are one-size-fits-all means that they truly fit no one. I'm not into gimmicks. They don't work. What I am into is teaching and coaching people about good, sensible nutrition. I'll help you learn about eating wonderful foods that make you feel your best, and help you develop positive habits that will last your whole lifetime.

I've had a lifelong fascination with food. When I was 12, I was diagnosed with severe hypertension, or high blood pressure, and spent 3 months in a hospital. None of the many doctors who treated me could understand why someone so young had such a rare—and critical—illness. Their answer was to prescribe numerous medications, none of which worked.

Because the doctors guessed that the illness originated in my kidneys, I ended up undergoing a kidney operation. The doctors assured my parents and me that my blood pressure would return to normal after the surgery. It didn't. I had to continue on medication because that was the best treatment my physicians thought they could offer me.

Fortunately, my parents didn't settle for that. They asked the doctors, "Doesn't diet play a role in high blood pressure? Don't Janine's emotions play a part in her high blood pressure? Isn't there anything we can do for our daughter other than give her medication?" Still, the doctors insisted that the only thing my parents could do for me was to make sure I got my medication.

My parents did a ton of their own research and changed our whole family's diet. They cut way down on processed foods and eliminated fast food. (I was devastated.) There were no more salty canned foods (like soups and vegetables), no more pickles (my favorite), no more chips, no more frozen dinners, no more processed meats (I especially loved salami).

I had been a salt addict and especially loved potato chips and other salty snacks much more than sweets. Before my illness, I used to buy very large bags of chips and eat them in private or, sometimes, with a friend. I used to salt everything I ate, including Burger King burgers and fries. Because of this addiction, cutting salt out of my diet was an especially hard adjustment for me to make.

My mother eliminated all salt from her cooking and started using a lot of garlic (she read that it could help lower blood pressure) and other herbs and spices. We ate many more fresh fruits and vegetables. In addition to the vitamins my parents thought might help me, we started buying a lot more of our food from the health food store, particularly bread (many supermarket brands can be surprisingly high in sodium), cereals (much cereal is high in salt as well as sugar), and low-sodium soup stock (to make fresh vegetable soups). Nowadays, healthful, low-sodium foods are widely available in supermarkets.

We ate a lot more fatty fish because my parents read that fish has a high water content and contains omega-3 fatty acids that may help to reduce blood pressure. We also ate much less red meat. This was pretty hard because my father is from Argentina, where they eat beef every day. Margarine was banned from the house completely, and we had butter only on rare occasions. We used olive oil and canola oil instead (again, because my parents read that it may help reduce blood pressure). When we went out to dinner at restaurants, my whole family would order food *without salt, please!*

My mother took me to weekly biofeedback sessions so I could learn how to relax and deal with my emotions. My parents suspected that emotions affected my blood pressure even though the doctors insisted that emotions had nothing to do with it (remember, this was 1980). I went to biofeedback for a few years. What I learned proved helpful when I had to go to regularly scheduled doctor's appointments to get my blood pressure checked. Though I would initially get very upset, I was able to successfully use the biofeedback techniques to help calm myself down and lower my blood pressure.

The life changes my family and I undertook worked—and they're still working. My blood pressure finally became manageable through a changed diet and a new consciousness about food. The experience resulted in my whole family getting a better food life. We all became aware of how foods make us feel physically and emotionally; how important fresh fruit and vegetables are to feeling good; how more fiber and less meat gives us more energy; how cooking is a nurturing and nourishing family activity; how to speak up for our food needs when we're out to eat; and how to listen to our bodies. It also led me down the path to where I am today: helping people get Real Food Lives, with the understanding (and personal knowledge) that emotions play into people's eating habits and health.

After receiving my master's degree, I ran the nutrition department for the United Kingdom's largest sports club. It was there that I discovered that people want delicious, satisfying foods that are also good for them. And it was there that I realized the profound way in which people's food choices are wrapped up with their emotions. I began creating a down-to-earth philosophy toward food that really helps people to come to grips with out-of-control food lives. I even developed a wide range of recipes that I share with anyone who wants them (I've included more than 70 in this book).

Every strategy in this book—from the shopping lists, to the coping mechanisms, to the 8-Week Food Life Makeover Plan—is based on my 11 years of experience helping people just like you. My advice always takes into consideration the social, psychological, and physical aspects of food, with the clear understanding that eating well is so much more than what should or should not be eaten. After all, food is an integral part of our lives and culture.

What I'll Do for You

For each client I work with, I create individual, daily food strategies. We are all unique and have our own sets of food issues: emotional, practical, and so on. In my experience, I've found it is vital that each person get his or her own distinct food plan that suits his or her particular lifestyle, eating habits, likes and dislikes, comfort foods, and schedule. Likewise, I'll help you to create a personalized nutrition blueprint. This book will educate you on the right way to eat for your way of life. Whether you're a college student away from home for the first time, a junior executive working your way up the ladder, a busy parent, a fiftysomething, or a person looking forward to the lifestyle changes that retirement might bring, this book will help you shape a sane food program suitable for your own lifestyle.

I like to tell my clients that by working with me for 8 weeks, they will become empowered about their food choices and, in effect, become their own personal nutritionists. So will you. Even if you can barely boil a pot of water or don't know the first thing about grocery shopping, this book will guide you toward the most fundamental and beneficial ways to eat in order to feel great.

Shedding Unhealthy Food Habits

Over the past 2 decades, way too many gimmicky diets have been sold as life-changing panaceas. And while some short-term weight loss can be had from these "diets du jour," people inevitably put the pounds back on and then some (mainly because many fad diets slow

BEST BITES

Super Foods for Women

A lowered risk of breast cancer. Protection against anemia. Sharper brain functioning. The following foods truly are superstars when it comes to their health benefits.

- Fatty fish, including salmon, sardines, tuna, herring, mackerel, and trout, are great sources of omega-3 fatty acids and high-quality protein. Omega-3's have been linked to lowered blood pressure and reduced risk for stroke and heart attack.
- Eggs contain choline, which is important for brain functioning and development. They're also an excellent source of protein and nutrients. For additional benefits, choose eggs enriched with omega-3's, which are now available in many supermarkets. Enjoy up to seven eggs a week. (Limit yourself to no more than four eggs a week if you have diabetes or high cholesterol or are overweight.)
- Beef is loaded with heme iron, which is crucial in protecting against anemia. Eating lean beef such as filet mignon or flank steak with iron-rich vegetables (such as spinach and Swiss chard) will help increase the absorption of the vegetables' iron.
- Soybeans are high in protein, fiber, B vitamins, and iron. They also contain phytoestrogens, which the body converts into hormonelike substances that act like a weak form of estrogen. For premenopausal women, this can mean a lowered risk of breast cancer and possibly heart disease. In older women, phytoestrogens can ease menopausal symptoms such as hot flashes. Soy is delicious, versatile, and available in many forms—from tofu to soy nuts to boiled edamame.
- Dark green, leafy vegetables are a great source of calcium, fiber, B vitamins, phytochemicals, and antioxidants such as beta-carotene.

the metabolism by at least 10 percent). Not only do these fad diets have no positive long-lasting effects, but most people who use them don't even realize that they are nutritionally unsound. Where three square meals, the four basic food groups, and family dinners once reigned, many people today never learned how to eat properly in the first place, either at home or as part of their grade school curriculum.

The modern world is filled with all kinds of shortcuts, quick fixes, and immediate grat-ification. In a world with so many high-tech conveniences, people want their food in-stantly, too. Add to this the media hype pro-moting what often turn out to be unhealthy diets, irresponsible and often incorrect re-porting on nutrition topics, and not learning how to eat properly as children, and no one knows what's good for them anymore.

By using this book, you'll learn to shed old, unhealthy food habits and adopt healthful new ones. You will learn to listen to your body—not some celebrity with a quick-fix weight-loss program—to find out what it needs from you. Many of us have become so used to punishing our bodies through restric-tive diets, overeating, bingeing, or regularly eating foods filled with saturated fats, sodium, and chemicals—such as fast food—that we don't even know how our bodies *should* feel.

Your first step toward your Real Food Life will be to keep a food journal. This will be your companion for at least 8 weeks. By keeping an honest account of everything you put in your mouth, and how you feel before, during, and after eating, you'll learn to listen to your body. And by listening to your body, you'll hear if it's thirsty, tired, or hungry. When you listen to your body, you'll start to understand which foods suit your body and make you feel alive, energetic, and satisfied. You'll also discover which foods make you feel bloated, lethargic, and mentally fuzzy.

Toward the Good Food Life

In the chapters that follow, I'll help you cus-tomize your strategy for getting a Real Food Life. To get you started, though, here are some broad tactics to employ on your journey.

Create Food Sanity

If you want a Real Food Life, you'll have to rid yourself of your food obsessions. Con-stantly thinking about *anything*—including food—will consume you and drag you down. Food is there to nourish your body and sat-isfy your soul. If you are obsessing about food, you aren't enjoying a necessary and pleasurable aspect of your life.

What brings on food obsessions? In my experience, they're often a result of people depriving themselves by over-restricting their diets and trying to "control" their food. Other times people simply don't eat enough;

they try to be "good" with their food (they're usually trying to lose weight), so they eat too little of it. But eating too little promotes obsessive food thoughts, interferes with your brain chemicals, and can lead to binges and eating disorders. When you eat too little, your levels of cholecystokinin (CCK)—a neurotransmitter whose function is to send signals to stop eating, switch off the appetite, and activate feelings of fullness—become unbalanced. Conversely, when you eat a healthy, balanced diet, your CCK levels are balanced and your body will naturally tell you when it has had enough food.

Here are some tips to help you get started on eliminating food obsessions and working toward getting a Real Food Life.

Listen to your body. When you start listening to your body and hearing what it really needs, food will become less of an issue for you. Begin by simply noticing how you feel after eating. Are you tired, or do you feel energized? Do you feel bloated and a bit queasy? Or ready to take on the world? Tune in to the connections between what you feed your body and how your body feels afterward.

Keep busy. Do whatever it takes to have an active and full day, both physically and mentally. It may sound simplistic, but when you're busy and involved with other activities, you're not going to be thinking about food all the time.

Shop and cook. Going grocery shopping and cooking for yourself—rather than simply picking up a meal at the local fast-food drive-thru or heating up a frozen dinner—are proactive ways to stop food obsessions. Not only do they make you more conscious of your food choices, but they also give you a sense of accomplishment since they help you to connect with what you're putting in your body. The simple act of preparing a meal also helps you to take time to nourish and provide for your soul.

Create an action plan. An action plan is a food life schedule where you write down what you will probably eat for the whole day. If you plan your "food intentions," you can move on with the rest of your daily life. Don't worry if the plan doesn't work out exactly; just the act of creating a plan will help you think less about food.

Eat deliciously. All the food you eat, whether it's a snack or a meal, should be very tasty and gratifying. If you choose delicious foods every time you eat, rather than trying to choke down foods you don't like but you think are good for you, you'll be much more satisfied. And if you're always satisfied with your food choices, you are much less likely to obsess about food. Fortunately, there are literally hundreds of delicious *and* nutritious food choices out there, including many varieties of fruits and vegetables that you've probably never even tried.

Undo damaging thoughts. You have to put an end to negative thoughts about your-

(continued on page 14)

LIVING A REAL FOOD LIFE

She Ditched the Dieting Mentality— And Gained Confidence in Return

Name: Chelsea

Real Food Life Issues: PMS, diet mentality, family food pressures

Chelsea is a 30-year-old single lawyer who often works until midnight. On her evenings and weekends off, she's usually on dates or out with friends, eating and drinking into the wee hours. When we met, she suffered from acute PMS, which contributed to her anxiousness and chronic low energy. She was "addicted" to caffeinated drinks and sweet foods and used them as energy- and mood-boosters. Here's where I found her:

December 2

I'm drowning in holiday spirit. Things are getting a little out of hand on the social front. I'm expected to turn in about 200 billable hours in the next 3 weeks and I have no clue how this will be achieved at the peak of the party season. Will have to rely heavily on the talents of my good men Johnny Walker and Juan Valdez.

Dreading the trip home. My (s)mother is gearing up to lay it on super-thick, I can feel it. She's been coming out with some real winners lately. A current fave: "Did you get a flattering dress for the party this time?"

Vicious cramps today. Face broken out into a connect-the-dots in the shape of Raggedy Ann. Am seriously considering seeking solace in some chocolate cupcakes washed down with a pint of butter pecan.

Ever since she was a teenager, Chelsea felt "too heavy." Throughout her life, she had tried every new diet available—but eventually "flunked" all of them. Chelsea would always feel guilty about everything she ate, and despite her professional and personal successes, she felt like a failure with food and out of control with her food life.

First, we worked on getting rid of her diet mentality. I explained that restrictive diets don't work and will only make her crazy. She couldn't even remember how many diets she had tried. When I asked how many of them worked, she replied, "None." I think that was the turning point:

After that conversation, she started thinking that maybe the information I was sharing was right.

Next, we weaned her off caffeine. Instead of three cups of coffee and four daily colas, she started drinking water, green tea, and a single cup of decaffeinated coffee each day. Within 2 weeks, her anxiety was evaporating. When she recognized that caffeine made her feel more anxious than she actually was, she was relieved. To deal with the PMS, we upped her calcium intake. She started taking a calcium supplement and ate a few servings of low-fat dairy foods every day. She also started eating fatty fish three times a week, which was an easy change because she loved tuna and salmon. In addition, she incorporated some other foods that are high in essential fatty acids into her diet: She dressed her salads with olive oil and ate nuts and seeds for snacks. She also started taking vitamin B_6 supplements daily.

She became aware that the candy and other sweets she ate simply because they were available at work just made her feel sleepy. I suggested she try more wholesome snacks, so instead of miniature candy bars and cookies, she began to eat more whole grains and fruit. I also encouraged her to keep healthful snacks in her desk so she'd be prepared when hunger did strike.

Chelsea and I talked extensively about how her emotions were wrapped up with her food. Her mother, a demanding, opinionated, and very slender woman, had always been critical of Chelsea's weight. We came up with specific ways to cope with the emotions and the calories of the big upcoming holiday meal. One strategy she particularly liked was to eat small portions of the foods she loved—like sweet potato and marshmallow casserole and cranberries—so she wouldn't feel deprived, along with larger portions of vegetables and salads.

We also worked on her food intentions with all the other meals. She knew she would have a whole grain with a little protein for her breakfast, such as oatmeal with a few walnuts, cinnamon, a drizzle of honey, and fat-free milk. The basis of her lunches and dinners would be lots of vegetables, with some good protein and grains. She could eat leftovers, but instead of leftover cookies, she ate the Brussels sprouts, the green beans, a small serving of cranberries, and some turkey, surprising herself with how satisfied she felt.

When her mother made comments about her food, Chelsea asked her to respect her food choices and leave her alone. And much to Chelsea's surprise, her mother made an effort to stop. Afterward, she was amazed how much calmer she felt around her family and food.

After 8 weeks, Chelsea's PMS symptoms improved. She was thrilled to finally get over the "need" to go on a diet. Mostly, though, she felt more secure with herself and her ability to confront her negative emotional issues with food.

self. If you keep telling yourself things like, "I'm always going to be large," "I'll always be a mess with food," or "I have no self-control," you'll sabotage your own efforts to achieve a Real Food Life. It's imperative to find a way to eliminate these types of phrases from your mind. The next time you catch yourself saying something negative, consciously replace the thought with a positive one. For example, visualize yourself eating in a more wholesome and healthy way, imagine yourself cooking a nutritious meal that makes you feel great, or picture yourself full of energy and able to conquer anything.

Ditch the "Good" Food/ "Bad" Food Syndrome

In a Real Food Life, there is no such thing as "good" and "bad" foods. Instead, no foods are forbidden. I've found that labeling foods as "good" or "bad" leads to feelings of guilt. The interesting thing about guilt, though, is that it's a self-imposed emotion; you are the only one who can make yourself "feel guilty."

Did someone ever say to you that the chocolate you were eating "will make you break out" or "will go straight to your hips" or that those potato chips "will make you fat and crave more"? These types of comments make people afraid of their food. In fact, many of us take to heart the criticism inherent in comments like these. But, once again, realize that only *you* can make yourself feel guilty about the food you eat. It is no one else's business what you choose to eat, and no one has the right to say anything about what you're eating—unless, of course, they want a bite.

To start on the path to overcoming the "good" food/"bad" food syndrome, keep these general points in mind.

Realize that no food is off-limits. When you set limits, you'll break them—it's human nature. If you tell a child not to touch a certain lamp, he'll make a beeline for that lamp. By the same token, if you tell yourself you can't eat something, that something will be the only thing you want to eat. Permit yourself to eat any food—after all, savoring delicious, mouthwatering foods is one of the greatest joys in life.

Erect food boundaries. Just because no food is forbidden doesn't mean that there shouldn't be boundaries. Obviously, you do your body no good when you feed it a steady diet of colas, chips, ice cream, and hamburgers. Know that you can have any food, but have a controlled, contained amount. For example, if you love chocolate, have a few Hershey's Kisses rather than the whole bag. No doubt you'll come to realize that a taste of the chocolate candies satisfies you and is really all you want. Boundaries don't limit food; they put it into perspective.

Fortify your food boundaries. To keep from overindulging, write down the food you most crave and the amount you will eat (a small portion should do it). Then buy the food and eat just that amount. It's a good idea to buy a small, single-serving package of the food you crave. If you can get it only in large sizes, though, throw the rest away after you've eaten the amount you specified; don't bring it home or keep it around you. After a few attempts, you may be able to keep the remainder of that food around, but if not, that's okay.

Accept Your Body

There's a lot of self-hate out there, and it's usually about body size. While many men have low self-image issues, this seems to be a problem that most affects women. Remember this: There is no such thing as a perfect body. The perfect body is a fantasy created and perpetuated by the media. The average American woman is 5 feet 4 inches tall, wears a size 14, and weighs in the 150-pound range. One-third of all American women wear a size 16 or larger. The average model, on the other hand, is 5 feet 9 inches tall and weighs 110 pounds (and usually wears a size 4).

To be female means to have curves, a rounded butt, and larger hips and thighs. Women have more body fat than men do, and there's nothing you can do to change that biological fact. More curves—and fat—are how women were created and have evolved; they need their curvy bodies for their hormones to work properly, to be able to get pregnant, to hold on to a pregnancy, and to give birth.

Male or female, if you spend your life at the gym, you will become fitter and more toned, but you'll probably never achieve the body of somebody you see in a magazine. Most models are very tall and very lean due to their genes; some eat, some don't. Their bodies are the exception to the rule; they are genetic eccentrics. The majority of people in the world don't look the way models do and never will. Ever.

Work with your body. The key to getting over your notion of a "perfect body" is to accept what you have. If you hate your body, it won't work with you. Your poisonous thoughts about your body will always sabotage your efforts to have a great food life. If you accept your body—and even learn to like it—you can achieve peace with your food life. When you accept your body, you will realize that having a good food life leads to the body that is perfect for *you*.

Step Away from the Scale

You are not a number on a scale. What is important is how you feel—not what you weigh. If you place all your importance on what a scale says, you risk becoming controlled by it.

Your body is constantly changing, and you'll weigh something different every day. If, for example, you ate a salty dinner last night, your body may be retaining anywhere from 3 to 5 extra pounds of water weight. With variances like these, why live and die by what a mechanical numbers machine tells you?

It simply isn't fair to your body to choose an "ideal" weight and then struggle to reach it. Any number you pick will be arbitrary, and there are many factors, not the least of which is genetics, that will or won't let you reach that number. Instead, your "ideal" weight should be what makes you feel most comfortable in your skin. It's the weight at which you feel the healthiest, the most energetic, the most *alive*.

Let your clothes be your guide. The most accurate indication of whether you've "gained" or "lost" weight is how your clothes fit. If you've noticed that all your clothes are becoming tight and you've considered buying clothes in a larger size than usual, it's probably a sign that you need to reevaluate what you've been eating and exercise a bit more often.

Calculate your BMI. If you absolutely must have some form of size measurement, I recommend using the Body Mass Index (BMI) instead of scale weight. Doctors, nutritionists, and other health professionals use

Your Body Mass Index (BMI)

Height	Weight (lb.)													
4'10"	91	96	100	105	110	115	119	124	129	134	139	143	148	153
4'11"	94	99	104	109	114	119	124	128	133	138	143	148	153	158
5'0"	97	102	107	112	118	123	128	133	138	143	148	153	158	163
5'1"	100	106	111	116	122	127	132	137	143	148	153	158	164	169
5'2"	104	109	115	120	126	131	136	142	147	153	158	164	169	174
5'3"	107	113	118	124	130	135	141	146	152	158	163	169	175	180
5'4"	110	116	122	128	134	140	145	151	157	163	169	174	180	186
5'5"	114	120	126	132	138	144	150	156	162	168	174	180	186	192
5'6"	118	124	130	136	142	148	155	161	167	173	179	186	192	198
5'7"	121	127	134	140	146	153	159	166	172	178	185	191	197	204
5'8"	125	131	138	144	151	158	164	171	177	184	190	197	203	210
5'9"	128	135	142	149	155	162	169	176	182	189	196	203	209	216
5'10"	132	139	146	153	160	167	174	181	188	195	202	207	215	222
5'11"	136	142	150	157	165	172	179	186	193	200	208	215	222	229
6'0"	140	147	154	162	169	177	184	191	199	206	213	221	228	235
BMI	19	20	21	22	23	24	25	26	27	28	29	30	31	32

the BMI to gauge an adult's weight-related health risk. The BMI is a ratio of height to weight, and it's a fairly accurate standard for determining if someone is at a healthy weight, or if the person is overweight and at risk for weight-related problems such as high blood pressure, high cholesterol, and diabetes.

Take a look at the chart to calculate your BMI. Find your height in the left-hand column, then move across that row to find the number closest to your weight. Now follow that column to the bottom of the chart, where you'll find your BMI.

A BMI between 19 and 22 is considered desirable. If your BMI is between 23 and 25, you are slightly overweight and may be at risk for weight-related health problems. Your disease risk begins to increase at a BMI of about 26. (Bear in mind, however, that some women with BMIs of 25 to 27 are perfectly healthy. Take into account other risk factors, including your age, level of physical activity, family history, and eating habits, before becoming alarmed.) If your BMI is 30 or above, you are obese and have a substantially increased risk for developing disease. In one study, for example, scientists found that women with a BMI higher than 29 had a 230 percent greater risk for heart disease.

Spin a Social Web

I believe that social isolation is an epidemic and a major reason why our whole country is generally unhealthy and out of balance with their food. Humans are inherently social beings; we have been created to be with people, to live in close communities, to interact with each other, to belong.

In our hectic lives, we work long hours, get too little sleep, and don't have enough time to look after ourselves and create and nurture friendships. In addition, many of us now spend countless hours surfing the Web or writing e-mails rather than having face-to-face contact with others.

For some people, the problem is shyness. Others have crippling insecurity and are afraid of being judged, so they avoid interacting with others.

When we don't have meaningful contact with other people on a daily basis, we begin to feel isolated. We lose our support systems and feel we are alone in this world. The side effect for many people who feel lonely and isolated is overeating. They eat for company, they eat to feel less alone, and they eat to cope with the pain of their loneliness.

For your own good health, work on developing bonds with other people. Not only will these relationships help to strengthen your resolve as you work to get a Real Food Life, but they'll also enrich you emotionally.

Find fun. A great way to meet people is to join your local gym or take a class at a college or community center. Go to a lecture series. Do you have a hobby? Find a club and explore it further. At these types of venues there are people who share your interests, so building a friendship is easier since you have a basis of similarity. Once you get involved, keep going regularly; that way people get to know you and you get to know them.

Buddy up. Ask someone who seems approachable and friendly—perhaps a family member or someone at work, school, or your place of worship—to go through the 8-Week Food Life Makeover Plan with you. Working with someone who is helpful and not judgmental can make the whole process easier, more fun, and more social.

Give away your time. Find an organization that you admire and ask how you can help. Doing volunteer work is a great way to meet people, plus you're doing something good for the community at the same time. Giving your time and talent is the best way in the world to fill yourself up without eating a thing.

2 The 24 Most Common Food Issues

For me, being a personal nutritionist is, in some ways, like being a detective. Sure, it would be simple enough to just give my clients a diet, tell them to follow it, and send them on their way. But not only do I think that's professionally irresponsible, it's not how I work. Instead, I investigate my clients' eating habits and try to uncover their hidden food issues, because these issues directly relate to what they put in their mouths. I'll do the same for you, my newest client.

Everyone has food issues. Most stem from childhood experiences with food—when eating patterns are etched, when we're indirectly taught to ignore natural hunger cues, when we start using food as something other than a way to nourish our bodies.

In order to have a healthy food life, it's important that you honestly assess your eating patterns and come to understand your food issues and their source. When you know what your food issues are, you will be able to implement strategies to make permanent changes.

In this chapter, I've identified the 24 most prevalent food issues. I've also included proven strategies that will enable you to overcome these food issues and help you to take greater steps toward getting a Real Food Life.

This chapter is quite lengthy, so feel free to glance ahead at the titles of each of the 24 issues. Carefully read the descriptions and strategies for those issues that affect you. You might also want to skim through the others, though, since there could be subtle issues that affect your eating patterns without your even being aware of them.

1. I Am Always on a Diet but Can Never Stick with It

▶ Do you obsess about your body?

▶ Do you think that if you become thin, your life will be perfect?

▶ Do you find it difficult, if not impossible, to stick with diets?

▶ Do you feel that you lack the willpower to stay on diets?

▶ Are you "good" for the first half of the day but then usually end up "cheating" later in the day?

Restrictive diets are the bane of our existence. Lots of people spend the better part of their lives on them. Even before adolescence, many girls start obsessing about their bodies and comparing themselves unfavorably to the very thin actresses, models, and celebrities they see on TV. Lots of women think that being a size two is an obtainable goal—if only they just keep dieting.

Low-calorie or restrictive diets are difficult, if not impossible, to stick with. It's hard work to be constantly counting calories, reading diet books, and limiting yourself to a highly regimented daily food intake. Plus, dieters often are left with a feeling of failure when they "go off" the diet. They may binge in private or become consumed with the "If I just lose (fill in the blank) pounds, my life will be fabulous" mentality. When you spend your life on a diet, there is no way you can get a Real Food Life.

Strategy: If you're constantly following low-calorie diets, the first thing you need to do is stop. Restricting your diet is the worst thing you can do to your body and mind. If you diet, you're depriving yourself—physically and emotionally. Deprivations lead to obsessions, and having obsessions leads to binges and "failed" diets.

Simply put, the diet industry wants you to fail. The more times you attempt various diets, the more money the $34-billion-a-year industry makes. Because they're too restrictive in both food choices and calorie intake, most low-calorie diets set you up to fail. Also, most diets are not for the long term—they're for the quick fix and don't teach you how to eat for the rest of your life.

Restrictive dieting typically means severe calorie deprivation: consuming fewer than 1,200 calories a day. Regardless of what diet you're on, low-calorie diets have the potential to slow down your metabolism and reduce the amount of lean muscle tissue you have. This means that the calories you consume burn more slowly. Very restrictive dieting slows down your heart rate, lowers your body temperature (making you feel cold all the time), reduces your intake of vital nutrients your body needs to function properly, and ultimately promotes an increase in body fat. This type of dieting causes moodiness, lack of energy, food cravings, and food obsessions. It also disrupts your body's chemical balance and wreaks havoc on nerve chemicals, which could cause you to binge—especially on fat and sweets, which, of course, leads to weight gain.

Diets with fewer than 1,200 calories per day put your body into starvation mode. The body will naturally try to take care of itself, so if it thinks it's starving, it will slow down all functions and hold on to its fat stores to carry out essential body functions. If you normally consume 2,000 calories a day but then begin consuming only 1,200, your body will stop burning calories just to keep itself functioning. If your metabolism slows down, you will need only 1,200 calories to maintain your "starting weight" and will need much less to lose any weight. Basically, your body needs fewer and fewer calories to keep itself running, and permanent weight loss becomes almost impossible. If you go back to consuming 2,000 calories, those extra 800 calories will be stored as fat. It can take up to a year for your body to readjust itself and raise its metabolism back to where it used to be.

Now you see why low-calorie restrictive diets don't work. In order to begin your new food life, you have to start listening to your body. The first step to doing this is to start keeping a food journal. In it, you'll write down everything you eat and drink in the course of a day—as soon as you eat or drink it. You'll include the amount of food or drink you consumed, and how you felt before, during, and after eating. From these details, you'll learn about your food preferences, your cravings, your eating triggers, and your hunger levels. When you pay attention to your hunger levels—and this is key—you usually don't eat when you aren't hungry. You'll learn all the specifics of journal-keeping and get started on one in the first week of the 8-Week Food Life Makeover Plan (see page 142).

By using this book, you will learn how to have a great food life that suits you as an individual. In the chapters to come, I will help you create a food program that takes care of your personal food needs. It's time to start taking care of yourself, stop looking for the shortcut, and stop the dieting syndrome.

2. I'm Always Bingeing

▶ Do you try to have "perfect" food days, and when that doesn't happen, you stuff yourself until you feel sick (then feel out of control with your food)?

▶ Does bingeing make you feel "good" in the moment, but as soon as it's over, you're disgusted with yourself?

▶ Are you so used to bingeing that you never know when you're actually hungry?

▶ Is bingeing like a drug—whenever you feel you can't deal with life, you eat to relieve the pain?

▶ Do you starve yourself all day and then overeat wildly at night?

Many people who watch their weight wake up every morning saying, "This will be the start of my new diet program." By the end of the day, though, they're so hungry they binge—often in a big way. Bingers don't have to be dieters, however; bingeing is just some people's unhealthy and out-of-control way of eating. They may even binge twice a day, consuming a few thousand calories at a time. For many people, bingeing is like a drug: Whenever they feel they can't deal with life, they overeat to relieve the pain and stress they're feeling. The food binge becomes their coping mechanism.

If you're a binger, take heart in knowing you aren't alone. Twenty-two percent of all dieters say they binge at least once a week. Clearly, bingeing is a common practice. But if binge eating has always been your coping mechanism, you *know* it doesn't make you feel any better, especially when the binge is over.

Bingeing is terrible for your body. Bingers tend to be less healthy than people who don't binge; their immune systems tend to be compromised because they binge on junk food rather than on vegetables or healthier choices.

Strategy: In order to control your bingeing, you must stop blaming yourself and feeling like a failure if you do binge. But you also need to start reprogramming your body and mind not to use food as a drug or coping mechanism. To help with this, start keeping a food journal. By writing down how your body—not just your mind—feels before, during, and after eating, you can begin to reprogram your eating and start getting back to eating when you're actually hungry, not when you're feeling other things. Bingers tend to get to the point of starving before they will eat anything—then they eat everything. When you get a Real Food Life, you'll stop starving yourself and start eating when you feel real hunger. (See "Identify Your Hunger Level" on page 39.)

3. I Crave Sweets or Salt

▶ Do you feel that your sweet tooth is out of control?

▶ Do you love to snack on sweets, but usually feel dazed after the sugar binge is over?

▶ Do you salt your food before you even taste it?

▶ A week before your menstrual cycle, do you crave salt so much you have occasionally wondered if you're sodium deficient?

People who crave sweets are everywhere. They may crave sweet food only at night or all through the day with doughnuts for breakfast, chocolates for lunch, candy bars as

Healthy Substitutes for Sugary Snacks

The next time a sugar craving hits, reach for one of these tasty snacks. Not only are they more healthful than cookies, cake, or candy, they are also filling and will completely calm your craving. Unlike when you eat snacks filled with empty calories, you'll be so satisfied after you eat these foods that you won't find yourself foraging for more!

- 1 slice whole grain toasted raisin bread with 1 tablespoon of low-fat cream cheese (or 2 tablespoons whipped cottage cheese with 1 tablespoon all-fruit spread)
- 8-ounces low-fat vanilla yogurt mixed with one small box of raisins and 2 tablespoons of low-fat cottage cheese (for a protein boost)
- 1 chocolate sorbet bar (such as Häagen-Dazs or Sharon's Sorbet)
- 3 frozen Toffutti bars
- 2 whole grain crackers (Wasa or rice cake) with 1 tablespoon peanut butter and 1 tablespoon jam or all-fruit spread
- 2 whole grain crackers or 2 brown rice cakes with 2 tablespoons low-fat cream cheese and 1 tablespoon jam
- 1 Lifeline bran muffin (or 1 muffin from recipe on page 319) with 1 tablespoon jam or 1 teaspoon peanut butter or 2 tablespoons low-fat cream cheese
- 1 Thomas's honey whole wheat English muffin with 2 teaspoons cream cheese sprinkled with a dusting of cinnamon and 1 teaspoon sugar
- 1 medium packaged biscotti with 8 ounces low-fat hot chocolate or chocolate milk
- A ½-ounce piece of best-quality semisweet or bittersweet (dark) chocolate (such as Scharffenberg, Callebaut, Vahlrona, or Ghirardelli)
- 1 cup Honey Puffed Kashi or Good Friends Kashi or Kashi Go Lean cereal with ½ to 1 cup fat-free milk or soy milk or ½ cup vanilla yogurt
- 1 baked apple (see recipe on page 321) with 2 tablespoons low-fat vanilla yogurt
- ½ cup vanilla frozen yogurt scooped into 12 ounces diet root beer
- 2 Oatmeal Raisin Cookies (see recipe on page 317)
- 1 slice Blueberry Angel Food Cake (see recipe on page 322)

a 4:00 pick-me-up, and pudding after dinner. They're the ones who will go out in a hurricane for their chocolate fix. They are practically addicted to sweets, but usually feel dazed or nervous after their sugar binges.

Then there are the people who crave salty foods, such as fast food, French fries, potato chips, and pretzels. After consuming salt, though, they often feel bloated. Their eyes get puffy and their hands swell, making it difficult to put on or take off their rings.

Cravings for sweets usually stem from a desire for fat. It's actually sweetened fats—rather than plain sugar—that people crave. Cakes, ice cream, and cookies have almost as much (and sometimes more) fat as they do sugar. It's the combination of fat and sugar (creamy and sweet) that ignites sweet cravings. Fat on its own has very little flavor, but when combined with sugar, its taste is qualitatively better. Fats make food flavorful and contribute to wonderful aromas and tantalizing "mouth feels." Think of the butter in cookies: It makes them smell great, bake up crunchy, and, of course, taste delicious. Studies have shown that people are less likely to crave low-fat sugary foods such as gummy bears and hard candy than high-fat sugary foods such as brownies, ice cream, and candy bars.

The body needs fat—it's long-term fuel. Your appetite for fat (in the form of creamy, textured foods) is controlled by the brain chemical galanin. Galanin levels rise progressively throughout the day (which may explain the craving for creamy salad dressings at lunchtime or a creamy sweet snack, like a chocolate bar, in the late afternoon). Galanin levels also rise when estrogen levels are high, which may explain why women often crave high-fat sweet foods during their premenstrual cycles.

Strategy: Eat smaller but more frequent meals throughout the day, which will make your blood sugar levels more stable, and that may keep sweet cravings at bay. Also, eat a variety of complex carbohydrates all day long, but combine them with a protein whenever possible. The carbs keep serotonin (a brain chemical that regulates sleep, mood, food intake, and pain) levels normal, so you crave sugar less. The protein helps you to feel fuller longer. Good snacks to try include a slice of whole wheat toast with some peanut butter and a glass of fat-free milk, or baby carrots dipped in hummus with a low-fat yogurt. Also try increasing the amount of water you drink, since sugar cravings can be a sign that your body is dehydrated.

Putting on your sneakers and getting some exercise may also help you to avoid sugar cravings. Exercise releases the same "feel-good" endorphins that sugar does. Studies show that people who exercise regularly binge less and have fewer food cravings because they're getting their endorphin rush through exercise.

Finally, if you really crave a sweet, indulge yourself—if you try to ignore the craving, you'll eventually binge. But eat what you crave; don't opt for a diet product made with sugar substitute. Simply have a small portion of what you crave and then end it. You do not have to have the whole box of cookies to enjoy one.

While sugar cravings may be physiological, salt cravings are usually a learned response, a

Healthy Substitutes for Salty Snacks

Try one of the following snacks the next time you get a craving for a salty treat. Not only will you appease the craving, but you'll also be giving your body a more healthful alternative to other salty foods like full-fat chips and fast food French fries.

- 1 cup (1 small bag) Pirate Booty or Veggie Booty
- 1 small bag Harry's honey mustard pretzels
- 1 individual-serving bag of Terra chips or Terra olive oil and fine herbs chips
- 15 to 20 pistachios
- 6 to 8 walnuts
- ¼ cup sunflower or pumpkin seeds
- 1 cup unshelled or ½ cup shelled edamame soy beans (available in gourmet grocery stores, whole foods stores, Asian food stores, and Japanese restaurants)
- 1 cup Cascadian Farms oven-baked French fries
- Unlimited Roasted Vegetables with 1 to 2 teaspoons grated Parmesan cheese (see recipe on page 267)
- 1 cup Health Valley vegetable soup or Chunky Mixed Vegetable Soup (see recipe on page 281) sprinkled with 1 to 2 teaspoons grated Parmesan cheese
- 4 slices (2 to 3 ounces) smoked tofu on whole grain crackers with mustard
- 2 tofu sausages in a small whole wheat pita bread with mustard
- 3 tablespoons hummus in a small whole wheat pita with lettuce and tomato
- Shrimp salad (5 cooked shrimp chopped with 1 celery rib, chives, or red onion, and 1 tablespoon low-fat mayo) on 2 whole grain crackers or in a whole wheat pita
- Egg salad (1 hard-boiled egg and 2 cooked egg whites mixed with 1 tablespoon low-fat mayo and chopped scallions) on 2 whole grain crackers or in a whole wheat pita
- 1 pint (yes, a pint!) cherry or grape tomatoes dipped in 1 tablespoon Blue Cheese Dressing (see recipe on page 263)
- 1 small can water-packed tuna mixed with 1 chopped celery rib, 1 tablespoon raisins, ¼ teaspoon curry powder, and 1 tablespoon low-fat mayo on 2 rice cakes

habit. The more salt you eat, the more you want it. Sodium is necessary for survival, but we need fewer than 500 milligrams of sodium a day to supply all vital functions and maintain normal fluid levels, healthy muscle function, and proper acidity (pH) of the blood. Getting too little sodium is rarely a problem, but too much can lead to high blood pressure (hypertension) and fluid retention. It can also aggravate medical disorders such as congestive heart failure, kidney disease, and PMS.

If you are used to a high-salt diet and want to cut back, do so gradually. If you take salt out of your diet too quickly, it may trigger even fiercer cravings.

Salt cravings may also be due to a craving for food with stronger, fuller flavors. Lemon is a great salt substitute. Try adding a squirt of lemon to low-salt soups and meat and chicken dishes—you might not even miss the salt. You might also try dried herb mixtures such as Spike and Vegit, cayenne pepper, vinegars, fruit juices, mustards, garlic, basil, oregano, or curry powder. Of course, stop adding additional salt to food after it has been cooked.

Finally, read the "Nutrition Facts" label on packaged foods to discover how much sodium they contain (for more, see "Anatomy of a Label" on page 48). You'll probably be surprised to learn how much hidden sodium is in a lot of the foods you love.

4. I Sometimes Crash Diet

◗ Are you so desperate to lose weight that you'll go for days living on diet soda and cottage cheese?

◗ Do you buy clothes that are too small and hope you'll be able to fit in them in time for that big date?

◗ Do you try crash diets to be thin, thinking you'll be able to attract more men (or women)?

◗ Do you starve for a day or two and then binge wildly on the third day?

◗ Do you deny yourself most foods when you "feel fat" or have overeaten?

When I hear the phrase "crash diet," I get a little upset. It means that someone in our country of abundance is willing to forgo food in the hope that it will cause immediate weight loss. Starving yourself—and the binge that inevitably follows—is no way to have a Real Food Life. People have all sorts of reasons for wanting to lose weight really quickly; these reasons often have to do with dating, or a big event, or the misconception that a crash diet will jump-start a good food life.

Crash diets are truly one of the most unhealthy weight-loss options around. These diets drastically cut out most foods when, in fact, the body needs a variety of food. They dehydrate you (which causes lethargy and dizziness); they break down lean muscle mass (and that slows down the metabolism and heart rate); they can make you feel cold and irritable; and they can cause illness (because they impair the immune system). Since these diets advocate eating nearly nothing or only one type of food, they lead to food obsessions, then cravings, then binges. That, in turn, leads to depression, guilt, and even feelings of hopelessness. While people might lose weight on crash diets, they're not losing fat; they're losing water and muscle weight.

People who crash diet can end up with compromised immune systems and tend to be low in vitamin C (which comes only from eating foods rich in vitamin C or taking vitamin C supplements). Being deficient in vitamin C can lead to gum disease and gum bleeding, joint pains, low energy, poor digestion, slow wound healing, bruises, water retention, and an increased susceptibility to infection, such as colds and bronchitis.

In addition to all this, starving yourself will only cause you to overeat eventually. It doesn't work as a weight-loss program and never will.

Strategy: You need to develop and maintain an eating program that's specifically tailored to you. This program must allow you to eat nutritious foods consistently and throughout the day. Only then will you be able to end the cycle of starving and bingeing and develop a Real Food Life. You'll learn how to create an eating program that will suit your lifestyle when you begin the 8-Week Food Life Makeover Plan, starting on page 131.

5. I'm Addicted to Junk Food

▶ Are you obsessed with junk food? Do you sometimes wake up in the middle of the night just to grab some?

▶ When you drive past a fast-food restaurant, are you compelled to order something even when you're not hungry?

▶ When you're at the supermarket with your kids, do they beg for junk food and you give in to them—and end up eating it, too?

Junk food is a hot-button issue in our culture. It's available almost everywhere, advertised almost everywhere, and consumed practically everywhere. But, ironically, everybody knows it's "no good for you"—that's why it's called junk food.

Because of its accessibility, junk food is an easy way to eat, which leads many people to indulge in it even if they don't intend to. But other people crave it. They love the taste (which is better: a cheeseburger or carrot sticks?), and they never seem able to say no. Having children makes the junk food situation especially tricky, since most kids love the stuff and it's hard to deny them because it's always on hand. One thing about junk food: Once you've had a taste, it's difficult to stop eating it, try as you might.

Strategy: Junk food is practically a constitutional right. You can't avoid junk food, and if you love it and completely ban it from your diet, you will likely crave and obsess over it. Having something small (and decadently satisfying) may help you get through the initial cravings if you're trying to cut back. Not everyone can live with the discipline, but if you can limit yourself to just a taste, then end it, you can move on from your craving.

Many people simply don't eat enough during the day, so by 4:00 in the afternoon their blood sugar levels are as low as the South Pole. This is a prime time for cravings to hit. Not surprisingly, chocolate is a very common afternoon treat—especially for women—because chocolate satisfies many of the body's natural cravings: sugar and a little caffeine for an afternoon pick-me-up and creamy fat, because the body naturally craves fat later in the day. Eating small meals throughout the day can help to curb cravings because it stabilizes your blood sugar and in-

The Cleanse and Flush Plan

If you have severely overindulged and want to reduce that bloated, lethargic feeling, you can use the following plan. You will drop a pound or two, but be aware that the loss is temporary—because it's only water you're losing, the weight will come back. You can safely stay on this program for 3 days, but you should resume your new eating program as soon as you feel better. The plan is loaded with fresh fruits and vegetables and fish because they all have a high water content, which means they'll fill you up and flush you out. And, yes, you do eat the same things every day.

First thing in the morning:
2 glasses of warm water with lemon

Breakfast:
1 cup green tea
Fruit salad made with half a cantaloupe, ½ cup raspberries, and ½ cup blackberries
½ cup plain fat-free yogurt with a sprinkle of cinnamon
1 whole hard-boiled egg

Midmorning snack:
2 glasses warm water with lemon
1 pear
5 walnut halves

Lunch:
2 glasses warm water with lemon
Large mixed vegetable salad (try to include all or some of the following vegetables: cucumbers, spinach, broccoli, tomatoes, romaine lettuce, peppers, watercress, shredded carrots, cooked beets, cooked asparagus) with 2 teaspoons olive oil

sulin levels, so you'll feel less hungry and less apt to crave junk.

Junk food is a habit that you can learn to break. There are many foods that you can prepare at home in nearly the same amount of time it takes to stop at a fast-food restaurant, but that are cheaper and much more whole-some than fast food. For nearly instant at-home meals and snacks, consider veggie burgers or veggie hot dogs (both cook in min-utes), edamame (fresh soybeans that cook in 5 minutes), dried fruit or a handful of nuts (in-stant), or lower-sodium canned soup or bean chili (merely heat and eat). You might also

¼ avocado

4 ounces cooked (grilled or baked) fresh fish, such as salmon, tuna, herring, sardines, mack-erel, pompano, shad, trout, whitefish, or sable; or any canned fish (but make sure it's packed in spring water or olive oil, and then drain it well)

Lemon (as much as you want on the fish and the salad)

½ cup fresh or canned beans (any type, rinsed very well)

Afternoon snack (spread throughout the afternoon):

2 glasses warm water with lemon

½ cup mixed berries

½ cup 1 percent cottage cheese (whipped cottage cheese is especially good) mixed with ½ cup salsa and (unlimited) baby carrots to dip

1 steamed artichoke with lemon

Dinner:

2 glasses warm water with lemon

Large mixed vegetable salad (same as lunch) with 2 teaspoons olive oil and as much lemon as you want

¼ avocado

1 cup Roasted Vegetables (see recipe on page 267)

4 ounces fish (same as lunch) or 4 ounces grilled or baked chicken breast (see recipe on page 311)

1 small baked potato (3½ ounces)

½ melon (any type)

Great "Junk" Food

Not all junk food is created equal. Check out the following items—they will likely satisfy your cravings, but they're kinder to your body than many other types of junk food. Pay attention to the serving size: When they're available, individual-serving-size containers can mean the difference between a snack and an out-of-control feast.

Crunchy and Salty
1 small bag barbecue Baked Lay's potato chips
1 small bag fat-free tortilla chips
1/4 cup roasted, salted mixed nuts
1 small bag Smartfood cheese popcorn

Crunchy and Sweet
2 Fig Newtons
10 animal crackers
2 Oreos
1 Dream Bar candy bar
1 cup frosted flakes with 1/2 cup low-fat milk
5 lollipops
2 pretzel rods with 1 tablespoon honey to dip
1 waffle drizzled with 1 teaspoon chocolate syrup

Creamy and Sweet (and Chocolaty)
1 Milky Way Light bar
5 Hershey's Kisses
5 bite-size Tootsie Rolls
5 chocolate licorice sticks
1 Fudgsicle
20 chocolate-covered raisins
1 York Peppermint Patty

want to try a piece (or two) of fruit before you reach for the junk food. If you have some fruit first, about half the time it will squash your craving for junk food.

A great strategy is to make exchanges. For example, try peanut butter and jelly on crackers instead of having cookies. If you wake up in the middle of the night craving something, have a small snack of crackers and cheese, or a small bowl of cereal, or a low-fat hot chocolate. If you fight the craving, you'll probably end up bingeing. But if you try eating a small amount of a more healthful food, the cravings may eventually stop. In my experience, stress is often the culprit in cravings, so make sure you note how you are feeling when your cravings hit.

Don't keep your favorite junk food in the house. If it's not around, you can't eat it. I've found that the occasional bag of potato chips always calls me into the kitchen, where I usually can't shut it up until I've finished the bag. So, to keep my Real Food Life in check, I don't keep chips in the house. Or, if I do buy them, I purchase the small bags that can be easily managed.

Finally, set limits on your children when they accompany you food shopping—this also sets limits on yourself. Before you go food shopping, tell the kids that they can pick out only one "junk" item. Then stick with the plan when you're in the store, even if they start to complain and beg for other items.

6. "I'll Start Tomorrow"

▶ Have you ever tried to be "good" with your food day, but when you overate at lunch, you gave up for the day, figuring you'd "do better" tomorrow?

▶ Do you constantly "diet" but then get bored and spend the day eating all sorts of junk food, knowing you can always "make it up" tomorrow?

▶ Did you have an extra-busy day and end up eating whatever was easiest since you figured you could eat right starting tomorrow?

Many people put off healthful eating until "tomorrow" (or later). They want a fresh start if they feel they "messed up"—perhaps they ate a big, high-calorie meal or had a mini-binge. They feel they can't keep their food lives together if they indulged, and psychologically they can't move on until they have a clean slate.

Typically, people who procrastinate about improving their food lives get caught up with the idea of perfection. This type of person believes that unless her food life is perfect, she can't have a good food life at all. Anything can trip up a so-called perfect day—it could be a busy day at work or school, a deadline, traveling, problems with the children, or just life in general.

Strategy: The solution isn't "starting tomorrow." It's saying to yourself "I binged," or "circumstances got the better of me," and moving on. You need to start eating sanely at your next meal—not the next day. Getting a Real Food Life means losing the procrastination mentality. Every single day you'll encounter all sorts of obstacles at home, at work, and with food. That's okay. Not only is it okay, it's life, and it's normal. There's no such thing as a perfect food day.

The key is knowing how to manage *your* food day and not getting caught up with how you are "supposed to eat" or what your friends or family are eating. Everyone is different, and you need to find food strategies that work for you, that you can live with, work with, and play with.

When you get a Real Food Life, you realize that you don't need to eat perfectly, so there's never a need to have a clean slate. If you binge or indulge, or if circumstances get the better of you, don't beat yourself up about it or think that you need to delay eating well until tomorrow. A Real Food Life is forever.

7. I'm Always Hungry, Especially at Night

▶ Do you go through the day making sensible food choices, but as soon as it's dark outside—even if you had a good dinner—your good food sense seems to fly out the window?

▶ Are you worried that getting a Real Food Life means you'll never be satisfied and always be hungry?

▶ Do you feel that because you are hungry all the time, food is always on your mind and you're obsessed with food?

▶ Are you always dieting, but you don't find food satisfying, and you're always hungry?

▶ Do you always feel hungry at work?

Don't Ignore the Signs of Extreme Hunger

Many people—especially those who have been on various fad diets—have become so out of touch with their bodies that they no longer recognize signs of extreme hunger. Others, desperate to lose pounds, ignore the cues their bodies are sending them. The symptoms below are all signs of extreme hunger. Try never to allow yourself to get to this point before eating, because chances are you'll be so famished that you'll make poor food choices. If you do have two or more of these symptoms, you're probably overdue for a meal.

- You feel faint.
- You're lightheaded.
- You have difficulty concentrating.
- You have a headache.
- You feel irritable.
- You have noises in your stomach.
- There's a gnawing feeling in the pit of your stomach.

Is It Hunger or Thirst?

If you think you're hungry but have the following symptoms of dehydration, you may simply be thirsty. Try drinking a glass of water before reaching for something to eat.

- You have recently eaten a reasonably sized meal but are still hungry.
- Your urine is dark (it should be almost clear).
- You have a dry mouth.
- You feel very tired—mentally and physically—and don't know why, since you had a decent night's sleep.
- You're constipated.
- You're excessively thirsty. (Keep in mind, though, that you can be dehydrated and not feel thirsty.)

Many people never feel satisfied with their food, so they always eat because they feel hungry all the time. Maybe they're always hungry in the late afternoon, or maybe, for women, they're especially hungry right before their periods. Maybe they're always hungry at night, even if they ate sensibly during the day. People who are chronically hungry inevitably have food on their minds and become obsessed with food. Often, it's the fear of hunger that prevents people from eating more healthfully; they incorrectly equate a Real Food Life with dieting and deprivation.

Strategy: There are a few ways to cope with the "I'm always hungry" syndrome. The first step is to learn to recognize whether you're actually hungry. You need to listen to your body, and this takes some practice. Is it hunger pangs you are experiencing, or is it really your mood that's making you turn to-

ward food? Are you angry, stressed, depressed, nervous? Food is often used as a stress reliever and a balm to troubling emotions.

Another way to combat this syndrome is to eat small meals all day long. It's that easy. Eating smaller amounts of nutritious foods throughout the day (instead of just three larger meals) helps your metabolism stay active, gives you the sensation of fullness, and produces less insulin after you eat. What that means is that the calories you eat are burned more efficiently, and if they are burned more efficiently and don't exceed your energy needs, they're not stored as fat. Eating smaller meals more often gives the power of food back to you. It keeps your blood sugar levels balanced and keeps your mood in check. If you spread out your meals, you can learn to have small portions of food that you love

"Free" Foods

The following foods are low in calories and high in nutrients. They're pretty much all-you-can-eat foods. They do have calories, however, so you might think twice if you plan on eating a pound of each of these every day.

- All vegetables (except starchy ones such as corn, peas, and potatoes), including artichokes, asparagus, beets, bok choy, broccoli, broccoli raab, Brussels sprouts, cabbage (any color), carrots, cauliflower, celery, celery root, cucumbers, mushrooms (any variety), parsnips, peppers, tomatoes, and turnips
- Eggplant, zucchini, and other squash such as acorn, butternut, hubbard, and spaghetti
- Beet greens, endive, fennel, kale, mustard greens, radicchio, romaine, spinach, Swiss chard, and any other type of lettuce
- Grapefruit and watermelon

(where a large portion might have too many calories for your eating plan).

If you're truly hungry, you should eat; but whether it's a snack or a meal, try to make everything you eat count. All the food you eat should be both delicious and nourishing. When you can, make sure you have a balance of protein, carbohydrates, and good fats, such as those found in fish and peanut butter.

If you're always hungry, you can eat "free" foods like vegetables all day long. I consider them "free" because they have almost no cost when it comes to calories. Further, they're filled with fiber, so they fill you up; they're also high in vitamins and minerals. Eat as much of these foods as you desire, and make soups and other veggie dishes from them to have in your refrigerator at all times. See " 'Free' Foods" for the complete list.

When you develop an eating plan, it should include plenty of low-calorie, healthful snacks. (For some suggestions, see "Healthy Substitutes for Sugary Snacks" on page 23 and "Healthy Substitutes for Salty Snacks" on page 25.) If you're always hungry, be sure to create an eating plan with flexibility—build in some days that are "foodier," where you eat more than other days. If you have some lighter food days, those will balance the heavier ones. By the same token, if you're always hungry at night, plan for that. Pick out some sensible snacks that fit into your eating plan. Determine what you really crave and what will really satisfy you: Sweet? Salty? Creamy? Crunchy? There are lots of low-calorie snacks available that will satisfy these cravings. Check out "Great 'Junk' Food" on page 30 for some ideas.

Finally, be sure to drink water—lots of it. In fact, it's a good idea to drink one or two glasses of water before each meal. You should strive for at least eight 8-ounce glasses of water each day, but there's practically no such thing as drinking too much water. Water helps to fill you up, and it also flushes you out.

8. I Eat When I'm Stressed Out

▶ Do you eat when you are under deadline?

▶ When you're at a party and you're uncomfortable, do you hover around the snack table?

▶ Do you eat when you feel overwhelmed?

▶ Do you use food as a coping mechanism?

Stress comes in many forms: deadlines, demands, crises, kids clamoring for attention or getting into trouble, the feeling that you have to please everyone, nervousness (social, financial, career, or otherwise), and even worries about your food life. Whatever its origin, feeling stressed out often leads to eating. We use food to soothe our anxieties. For many of us, food is a coping mechanism, a comfort, a release.

The thing is, stress-eating is mostly unconscious eating. It's reaching for food without even thinking about it; it's eating whatever is placed in front of you or whatever you can find—and often when you're not even hungry.

Strategy: The first way to cope with stress-eating is to *not* deny yourself some edible stress outlets. If you deny yourself, you'll start to obsess about food. Keeping a food journal is critical when you're learning to calm your stress-eating because it makes you accountable for what you eat—and when you're accountable, you can help keep your food life in check.

You won't always know when you're going to be under a lot of stress, but if you build in to your eating plan foods that help you get through the day (a small portion of your favorite chocolate, a small bag of lower-fat chips, or a few sorbet bars, for example), these can be your go-to goodies in times of stress.

In addition, exercise is an amazing stress reliever. When you work out, your body releases endorphins (feel-good brain chemicals) that make you feel better and calmer and also stimulate T lymphocytes (cells that play a crucial role in attacking pathogens within the body). Since stress can compromise your immune system and make you more prone to getting colds and infections, exercise is a great option. Even a moderate walk will help. And if you just can't find any time to get those endorphins flowing by exer-

How Stress Sabotages Your Health

Unless you live in a fantasy world, chances are you've felt the effects of stress in the form of a nagging headache or upset stomach. But did you know that stress can affect your body in many other ways as well? Here's a laundry list of the ways stress can affect your health. Use it as motivation to incorporate some stress-reducing activities, such as exercise, meditation, or even yoga, into your day.

- Stress can cause fatigue, chronic headaches, irritability, changes in appetite, memory loss, cold hands, and gastrointestinal problems, including irritable bowel syndrome.
- Stress slows down the healing of cuts and the recovery from colds.
- Researchers say stress causes at least 80 percent of all major illnesses, including back problems, heart disease, infections, and skin disorders.
- When a person is under stress, major body changes occur, including increased blood pressure and heart rate, increased cholesterol levels, and decreased immune system functioning. In addition, digestion may slow, fats and sugars may be released from stores in the body, and blood may tend to clot more easily.
- Stress can lead to nutritional deficiency caused by an increase in production of the adrenal hormones. These hormones cause the body to step up the metabolism of protein, fats, and carbohydrates. What this means is that stress causes your body to burn the nutrients it needs more quickly, so your body can't absorb those nutrients as well as when you're not stressed.
- When you're stressed, your body excretes amino acids (building blocks of protein that are needed to build muscle), potassium (a mineral important for a healthy nervous system and regular heart beats), and phosphorus (a mineral important for bone and teeth formation, cell growth, and heart and kidney functions). All this depletes magnesium, and if magnesium is low, it will lower the amount of calcium in your body (because magnesium helps calcium uptake).
- Stress may cause a B-vitamin deficiency. Since the B vitamins are needed for the proper functioning of the nervous system, and the nervous system kicks into overdrive during times of stress, the body has greater requirements for B vitamins during these times. In times of stress, people tend to overeat and overdrink—or, conversely, undereat—which will also compromise their B-vitamin stores. Symptoms of a B-vitamin deficiency include irritability, lethargy, and depression.
- Stress can set off food cravings because the stress hormones norepinephrine and corticosterone raise levels of the brain chemical galanin, and increased galanin levels lead to an increased appetite for fat, overeating, and possible weight gain.

cising, a quick fix can be a glass of fat-free or 1% milk with a tablespoon of cocoa, since both lactose and fat may help release endorphins as well.

There's no magic bullet, but some foods can actually help in the battle against stress.

Fruits, vegetables, and whole grains all contain carbohydrates, which release serotonin, a brain chemical that makes you feel more relaxed. (The corollary is that stress may actually stimulate the breakdown of serotonin.) If you have a breakfast that includes carbohydrates, it may

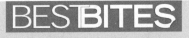

Foods That Soothe

When you're feeling particularly stressed, reach for one of the following foods. They're all known for their ability to soothe and calm you, and each contains about 100 calories.

3 fresh apricots, or 1/2 cup dried

1 medium banana

1 cup fresh blueberries

1 small baked apple

1/2 cup dried fruit

2 medium fresh figs

1 cup grapes

2 cups honeydew melon

2 medium kiwifruit

1 cup fresh mango

2 cups diced papaya

1 large orange

1 pink grapefruit

1 large peach or nectarine

1 cup fresh cherries

4 dried dates

4 tablespoons Guiltless Gourmet black bean dip with unlimited baby carrots

1 cup Health Valley split pea soup

1/2 cup low-fat vanilla yogurt sprinkled with 1 tablespoon wheat germ

1 ounce low-fat Muenster cheese on 1 whole grain cracker

1 cup low-fat whipped cottage cheese

The Antioxidant All-Stars

Antioxidants help to protect the body from attacks by free radicals, unstable oxygen molecules that play a role in the development of cancer, heart disease, and aging. Fortunately, there are numerous foods that are good sources of antioxidants.

Green tea, dark chocolate, soy beans, and tofu are antioxidant all-stars in that they contain high levels of many different antioxidants. Below are other members of the all-star team. These foods have made the cut because they contain particularly high levels of a certain antioxidant.

Beta-carotene: Asparagus; broccoli; Brussels sprouts; dark green, leafy vegetables (including cooking greens like beet greens, collards, kale, and spinach); orange and yellow vegetables (including apricots, carrots, nectarines, peaches, squash, and sweet potatoes)

Coenzyme Q$_{10}$: Beef, mackerel, peanuts, salmon, sardines, spinach

Selenium: Brazil nuts, broccoli, brown rice, chicken, dairy foods, garlic, salmon

Vitamin C: Asparagus, avocados, beet greens, berries, broccoli, Brussels sprouts, cantaloupe, citrus fruits, green leafy vegetables, mangoes, papaya, potatoes, red and green bell peppers, spinach, tomatoes

Vitamin E: Avocados, brown rice, canola oil, cereals and breads made with 100 percent whole grain, eggs, extra-virgin olive oil, green leafy vegetables, legumes, milk, nuts, oatmeal, seeds, soybeans, wheat germ

Zinc: Egg yolks, fish and shellfish, lamb and other meats, legumes, lima beans, mushrooms, oysters, pecans, poultry, pumpkin seeds, soybeans, sunflower seeds, whole grains

help set a mellower mood for the whole day.

In addition, try to eat foods that are high in antioxidants, such as vitamins C and E and the B vitamins. (See "The Antioxidant All-Stars" for a list of some of these foods.) Antioxidants are a group of vitamins, minerals, and enzymes that protect the body from free radicals, atoms that attack the immune system and can cause cell damage, infections, heart disease, cancer, and aging.

There's no getting around it: Our lives are filled with stress. But by eating right, exercising, and having snacks on hand that you can turn to in difficult times, you no longer need to be its victim.

9. Food Cheers Me Up (and Is My Companion)

▶ Do you soothe your sadness, unhappiness, or depression with food?

▶ When you've suffered a disappointment, do you eat?

▶ If you're upset about working too much, or not working enough, do you eat?

▶ Do you use food to cope with loneliness?

▶ Do you eat more when you're alone—and you're alone a lot, so you eat a lot?

Sadness, depression, and feeling alone often lead to overeating. Whether you're struggling with a professional disappointment, a scholastic setback, wintertime sadness (clinically referred to as Seasonal Affective Disorder, or SAD), a personal frustration, or social isolation, it's common to try to soothe yourself with food.

You might use food as a comfort, a diversion, or a friend substitute. But using food in this way is a cycle that repeats and repeats with the same consequence: mindless overeating.

Strategy: Using food as comfort and company is a way of nurturing yourself. You probably learned early in life that eating makes you feel better, so you turn to this strategy even as an adult. Eating to deal with loneliness or sadness is rarely about being physically hungry. By learning the triggers of emotional eating, you can stop yourself before you pig out and ask, "Am I truly hungry or emotionally hungry? Is it really depression, anger, or loneliness that I'm feeling?"

Head hunger is the need for something else that is not food, but food is a comfort-

Identify Your Hunger Level

When you listen to your body, you'll learn how hungry you are (or aren't). By helping you to tune in to the feelings in your stomach before, during, and after eating, the following scale can aid you in gauging your hunger level. You should start eating when you drop to level 3 and stop eating at level 7.

Level 1: Empty stomach—can't function; in pain
Level 2: Functioning barely; serious unease
Level 3: Functioning, but very hungry; tolerable unease
Level 4: Functioning, but can't wait to eat
Level 5: Neutral
Level 6: Still hungry, but aware of food in stomach
Level 7: Still some room in stomach, but satisfied and comfortably full
Level 8: Slight unease; somewhat overfull
Level 9: Uneasy; much too full
Level 10: Can't function; in pain

able stand-in. Head hunger is used to keep emotions that you think you can't cope with at bay. The problem, though, is that you're not facing the actual issues that made you feel upset in the first place. Food is used as self-medication—it's numbing and makes you feel good instantly.

This type of eating often occurs because people wrongly believe they're bad or weak. If this is true of you, ask yourself what you are hiding from. Facing issues such as loneliness or depression is painful, but it has to be done if you want to get out of the cycle of overeating. You have to get in touch with your feelings—not mask them by eating. For example, if you're bored or lonely, call up a friend and try to brainstorm things you could do together. Even if you end up just going for a walk around the block, the change of scenery may be enough to keep you from reaching for food. If you're sad, know that it's okay to cry. And if you're lonely, make some positive step in interacting with people, such as volunteering, joining a club, or going to a lecture. If you're feeling really low and cripplingly shy and you can't find a way to help yourself, seeking professional counseling is probably the best thing you can do for yourself.

Interestingly, depression can be caused by your diet. Eating large quantities of simple carbohydrates like sugar and refined grains (such as white bread) causes your blood sugar level to rise and then fall very rapidly, creating a "high" followed by a severe crash that induces feelings of depression. Cutting back on sugar, refined grains, and caffeine, which also raises and drops your blood sugar level very quickly, can help to regulate your mood swings.

Another possible cause for depression is inadequate vitamin B_6, which is needed for proper functioning of the central nervous system. Low B_6 can be a result of too much exercise, constant dieting, or too much alcohol. To increase your level of B_6, eat more carrots, chicken, eggs, walnuts, fish, meat, cheese, spinach, sunflower seeds, and wheat germ.

To deal with mild depression, try eating complex carbohydrates, which increase levels of tryptophan (mellowing brain chemicals) and serotonin (feel-good brain chemicals). These chemicals can help brighten moods and decrease irritability. Crackers, fruit, and even potatoes can provide temporary relief for low moods. Niacin can also help fight depression, but you should get it only through food, not supplements. Particularly good sources of niacin are broccoli, carrots, cheese, dandelion greens, dates, eggs, fish, milk, potatoes, and whole wheat products.

A good way to learn about the causes and effects of head hunger is to keep and analyze a food journal. By jotting down what you eat, when you eat, and what your mood is before, during, and after eating, you can learn if it's your diet that's making you feel down, or if you feel down regardless of your food intake. If you discover your depression isn't diet-related, discuss this with your doctor, who can identify other causes for your depression and refer you to a specialist as needed.

10. I Love to Snack

▶ If you could snack all day without gaining weight, would you?

▶ Do you think that snacking is bad?

▶ Do you munch on your kids' leftover chicken nuggets, mini pizzas, and macaroni and cheese?

Snacking is an American obsession. Lots of people would opt to snack all day if they knew they wouldn't gain weight. Snacking has gotten a bad rap: People think that they should eat only three "proper" meals a day with nothing in between. But when chosen wisely, snacks can be part of a healthful eating plan.

Of course, if you snack all day long, that's basically a binge. And if you snack only on junk food such as potato chips and candy bars, that's not good snacking. If you're emptying the vending machine, chowing down at fast-food places, or munching on your kids' leftovers, that's not smart snacking either.

Strategy: Snacking can be healthy, but you have to be smart about it. Snacks need to fit in with your individual eating plan; they can't simply be mindless eating without hunger. If you love to snack, you should be snacking smart.

Smart snacking is a very efficient way of burning calories. You get the same benefits that you do when you eat small, frequent meals—less insulin is released and your metabolism is more active. Smart snacking keeps blood sugar levels balanced, it relieves that "starving" feeling so you don't overeat at your next meal, and it helps you feel less obsessed with food because you know you can eat when you feel hungry.

Unsmart snacks tend to be foods high in simple, or refined, carbohydrates, such as pretzels, potato chips, popcorn, white bread, and cookies. These foods raise and lower your blood sugar levels very quickly and cause tiredness, hunger, and cravings. They're also emptied from your stomach quickly, so they don't keep you satisfied for very long.

When you snack, try to have a protein combined with a carbohydrate. That way, the food stays in your stomach longer than if you ate a carbohydrate alone. Fat also delays emptying of the stomach and keeps you fuller longer. Having a snack of a small handful of nuts, which will provide protein and fat, with a low-fat yogurt or a slice of whole grain bread with hummus (mashed chickpea spread) will likely keep you full and satisfied for a few hours.

It takes time to find the snacks that really suit you—both body and mind. Be aware that snacking is not for everybody. Some people find that snacking leaves them feeling out of control with food. If this is the case for you, larger meals spaced farther apart should help you feel satisfied and in control.

11. I Eat When I'm Bored

▶ Do you eat to pass time when you're bored?

▶ When you're working long, tedious hours, do you eat?

▶ When you're watching TV or working on the computer, do you finish a whole bag of chips or cookies without even realizing it?

When you're bored, eating can be a (temporary) savior. Food becomes the focus of entertainment, and eating keeps you busy. And while the TV and computer can connect us to nearly anyone around the globe, they're also passive activities, and mindlessly eating while watching or working on them is natural.

Strategy: Eating can be a coping mechanism to deal with boredom, whether you're at work, school, or home. When there is no other emotional arousal, eating gives you something on which to focus.

Boredom-eating usually has nothing to do with hunger. It is mindless eating, eating whatever's there, eating without taking into account your actual hunger level. (Mindful eating, on the other hand, is eating consciously and only when you're hungry, with awareness that your food life is nourishing for your body and your emotions.)

An effective way to monitor mindless eating is to keep a food journal. When you write down everything you eat, when you eat, and how you feel as you're eating, you'll discover that you're not actually hungry every time you eat. (For specific information on how to start a food journal, see page 142.) After just a few days of keeping a food journal, you'll start to notice how often you engage in mindless eating. You'll soon be able to determine if you are actually hungry, or if you are simply in the habit of eating to get through a situation (even if that situation is watching TV or working on the computer).

One of the best ways to keep yourself from turning to food when you're bored is to find what I've dubbed anti-boredom activities. For at least 10 minutes out of every hour you're on the computer or watching the tube, move. Try dancing, jogging in place, doing jumping jacks, or walking. Or, instead of just surfing the channels and not really watching any one show, buy workout tapes and use them. Once you've memorized some exercises, you can even work out while watching a favorite show. You might want to keep a pair of weights next to the sofa and do lifts during the commercials. On days when you're feeling less ambitious, just getting up and getting a drink of water during the commercials is better than nothing—you'll increase your daily water consumption and get a bit of exercise, too.

Although incorporating some movement

while you watch TV will help, also try to find activities that get you off of the couch and limit the amount of time you have available to watch the tube. Instead of watching TV for hours each week, read, practice a hobby, or try physical activities like walking, jogging, doing yoga, or even cleaning the house. These will help to relieve boredom, get you away from food, and get your body moving. As a bonus, physical activities help reduce depression and anxiety because they release endorphins that help you to feel more relaxed.

Even with these safeguards, all of us eat out of boredom occasionally. When this happens to you, simply choose your boredom-foods wisely. Try to have healthful snacks nearby, and throw out food that leaves you feeling out of control, such as huge bags of potato chips and supersize candy bars. Challenge your cooking skills by making nutritious *and* delicious snacks for yourself and your family. (Check out the recipes beginning on page 259.) Finally, stock up on a variety of vegetables, which are considered "free" foods, in that you can eat as much as you want without consequence. (See " 'Free' Foods" on page 34.)

12. I Make Deals with Myself to Eat What I Want

▶ If you're "good" during the day, do you feel you deserve a pint of ice cream at night?

▶ Are you "good" for the week and then pig out over the weekend?

▶ If you overindulge one night, do you rationalize that you'll work "extra hard" at the gym the next day (but of course you're either too tired or too hung over to work "extra hard" when the day comes)?

Bargaining with yourself about food is no way to have a healthy food life. I see this fairly often: People have a deal-making mentality that if they are "good" (which usually means eating too little), they "deserve" a food reward (and then wonder why they're gaining weight). Or they rationalize that since they're working long, hard hours, they deserve to eat what they want today, and they vow to eat better the next day (but that never happens and then they get depressed).

Strategy: Making deals never works. Negotiating your food intake with yourself only makes you feel angry and frustrated. Food isn't a business transaction. Making a "deal" with your food continues the cycle of not trusting yourself and sets you up for failure.

Allow yourself to have some of the foods you crave. This helps to keep food from becoming an emotional issue. If you feel you need some chocolate, or chips, or fries, have a small quantity and then move on. You don't have to binge to indulge a craving. You can allow yourself to splurge once in a while. So once a month, say, indulge in an extraordinary meal.

In the 8-Week Food Life Makeover Plan beginning on page 131, I'll help you to create a program that works with your lifestyle and makes you feel good. Then you'll be able to stop making deals with yourself and get a better grip on your food life.

13. I Can't Get Organized to Eat Regular Meals

▶ Do you feel so overscheduled with work, school, or your family responsibilities that you can't eat right?

▶ Are you so busy that it's easiest to "just grab something" on the road, from a vending machine, at a fast-food joint, or from the cupboards?

▶ Do you find it too overwhelming to prepare three proper meals for the day, so you go to the other extreme and eat mindlessly throughout the day?

Many clients tell me the same thing: "My life is so fast-paced that I can never 'eat right' or sit down for a regular meal." They're not even sure what a "regular" meal is, since they're used to having "irregular" meals. They spend their days picking at food (rather than having meals), or they feel so full after a "regular" meal that they need to unbutton their pants. They're tied up with work, school, or the kids and don't have the focus or time to have a balanced, nourishing meal, so they grab whatever they can find. And then they feel guilty for not sitting down to eat "actual" meals.

Some people never learned how to cook: how to prepare a simple omelette or baked potato, or how to stock the refrigerator. They think the only way to get organized with their eating is to hire a nutritionist, a food shopper, a cook, and a maid to clean up. (Like that's a practical solution!) They want a quick and easy "no-brainer" way to eat well.

Strategy: It's time to get back to food basics. Sure, it takes a little time, practice, and patience to get organized to eat smart, but it is doable. This book is filled with ways for you to get organized with your food. In part 3, I'll take you step by step through my 8-Week Food Life Makeover Plan. As part of that plan, I'll give you directions for doing a kitchen makeover (see page 176), a shopping list (see page 186), and many other strategies and new ideas for getting a Real Food Life. There's even a whole chapter with simple and quick recipes (see page 255).

A regular "meal" doesn't have to mean a three-course dinner. It can mean small but frequent "meals" throughout the day, which is a healthy way to eat. When you "graze" on small but frequent meals, less insulin (a hormone that helps regulate blood sugar) is released into your body, so your metabolism is more active.

Finally, grazing on healthy foods all day can actually make you feel more comfortable. Whereas a larger, "regular" meal may leave

Caffeine Quotients

Caffeine is most often consumed in beverages, where it is either naturally occurring, as in tea and coffee, or added to the final product, as in colas. To find out how much caffeine is in some popular drinks and foods, check out the following table.

Item	Amount of Caffeine (mg)
Coffee (10 oz)	120–270
Instant coffee (10 oz)	60–240
Decaffeinated coffee (10 oz)	2–10
Brewed tea (5 oz)	20–110
Iced tea (12 oz)	65–80
Green tea (5 oz)	12–60
Instant tea (5 oz)	25–50
Semisweet chocolate (1 oz)	5–35
Hot cocoa (8 oz)	2–20
Chocolate milk (8 oz)	2–8
Mountain Dew (12 oz)	55
Coca Cola Classic or Diet Coke (12 oz)	47
Shasta Cherry Cola (12 oz)	45
Dr. Pepper (12 oz)	40
Pepsi Cola (12 oz)	39
Diet Pepsi (12 oz)	37

you feeling too full, grazing makes you feel full but not stuffed. It also gives you greater control over your food, thereby making you less obsessed with food.

14. I Can't Live without Caffeine

▶ Do you find it hard to think straight until you've had a cup of strong coffee?

▶ Do you go through at least a liter of cola a day?

For many people, coffee and colas are an addiction. They can't lift their heads in the morning unless they know they'll have their fix. Many have been doing it for years and are certifiable caffeine junkies, drinking up to 10 cups of caffeinated beverages each day. Some use caffeine only to get through the morning and over the afternoon hump. Some prefer cola and other caffeinated sodas. They'll start their day with a pop and don't stop until after dinner. They might believe that as long as they drink "diet" soda, it's okay.

Strategy: Coffee is America's second

most popular drink, right behind soda, which is number one. Americans consume half the world's coffee crop, averaging 450 cups per person per year. We each also drink 450 glasses of soda each year!

Caffeine is absorbed into your blood within half an hour of consumption and affects your brain, heart rate, respiration, muscle coordination, and central nervous system almost immediately thereafter. It stays in the body for up to 4 hours. Coffee drinkers take longer to fall asleep, they don't sleep as well, and they wake up not feeling as refreshed as people who don't drink coffee.

Coffee (and the caffeine in it) is not "bad" per se—it does help people to think faster, elevates the mood, and improves motor skills and short-term memory. But too much has the opposite effect: It causes fatigue. Because caffeine is a diuretic, excessive consumption may cause dehydration, and one of the results of dehydration is fatigue. In addition, dehydration can potentially lead to constipation. Further, caffeine consumed in excess may decrease your body's iron stores, which in turn may compromise your immune system, making you more prone to colds and flu. Unfortunately, these symptoms often begin a vicious cycle: The coffee junkie ends up consuming more caffeine to fight fatigue, and soon she needs to drink more and more to get the same results.

You don't have to stop drinking coffee altogether—just cut back. The average 10-ounce mug of coffee has about 200 milligrams of caffeine. Try to limit yourself to one and a half mugs (15 ounces total) or less in the morning. (Of course, you'd want to limit your intake even more if you are highly sensitive to caffeine, but in that case, you would probably know this already.) You can try decaf, but be sure to buy coffee that is "Swiss water process" decaf—a safer decaffeination process than others.

It's not wise to try to replace your coffee with cola or tea. It's true that both have less caffeine than coffee, but ingesting more than 300 milligrams of caffeine per day—whether it's from coffee, tea, or colas—isn't a good idea. Since many people use colas or tea as their replacement "fix" from coffee, they'll typically just end up drinking more cola or tea to compensate.

You might try switching to decaffeinated green tea, which is filled with amazing amounts of antioxidants. In addition, you should drink plenty of water all day long to stay energized and hydrated (and to make up for caffeine's dehydrating effects).

If you want to try to kick the caffeine habit, reduce your intake slowly. Withdrawal symptoms from caffeine can include headaches and fatigue. You might try switching to a grain-based drink such as Pero, Postum, or Cafix. None of these products have caffeine, they're very low in calories, and they taste similar to coffee.

Finally, beware hidden caffeine. It is found in coffee ice cream, chocolate, and quite a few over-the-counter medications, including headache remedies, diet pills, and sleep suppressants.

15. I Don't Have Time to Shop (and Its Evil Twin: I Don't Know *How* to Shop)

▶ Are you so busy you can't possibly fit grocery shopping into your schedule?

▶ When you go shopping, do you get confused and overwhelmed by too many choices?

▶ Do you wonder what the labels on products mean?

▶ When you do find the time to go shopping, are you immediately overcome with the urge to eat everything in sight?

Food shopping can sometimes be a chore, but it doesn't have to be something you dread. Many people claim that they simply don't have the time to shop. And if you have kids, taking them to the market adds a major challenge to the process. As soon as you enter the market, inevitably the kids are screaming or bored, or they start tossing junk food into the cart.

Strategy: A motto of mine is "if you shop right, you'll eat right." Finding the time to shop and getting over the dread of food shopping are big steps toward getting a Real Food Life. One way to start is to create a shopping list. Even a couple of days before you go to the market, post a list on the fridge and get the family to add to it whenever they finish something. On page 186, I've created a shopping list for you. It includes the best, tastiest, and most nutritionally sound products I have found—and used—over the years.

You do need to set time aside for yourself to shop. While food shopping may not be glamorous, it can be fun. It doesn't have to take hours, especially if you have a list before you go that takes into consideration your meals and eating plan. One way of finding time is to employ a strategy many of my clients use: Split up the shopping. For example, shop for a few essential items on Monday at a small local grocer, and go to the big supermarkets on the weekend. If you do a really big shop, you're good for several days or even weeks. Take advantage of your freezer, your refrigerator, and your cupboards. Fill them with healthy foods for all occasions, meals, and snacks, and you'll have to go shopping less often.

If you live in or near a city, the Internet can be a boon. There are several Web sites devoted to online grocery shopping. Many offer a wide variety of fresh fruits, vegetables, meats, and fish as well as whole grain breads, cereals, and pastas. Some sites you might want to try include www.peapod.com and www.netgrocer.com.

Anatomy of a Label

If you take the time to learn how to read the Nutrition Facts labels found on nearly all packaged foods, you'll find that they can be treasure troves of valuable information. Here I've explained the most important elements.

Serving Size: The serving size tells the consumer what the nutritional values are based on. The serving size is recommended by the product manufacturer, who uses level measuring cups and spoons when determining this amount. Just because the manufacturer suggests a serving size doesn't mean it's right for you; it's a general guideline.

Amount per Serving: These are the total grams of fat, cholesterol, minerals, carbohydrates, and protein in a serving of the product. There's also an at-a-glance percent Daily Value column on the right, so you know if you are nutritionally on track.

Vitamins and Minerals: By law, labels must list sodium, vitamins A and C, calcium, and iron. If the product is fortified, meaning that vitamins or minerals are added, this must also be listed.

Calories per Gram: This is just a helpful fact. It simply means that 1 gram of pure fat has 9 calories, 1 gram of pure carbohydrate has 4 calories, and 1 gram of pure protein has 4 calories.

Calories from Fat: These are the total number of calories from fat per serving. If you divide the calories from fat by the total calories, you get the percentage of total fat. In this case, you divide 10 by 120 to get a percentage of total fat of 8 percent. Nothing you eat should have more than 25 percent of its calories from fat.

Percent Daily Value: These percentages come from the Daily Values listed below. For each serving, you want low percentages of:

- fat (less than 5 percent)
- saturated fat (less than 2 percent)
- cholesterol (less than 5 percent)
- sodium (less than 8 percent)
- sugar (no more than 7 grams)

For each serving, you want high percentages of fiber (at least 12 percent, or 3 grams) and as many vitamins and minerals as possible.

Based on a 2000-Calorie Diet: This section of the label is a reference tool for the consumer.

These numbers are the same on every label because they're the government's recommended daily allowances of nutrients based on diets of either 2,000 or 2,500 calories per day, which is an average calorie range for most people.

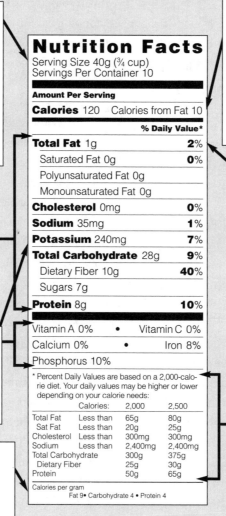

Nutrition Facts

Serving Size 40g (¾ cup)
Servings Per Container 10

Amount Per Serving

Calories 120   Calories from Fat 10

	% Daily Value*
Total Fat 1g	**2%**
Saturated Fat 0g	**0%**
Polyunsaturated Fat 0g	
Monounsaturated Fat 0g	
Cholesterol 0mg	**0%**
Sodium 35mg	**1%**
Potassium 240mg	**7%**
Total Carbohydrate 28g	**9%**
Dietary Fiber 10g	**40%**
Sugars 7g	
Protein 8g	**10%**

Vitamin A 0%	•	Vitamin C 0%
Calcium 0%	•	Iron 8%
Phosphorus 10%		

* Percent Daily Values are based on a 2,000-calorie diet. Your daily values may be higher or lower depending on your calorie needs:

		Calories:	2,000	2,500
Total Fat	Less than		65g	80g
Sat Fat	Less than		20g	25g
Cholesterol	Less than		300mg	300mg
Sodium	Less than		2,400mg	2,400mg
Total Carbohydrate			300g	375g
Dietary Fiber			25g	30g
Protein			50g	65g

Calories per gram
Fat 9• Carbohydrate 4 • Protein 4

Food shopping may not seem like such a chore if you view it as an opportunity to start your food life off on the right foot each week. Take the time to read food labels. This way, you'll be sure that you're buying only those foods that fit into your eating plan. By government mandate, nearly every packaged food now must have a "Nutrition Facts" label. In addition to serving size information, this label will tell you how much of certain nutrients a product contains. To learn how to decipher a Nutrition Facts label, see "Anatomy of a Label."

A great way to get the kids involved with the family's food life is to ask them to help you find new products that are good for them—and taste good. This is a great way to educate your kids about nutrition. Take this opportunity to teach them about Nutrition Facts labels.

Another way to make food shopping fun for kids is to involve them directly. Before you market, pick out a recipe with your kids, then go shopping for the ingredients together and have them help you cook it. This helps to foster great eating habits early on. If we involve kids in a good food life when they're young—by showing them how to shop and cook and eat—they will be healthier (and ultimately happier) children.

Finally, never go food shopping when you're hungry. This leads to overbuying and impulse buying (usually of the unhealthy foods that are at eye level, near the checkout counter). Have a small snack before you venture to the supermarket.

16. I Don't Know How to Cook (or I Don't Have Time to Cook)

▶ Are you too busy to cook?

▶ Are you scared of cooking?

▶ Do you think, "Can I really cook myself a good meal late in the evening when I'm tired from work or a day running around with the kids?"

▶ Do you read cooking magazines and watch cooking shows on TV and think, "If I can't cook that way, I don't even want to try?"

A lot of people don't know how to cook. Or if they do, they can't find the time. Maybe they never had the opportunity to see home cooking in action, or simply weren't interested in learning at the time. Whether you have a full-time job or course load or are a busy parent, carving out time to shop and cook can be a challenge.

Strategy: Cooking for yourself or your family doesn't have to feel like an overwhelming project. Even without much cooking experience, you can turn out quick, simple, and delicious meals that are satisfying to your body and soul.

Cooking doesn't have to be hard. I've

never taken a cooking lesson in my life, but I was able to learn how to cook by reading cookbooks (and making some mistakes). Once you try out a few simple recipes, you'll gain some confidence in your cooking skills—and a sense of empowerment over your food life. When you cook, you have control over the food you put on your plate and in your body. Cooking, like most things, takes a little preparation, patience, and practice. But once you start to squash your fears, you'll be amazed at what you can do. On page 186 you'll find a shopping list and strategies that will make your cooking life and food life easier.

If you lead a particularly fast-paced life, you might want to prepare food on the weekend that you can eat all week. Also, don't think that you need to prepare a three-course meal each night. I'm a big fan of simple, quick meals, such as Unfried Chicken Breasts (see recipe on page 311) with mixed sautéed vegetables. Or try a baked potato with Health Valley chili (it's in a can, and it's surprisingly good) and a mixed salad. In chapter 15, there are many fast and tasty recipes to help get you started.

17. I Always Eat More When I'm with My Family

▶ Do holidays with your family make you eat more because you're served one calorie-packed meal after another?

▶ Does going out to eat with your family mean going to an all-you-can-eat buffet?

▶ Does your family say you're "no fun" when you try to resist the family food traditions, so you always give in and eat?

▶ Do you take your family to fast-food restaurants since they're convenient and inexpensive, and your kids love them?

Families are great! We love them, need them, and for the most part, are lucky to be a part of them. But think about what brings us together most times—mealtime. We have so many traditions centered around food that it's hard and frustrating to have to think about what and how much you're putting into your mouth when you're just trying to have a good time with your family.

Strategy: There's no way around it: Most family visits and meals *are* emotionally charged, so overeating at these times is common. But you can change your behavior—especially if you're prepared. For example, if you're going home for the holidays, prepare ahead of time by writing down your meal plan before you leave—including what you'll eat for every meal and snack—and sticking to that plan.

A little less structured approach is to have a clear mental picture of your "food intentions." Know that the basis of your breakfasts, for example, will be whole grains, such as cereal or crackers, and some low-fat protein, such as yogurt or light cheese. Do this for all your meals: That way, you'll have a clearer plan for eating healthful foods at each meal, but you won't be tied down to a specific menu. Before the big family meal, exercise or go for a walk and visualize what you'll eat. Also, know that it's okay to change your food plan as you go along. If you're too rigid, you might inadvertently set yourself up for a downfall.

One good strategy is to eat what the family is eating—whether it's a holiday dinner, fast-food meal, or all-you-can-eat buffet—but have half the portions. This isn't an easy task, but it really does work. When you have a fast-food meal, order sanely: grilled chicken instead of a burger, a salad instead of fries.

If a meal will be served to you without your input, make sure you aren't starving when you sit down. This may mean that you eat before you go to your family meal. Try snacking on some "free" foods (see the list on page 34) prior to the meal. These are foods you can eat mindlessly, since they're high in nutrition and low in calories. If you're reasonably full before you sit down, the food served to you isn't such a big deal. You can simply have a taste of it and not blow your eating plan. Also, try having just a small portion of meat or fish and fill the rest of your plate with lots of vegetables. That way, you're taking in fewer calories by bulking up on the veggies, but still satisfying your eating needs.

Finally: Speak up. It may be difficult, but

muster your courage to talk to whoever is preparing the holiday feast. Tell her that you'll bring foods that you can eat, or ask her to put less on your plate. And when you go out for a meal with your family, tell them you want to eat at a more healthful place with food that everyone can enjoy. Ask them to respect your food choices and amounts. It's your body, it's your food life.

18. I Eat When I'm Tired

▶ Do you eat to stay awake?
▶ When you're sleepy, do you overeat?
▶ Are you so tired you don't care what you eat?

Whether you're an overscheduled student, an overworked employee, an overextended parent of a teenager, or a new parent of an infant, lack of sleep is an epidemic. The average American gets only 6 hours of sleep a night, but adults actually need about 8 hours. Sleep deficiencies are bad enough, but they also lead to mindless overeating. Further, recent studies suggest that people with poor sleeping habits are at a higher risk for developing diabetes.

Strategy: Though it might sound obvious, the key to dealing with this problem is to get enough sleep. (New mothers: I know from experience that this isn't always easy.) Everyone has his or her own sleep requirements, but generally, just trying to sleep more (and better) than you currently do is a good start. If you're one of those lucky people who can fit it in, try a 20-minute "power nap." A short nap will make you feel energized; a longer nap might make you groggy and grouchy.

Being low on B vitamins may be a cause for poor sleeping. B_6, in particular, is essential for the normal production of serotonin, a brain chemical that makes you feel calm and relaxed. Adequate amounts of folic acid and vitamin B_1 may also help you sleep better and increase your energy. If you're on a severely restrictive diet (less than 1,000 calories a day), you may be tired because you wake up hungry in the middle of the night (the most restful sleep tends to be continuous sleep). Making sure you consume enough calories for your body throughout the day may help you to sleep better.

Tiredness is also a symptom of both dehydration and iron deficiency. Make sure you're always well-hydrated by drinking at least 8 glasses of water a day. Iron brings oxygen to your red blood cells and is important for growth, a healthy immune system, and energy. Women, especially, are at risk for iron deficiency because iron is lost during menstruation. Try pumping up your eating plan with dark green leafy vegetables, lean red meat, and whole grains—all of which are excellent sources of iron—and see

Are You Sleep Deprived?

If you answer yes to four or more of the following questions, you're sleep deprived and need to get some shut-eye!

- Do you have problems waking up in the morning?
- Do you get really irritated with other people during the day?
- Do you get colds often (more than two in the past 6 months)?
- Do you fall asleep immediately after turning out the lights?
- Do you drink caffeine all day long to stay awake and have a cocktail at night to wind down from the day?
- Do you blow off social events or personal hobbies because you feel too tired for them?
- Do you have trouble focusing your eyes (or keeping them open) when you drive in the late afternoon or at night?
- Do you have trouble concentrating in the late afternoon and evening?
- When you go to the gym, do you feel too tired to have a good workout?
- On the weekends, do you sleep in really late and/or take lots of naps?

BEST BITES

Top 5 Drinks for Energy and Vitality

The next time your energy lags, reach for a cup of one of the following beverages. Consider it liquid energy!

- Water, water, water
- Green tea (hot or cold)
- Ginger tea (hot or cold)
- Seltzer with lemon or lime or a splash of orange juice
- Chamomile tea (for certain individuals, chamomile tea can actually cause sleepiness, so test it out)

if that increases your energy levels.

If you're eating to stay awake, you might actually be eating because you're bored or stressed. If so, turn to Issue 9 and Issue 11 (see pages 38 and 42).

If you're exhausted in the evening, after you come back from school or work or after a day with the kids, eat plenty of "free" food (see the list on page 34). Also drink at least two glasses of water before you eat everything in sight. The water will help to fill you up and help prevent dehydration.

19. I'm a Picky Eater

▶ Are the only vegetables you like corn, potatoes, and peas?

▶ Do you think fish belong only in the sea (or an aquarium) and not on a plate?

▶ Do you always eat the same foods because they're "safe" and you "trust" them?

▶ Do you prefer "plain" food without herbs or spices and live on meat, cheese, and pasta?

Everyone has different tastes, preferences, and food histories. While many people love all different types of food and all different types of cuisine, there are others who won't even look at certain dishes or food groups. They might have memories of being forced to eat something when they were kids. They may have been fussy eaters all their lives. They might be able to tolerate certain foods only if they're drowned in sauce. Or they may avoid new foods because they're scared of how they taste or are skeptical that they can be prepared to taste delicious.

Strategy: Let's get back to basics: If you're

in pursuit of a Real Food Life, you owe it to yourself to try to eat new things (assuming that you're not allergic to them, of course). You may be surprised by what you like. Eating a variety of foods is not only an amazing sensual pleasure, but a delicious and vital component of good health. If you have kids, it also sets a good example for them to follow. Being picky may not be a big issue now, but it could be in the long term. Are you always tired? Do you often get colds? Is your skin dry? Are you often cranky? These conditions may be due to the food you eat—or should I say, don't eat.

Learning to love vegetables, fish, or whatever you don't currently eat may take some time if you've spent your life avoiding them, but start slowly and try something new every week or two. If you open your mind and palate, you can learn to love new foods, and the benefits can be enormous. To get more comfortable with these foods, order them in a restaurant to learn how a professional prepares them. Explore your local farmers' market or gourmet store and ask the vendor for preparation tips. Also, refer to chapter 15 for lots of ideas for quick, easy, and truly tasty dishes.

You might also consider taking a cooking class to become more comfortable preparing a wide variety of food. Cooking classes aren't available only at cooking schools; many colleges and community centers offer classes on vegetarian cooking or Fish Preparation 101, for example. And once you see an instructor effortlessly whip up a dish, you're sure to have the confidence to try it at home.

20. I Eat What My Kids Eat (Yuck!)

▶ Do you always eat the same food as your kids?

▶ Do you sneak your kids' food after they go to sleep?

▶ Do you "snack" with your kids and then eat with your adult partner?

New and veteran parents alike are often surrounded by more junk food than they could have imagined before they became parents. Kids are growing machines and tend to eat all day long to keep up with their changing, hungry bodies. It's easy, then, for parents to become accustomed to eating with their kids, which often means a round-the-clock schedule of snacks and meals.

Strategy: Did you know that eating a handful of your kids' French fries twice a week can lead to a 5-pound weight gain in a year? One way to crack the eating-your-kids'-food dilemma is to limit the amount of junk food in your house. Also, find healthier foods that your kids actually like and buy those foods. For example, instead of regular potato chips, get baked chips, or better yet, have low-fat cheese with crackers. Get Häagen-Dazs sorbet instead of regular Häagen-Dazs ice cream; buy animal crackers instead of chocolate chip cookies.

Don't allow yourself to get in the habit of eating whatever your kids left on their plates. Take the leftovers and save them for your children's next meal, or simply throw them away. If you're cooking, make only enough food for that meal so there's no waste. (Or make extra and freeze the additional food for later.) Finally, eat when you feed your kids instead of later—even if that's at 5:00 P.M.

21. I Eat More When I'm Out with Friends

▶ Whenever you get together with friends, does it seem to turn into an out-of-control eating festival?

▶ When you're with friends, do you succumb to peer pressure to eat?

▶ Do you inhale the bread basket after you've had a few pre-dinner cocktails?

▶ Do you and your friends order fried or other high-fat foods "just to put something in your stomachs" while you're drinking?

▶ When you're at a party, do you find it hard to resist the hors d'oeuvres?

▶ Have you ever lost control with your food after you've had a few drinks?

Food and friends go together. And when you add alcohol to the mix, things can get even crazier. Just as alcohol lowers social inhibitions, it also lowers inhibitions with food. Eating at restaurants and going to dinner parties are inherently social activities. Whether you're a guest, a host, or just one of the gang, when you're in a social situation, it's easy to overeat.

Strategy: Eating with friends is definitely hard. Most people tend to over-order or cook too much. In fact, researchers at Georgia State University found that when people eat with one companion, they eat 28 percent more than if they were dining alone. When they eat with two companions, they consume 41 percent more, and when they eat with six or more companions, their consumption increases by a whopping 76 percent. And you're at even greater risk of overeating when alcoholic beverages are part of the festivities, since alcohol stimulates your appetite and lowers your commitment to being smart about food.

Fortunately, eating smart doesn't mean you have to become a hermit. Before going out, verbalize or write down your food (and booze) intentions. If you're seeing friends who drink and you're prone to eating after you've had a couple, promise yourself that you'll have only one drink. Do drink plenty of water or club soda, though, since it will help fill you up and hydrate you.

The key to drinking is moderation; for women that means less than 1½ drinks daily, and for men it means less than 2 drinks daily.

The risks of drinking to excess—liver damage, high blood pressure, cancer, and so on—aren't worth it.

Don't deny yourself food—this will cause you to feel deprived and you very well may binge when you get home. Before you go out with your friends, eat plenty of "free" foods (see the list on page 34) or have a bowl of vegetable soup. If you do this, you won't be starving when you arrive, so you'll be less tempted to overeat. If you're sharing food, family-style, choose two or three dishes and serve yourself half-size portions (don't let anyone serve you); that way you will satisfy yourself physically and emotionally.

22. Love Wreaks Havoc with My Food

▶ When you first fall in love, do weight concerns seem to melt away?

▶ When you're in a new love relationship, do you lose your appetite?

▶ Do you and your partner food shop, cook, and eat together?

▶ Does your love life revolve around going out to eat?

▶ Do you show your affection by sharing sweets with your sweetie?

Ah, love. We look for it for years (sometimes decades), and when it finds us, we're elated. The side effects are great: We're energized, excited, and busy, and food no longer is a looming issue. The flip side of new-love weight loss, though, is the added pounds that often come with a long-term relationship, whether it be marriage, cohabitation, or a committed partnering.

New love or old, lots of couples' lives together revolve around a shared love of food, including going out to restaurants and cooking and eating together. Sometimes women eat more because their partners eat larger portions. And often this leads to unwanted weight gains.

Strategy: Love works in mysterious ways, and it can decrease your appetite temporarily. When you're in love, your brain releases feel-good endorphins that may help to decrease your appetite. Further, being in love keeps your mind (and body) busy, so food becomes much less of an issue.

On the other hand, when things get comfortable between a couple, overeating often becomes a problem. We want to indulge, because food can make us feel special and, after all, food is an important part of our social lives. While overindulging on occasion is not a problem, when it becomes a daily habit, it can be detrimental physically and emotionally. Talk with your partner about your plans to have a better food life and ask for his or her help.

You need to create a plan of action for both of you every time you eat. Know your food intentions, and visualize yourself eating healthfully. If you two always go to a certain restaurant, continue to go, but have two appetizers instead of an appetizer and a full-size entrée. Say no to dessert, or share a dessert only once a week. Also, don't arrive at the restaurant starving; have a light snack before you leave so you can skip the bread basket.

When you're cooking together, eat only half of the portion you would usually have (save the rest for the next day). This way, you've cooked together and can eat together, but you'll just eat less.

If your partner refuses to help you in your quest for a healthy food life, you must speak up and tell him or her that you need to take care of yourself and do what is best for you. If your partner still refuses to help even after you've asked for support, enlist a friend or other family member to be your Real Food Life support system.

23. Lunch Is My Downfall

▶ Is the only lunch option at your school or workplace a cafeteria filled with high-fat or unnourishing food choices?

▶ Do you use the vending machine as your lunch stop?

▶ Do you work out during lunch and skip eating?

▶ Do you get confused about what to eat at the food court?

Being a slave to school or work geography is a drag. Perhaps your only lunch op-

tion is a cafeteria filled with greasy food, or the only lunch place within miles is fast food, or there's a food court nearby but you don't know what you should choose. Maybe your only lunch option is to order in, and you wonder what your best choices are. Or maybe you are one of those people who think endless cups of coffee are all the lunch you ever need.

Strategy: Eating a good lunch is important—it keeps your blood sugar levels balanced, keeps your metabolism burning high, keeps you energized, helps you to focus your thoughts, cuts down on afternoon sweet cravings, and keeps you from overeating at dinner.

An ideal lunch is heavier on protein such as fish, which is high in omega-3 fatty acids, the good kinds of fat, or lean meat, such as chicken or lean beef. It also includes a small amount of grains and some vegetables. Eating a high-protein lunch can help increase your energy level because protein ups the level of the amino acid tyrosine, which has been found to increase alertness, vigilance, and concentration.

A lunch high in carbohydrates has its pluses and minuses. Some people truly feel they have more energy after eating a meal with lots of carbohydrates such as bread, rice, pasta, and starchy vegetables. While women are more prone to feeling tired after a carbohydrate-rich meal than men are, people of both genders feel more likely to want a nap after a bowl of pasta than after a roast beef sandwich. Recent studies show that eating a lot of carbohydrates may decrease alertness. Of course, this doesn't mean you should stop eating them—carbohydrates are important— but you shouldn't have a whole meal of them. Listen to your body and note how you feel after eating certain types of food for lunch.

Finally, avoid high-fat lunches such as a cheeseburger with French fries. They will just make you feel more tired because they increase the levels of tryptophan (mellow brain chemicals) in your blood.

For specific ideas on what to have for lunch, see page 206.

24. I'm a Vegetarian

▶ Have you adopted a vegetarian diet but aren't sure what you should eat?

▶ Are you concerned that if you don't eat meat, you won't get all the nutrients your body needs (especially if you're not yet an adult)?

▶ Are you a vegetarian but hate vegetables?

▶ Is your meat-free diet causing you to be tired all the time?

▶ Are you worried that you won't be able to follow my eating plan if you're a vegetarian?

More and more people are becoming vegetarians. They may be sympathetic to the animal rights cause or to environmental concerns. Others simply don't like the taste of meat, or they've read that being a vegetarian is good for them. But even people who adopt a vegetarian diet are sometimes confused about what they should eat.

Strategy: You can get a Real Food Life and be a vegetarian. There are loads of vegetarian options throughout this book.

Many people think vegetarian diets are great for weight loss, but this isn't necessarily true. A vegetarian diet can be high in fat and calories, particularly if you rely on full-fat dairy products. By the same token, animal foods can be low in fat and calories and, when eaten moderately, can enhance your health. So don't become a vegetarian thinking it will help you to lose weight. Too many calories from *any* food will cause you to gain weight.

Getting enough protein is usually not a problem. The average person needs just 50 to 60 grams of protein a day—an amount that can easily be obtained even on a vegetarian diet. In recent years, increasingly more high-protein vegetarian foods have become available at supermarkets (see "Vegetarian Sources of Protein"). If you're a "vegetarian" who chooses to eat fish, know that fish is a great source of high-quality protein and is rich in good fatty acids (known as omega-3's) that are great for your hormonal system, your heart, your hair, and your skin and nails. If you're tired all the time and you think it's due to your vegetarian diet, you may be anemic and need more iron. Great vegetarian sources of iron include tofu; kidney, lima, or black beans; Swiss chard; acorn squash; spinach; green peas; and strawberries. Other excellent sources of iron are oysters, tuna, and lean beef. Eating foods high in vitamin C will help your body to absorb the iron in the foods you eat.

If you eat no animal products at all—no dairy, meat, or fish—you will need to take a vitamin B_{12} supplement every day, because B_{12} is found only in animal sources. Lack of B_{12} causes fatigue, impaired mental function, a shorter attention span, moodiness, agitation, and confusion. You should take a multivitamin as well. Personally, I believe everyone—vegetarian or not—should take a multivitamin daily.

Vegetarian Sources of Protein

It shouldn't be hard to get the necessary 50 to 60 grams of protein your body needs each day when you have the following tasty vegetarian options.

- Fresh tofu, plain or flavored (smoked, hot and spicy, lemon herb, Asian spiced, and so on)
- Edamame (soybeans)
- Nuts and seeds (raw or roasted)
- Soy cheese
- Low-fat yogurt or low-fat soy yogurt
- Chick'n Nuggets (soy)
- Boca Burgers or Gardenburgers
- Tofu Pups or other tofu hot dog
- Tofu sausages
- Tofu lunchmeats
- Veggie Soy Singles by SoyCo (they taste just like cheese)
- Hummus
- Black bean soup or dip
- Canned beans, such as black-eyed peas, chickpeas, and kidney beans
- Health Valley vegetarian chili
- Vegetarian baked beans
- Cascadian Farms vegetarian soy dinners
- Low-fat mozzarella, Cheddar, ricotta, or cottage cheese
- Alpine lace cheese (reduced fat and salt)
- Lentil Salad with Lemon and Feta (see recipe on page 284)
- Vegetarian Asian Tofu Sandwich (see recipe on page 299)

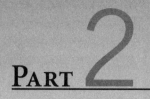
Nutrition
BASICS

3 NUTRITIONAL BUILDING BLOCKS

Whenever I work with clients, I give them handouts on the basics of healthy eating and good nutrition. Consider this section to be those handouts, but with even greater detail. I think it's absolutely crucial to learn some basics about what makes up certain foods and drinks and why they're good for you or should be avoided.

I've always found that this information serves as a good background and reference tool when people begin developing Real Food Lives of their own. My clients have found that by becoming familiar with the information in this section and understanding how the human body uses the fuel it is given, they are better able to stick to their Real Food Life plans. As you work through the 8-Week Food Life Makeover Plan later in this book, you might want to refer back to this section occasionally in order to bolster your food knowledge and remind yourself of why you are making certain choices.

Water

Unlike the other items discussed in this chapter, water is not a food group per se, but it is essential for maintaining good health and well-being. Water is vital to us because it is involved in almost every function of our bodies, including transportation and absorption of nutrients, body temperature maintenance, circulation, digestion, and waste excretion. Water is also necessary for lubricating joints and providing a protective cushion for the organs and tissues. While the human body can survive without food for 5 weeks, it cannot survive without water for more than 5 days.

Water is also vital because our bodies are made mostly of water. Men's bodies are composed of about 60 percent water (that's about 11 gallons), and women's are about 53 percent water. Women have less water than men because they have a higher percentage of body fat, and fat (about 23 percent water) has less water than muscle tissue (about 73 percent water).

Blood is made of about 90 percent water. Blood transports nutrients to the muscles and carries away waste such as carbon dioxide and lactic acid. When you're not getting enough water, your blood volume drops, which keeps your body from functioning properly.

Perspiration accounts for much of the water your body uses. Sweat prevents the body from overheating. Muscles in motion produce heat, and the body responds by sweating. The sweat then evaporates on the skin's surface and helps to cool the skin and muscles. Every day, the average person loses up to 2 cups of water through sweat (when not exercising); if you exercise, you can lose as much as 1 to 5 pounds of water, depending on the intensity and duration of your workout.

Water also plays an important role in digestion and waste control. The water in saliva and gastric (stomach) fluids helps the body to digest food. And without enough water, the colon can't process fiber as well as it should. Fiber without enough water makes solid waste too bulky and concentrated to pass comfortably and is a primary cause of constipation. My clients know if they don't drink enough water, food becomes like cement in their digestive systems—kind of graphic, I realize, but true.

Dehydration

Because our bodies are made mostly of water, even a little dehydration can be dangerous. If you lose just 1 percent of your body's weight in water, it can impair bodily functions and can cause a variety of ailments, including kidney stones.

Thirst is not a good indication of your body's water needs; by the time you feel thirsty, you're already dehydrated. Strenuous exercise can interfere with your thirst mechanism, as can hunger, too much caffeine, taking laxatives or diuretics, and having a bout of diarrhea. When you drink alcohol or excessive amounts of beverages with caffeine, both of which are diuretics, you may not realize how dehydrated you're becoming.

Water 101

Water, water, everywhere . . . but which kind should you drink? Tap water is the most convenient. But depending on where your water comes from, it could contain chemicals like chlorine and pesticides, or impurities like bacteria and parasites. More than half the cities in the United States add fluoride to their tap water to keep it clean, "soften" it, and provide anti-cavity protection. Some tap water is considered "hard," which means it has a high concentration of calcium and magnesium, minerals that can affect the taste of the water.

Filtering can improve your tap water because the filter removes contaminants and makes the water cleaner and, ultimately, better tasting. I happen to like filtered water; it's a cheaper alternative to bottled water and is very convenient.

If you prefer drinking bottled water, be aware that most states do not have laws governing the labels on bottled water, so they can be misleading or incorrect. Here is a mini glossary to help you understand the differences among a variety of waters:

Mineral water contains several mineral compounds and comes from natural springs usually in Europe or Canada. Mineral water must flow freely from the source (that is, it can't be pumped or forced from the ground) and must be bottled at the source. If you drink mineral water exclusively and aren't mineral deficient, you might be taking in more minerals than your body needs or can use. However, many Europeans drink only mineral water and claim it helps aid digestion. In America, most mineral water is prohibitively expensive to drink daily, but it is a delicious water option to enjoy on occasion.

There is no legal definition for **spring water**, and it may not actually come from a spring at all. But real spring water is unprocessed and originates in underground reservoirs that naturally rise to the earth's surface.

Sparkling water is water that is either naturally fizzy (generally from European mineral springs) or water to which carbon dioxide has been added to make it fizzy. **Seltzer** is simply filtered and carbonated tap water. Flavored seltzer or sparkling water may be made with sugars in addition to the flavoring agent, so always read the label. **Club soda** is filtered carbonated water that has added sodium in the form of bicarbonates, sodium citrates, and/or sodium phosphates. If you're cutting down on salt, stick with plain seltzer.

The best way to tell if you're well-hydrated is to check the color of your urine. If it is brightly colored or deeply concentrated and is low in volume, you're probably dehydrated. If it's almost clear and plentiful, you're probably well-hydrated. (Bear in mind, however, that vitamin supplements can make urine a darker yellow.)

How Much Water Do You Need?

I always tell my clients that water is instant energy. If you think of water this way, you'll want to drink it all day. If you're feeling tired or lethargic, a glass of water will often bring you back to life. That said, to keep your body functioning properly, you must drink at least eight 8-ounce glasses of water each day. If you are working out or feel bloated from eating a salty meal, go up to 12 to 14 glasses.

You don't have to drink only water to stay hydrated. Drinks that are equivalent to 100 percent water are fat-free or 1% milk, fruit juice, hot chamomile or ginger tea, and de-caffeinated hot coffee or tea. You can get 50 percent water from caffeinated hot teas, such as black and green tea, as well as iced tea. Alcoholic drinks count against your water intake since they dehydrate you.

You can add to your daily water intake by eating foods that have a high water content. Check out "High-Water Foods" for a list of these foods.

High-Water Foods

You can supplement your daily water intake by eating foods that have a high water content, but you still need to drink at least eight 8-ounce glasses of water a day. Here are some of the most water-filled foods around. The number following each is the percentage of water that makes up each food.

Cucumbers: 96%	Honeydew melon: 91%
Lettuce: 95%	Cantaloupe: 90%
Summer squash (all varieties): 94%	Carrots: 88%
Tomatoes: 94%	Artichokes: 87%
Watermelon: 93%	Brussels sprouts: 87%
Asparagus: 92%	Oranges: 87%
Cauliflower: 92%	Peaches: 87%
Collards: 92%	Raspberries: 87%
Mushrooms: 92%	Apricots: 86%
Peppers: 92%	Blackberries: 86%
Strawberries: 92%	Blueberries: 85%
Broccoli: 91%	Oatmeal: 85%
Grapefruit: 91%	Yogurt (plain, fat-free): 85%

Here are some strategies to help you get those 64 ounces of water each day.

▶ Keep a large (16-ounce) glass of water by your bed. When you wake up, you can start drinking immediately.

▶ Carry a bottle of water around with you. This will make it easier to get your water while you're on the run, and it's also a constant reminder to drink.

▶ Take bottled water with you in your car, especially if you're a commuter.

▶ Keep a bottle of water on your desk or near your work area and sip from it throughout the day (and keep refilling the bottle all day long).

▶ Bring a bottle of water to the gym— you'll drink more than you would if you relied on the water fountain.

▶ Log your water intake in your food journal. That way, you know how much you're drinking.

▶ Monitor your urine. You want a heavy flow of light-colored urine.

Carbohydrates

Carbohydrates should be an essential part of everyone's diet. Despite what gimmicky "no-carb" diets proselytize, for the human body to function optimally, more than half of the foods you eat each day should be carbohydrates.

Carbohydrates are the major fuel source for human beings; they provide energy and help the body function properly. Carbohydrates are composed of carbon, hydrogen, and oxygen and are found almost exclusively in plant foods like fruits, vegetables, beans, and whole grains. They're even found in sugar cane. Milk and milk products are the only foods that come from animals that contain significant amounts of carbohydrates.

There are two main types of carbohydrates: simple and complex. Simple carbohydrates are sugars; complex carbohydrates are also referred to as starches and are found in breads, grains, potatoes, peas, corn, rice, beans, pasta, and cereals.

All carbohydrates are the primary source of blood glucose, also known as blood sugar, which is either used as energy immediately or stored in the liver or muscles for future use. Stored glucose is called glycogen. When the body needs more energy, glycogen is taken out of storage and converted back to glucose. It is a major source of fuel for the body's cells and is the preferred source of fuel for the brain and red blood cells.

Carbo-Phobia?

The increasing popularity of high-protein/low-carbohydrate diets has given carbohydrates a bad reputation. People who have lost weight on these fad diets are afraid to eat any variety of carbohydrates because

The Glycemic Index

Every carbohydrate food has a different effect on blood sugar levels, and that effect is measured by the glycemic index (GI). The index measures how quickly a food is digested, turned into glucose, and absorbed into the blood—basically how much a certain food causes blood glucose levels to rise. The higher the glycemic index of a food, the faster the glucose is released into the bloodstream and the greater the outpouring of insulin. (Insulin is a hormone that controls the transport of glucose from the blood into cells.) Foods with a high glycemic index quickly enter the bloodstream and are quickly converted to blood sugar (that is, they provide fast energy that fades fast); foods with a moderate or low glycemic index enter the bloodstream more slowly and provide longer-lasting energy.

Most people don't have to be overly concerned with the glycemic index of foods. While many diet books are based on the premise that if the body produces too much insulin it causes the person to store fat, there is no scientific evidence to prove this. Studies have revealed, however, that a diet high in foods high on the glycemic index may lower HDL (good) cholesterol and increase the risk of diabetes, especially if someone is predisposed to diabetes already.

The index values shouldn't be too much of a concern for most of us, however, because they're calculated for individual foods, eaten alone. For example, potatoes are high on the index when eaten alone. But when they're eaten with a meal, they'll have much less of an effect on blood sugar because the meal will necessarily contain fat and protein and will affect the glycemic index of the potatoes.

they fear they will "get fat" from them.

High-protein/low-carb diets are usually extremely high in saturated fat, since the basis of this type of diet is meat and dairy. These high-protein diets overwork the liver and kidneys, dehydrate the body, leach calcium from the bones, and may compromise the immune system.

These diets do often cause you to lose weight because calories are significantly reduced in the long-term. The weight loss isn't particularly healthy, though, nor is it usually permanent. The glycogen stores of people on these diets diminish as their bodies try to maintain the blood glucose levels needed for proper body functioning. During this process, a lot of water is lost through urine as the glycogen storage tanks become depleted. This process happens fast, and dieters love what they see on the scale. However, since the weight loss is mostly water weight, especially in the beginning of the diet, it is always regained when the dieter begins to eat carbohydrates again.

Another reason people lose weight on these diets is because they're required to eat the same high-protein (and generally high-fat) foods all the time, so they literally become uninterested in eating. As a result, they will consume less than usual. Also, the body is more satiated with high-fat foods, but a high-fat diet can lead to high cholesterol and blood pressure levels. I am against any type of diet that requires people to forgo an entire category of food and that has the serious health implications of high-protein/low-carb diets.

What Kind of Carbohydrates Should You Eat?

About half of your daily calories should come from a variety of unrefined, or minimally processed, carbohydrates. Good choices include any carbohydrate that's as close to nature as possible, such as whole grains and fresh fruits and vegetables. Oranges, strawberries, peaches, and sweet potatoes are particularly high in carbs. A diet rich in these foods has lots of B vitamins, minerals, fiber, antioxidants, and phytochemicals. Even if you take a vitamin supplement, it can't compete with the benefits of eating these wholesome foods.

Refined carbohydrates, such as those found in cookies, candy, processed cereals, white bread, and white rice, on the other hand, often lack the nutrients crucial to good health. Refined carbohydrates can also be high in saturated fats and trans fats. Eating too many refined carbohydrates can ultimately increase your risk for diet-related diseases including diabetes, hypoglycemia, cancers, heart disease, and obesity.

Complex Carbohydrates

Complex carbohydrates are elementally different from simple carbohydrates. An easy way to think about it is that complex carbohydrates are made of three or more sugars, and simple carbohydrates contain two or less. In addition, complex carbs tend to be lower in fat than simple carbs. Beans, legumes, potatoes, rice, and whole grains are all rich in complex carbohydrates. Here's a quick rundown of two of the biggest sources.

Grains. Whole grains are a great energy-providing carbohydrate because they're instant fuel for the muscles. Grains are the seeds, or "fruits," of cereal grasses and, in their unrefined form, contain fiber, unsaturated fat, protein, iron, niacin, thiamin, and riboflavin. Refined grains (like those in white bread) have the bran removed. If you want the health benefits of bran, especially the fiber, you need to eat whole grain products. Studies have shown that people who eat a higher-fiber diet tend to weigh less than people who don't. Most likely this is because high-fiber foods fill people up, so they tend to be satisfied with less food. These foods also tend to be low in fat and calories. Some tasty whole grains are bulgur (cracked wheat), quinoa, buckwheat, pearl barley, and brown rice.

(continued on page 72)

LIVING A
REAL FOOD LIFE

She Learned the Truth about Carbohydrates

Name: Susan

Real Food Life Issues: gained weight after moving in with boyfriend, high-protein diet/fear of carbs

Susan is a computer programmer in her late twenties. She works hard but cherishes her time off, when she can hang out with her boyfriend and their dog, a cute black and brown mutt named Otis. She was thrilled when she moved in with her boyfriend 2 years back, but she has gained about 10 pounds since then—that hasn't thrilled her much. Here's where I found her:

> *January 27*
>
> *Okay, I know I have to do something about my diet. I'm craving carbs so bad, it's gotten to the point where Otis's dry food is looking good to me. Every time I pass the bakery section at the supermarket, I feel like I'm going to pass out with bread lust.*
>
> *On this score, Jason is no help. I tell him I miss carbs and he brings home an econo-size bag of tortilla chips and a vat of salsa. He thinks that's helping! He's a sweetie, but I feel like crying in frustration. I'm still struggling with these last 10 pounds, and I feel like I'm one chip away from blowing up into a ball of fat and bloat.*
>
> *Jason thinks an all-meat diet is as close to heaven as we're going to get. As close as we've become, I don't think he wants to hear about how my bathroom visits have become few and far between lately. For the first time in my life, I'm actually craving things like raw broccoli and cabbage. Oh, to eat something crunchy!*

When I met Susan, she hadn't regularly eaten fruit, vegetables, or whole grains in months. While she lost a few pounds on high-protein/low-carbohydrate plans, they were not the miracle diets she read about and was hoping for. On top of that, eating almost no carbs, simple or complex, caused her to experience major mood swings. She also had lower energy levels, constipation, and slight depression, and she felt that she hadn't had a good, focused, strong workout in months.

Since most of her diet consisted of meat, fish, and cheese, she began feeling physically ill at the sight of these foods. Also, she would have obsessive, uncontrollable urges for doughnuts and potato chips. She would then end up bingeing—eating an entire loaf of French bread or an entire large bag of chips at one sitting. Because she read about the "evils of carbohydrates," she was scared to eat them. She believed if she started eating carbs, they would cause her to gain more weight. Nevertheless, she missed fruits and vegetables and was ready to add them back into her diet. That's why she found me.

The first thing I did with Susan was reeducate her about the basics of a nourishing food plan. I explained that the body needs carbohydrates and cannot function properly without fruits, vegetables, and whole grains. I told her that she couldn't get her requirement of vitamins and minerals, much less important antioxidants and phytochemicals, without fresh produce in her diet. We worked hard to dispel her fears about carbohydrates and endeavored to add them back into her diet gradually.

Susan started off by adding one piece of fruit, a slice of whole grain bread, and a serving of vegetables to her daily diet. She did this for a week, but the bulk of her diet was still protein. The following week, she added more carbohydrates to her daily eating plan. Slowly, she continued upping the amounts of fruit, vegetables, and whole grains she ate, until she was eating a healthier balance of protein and carbohydrates.

Susan started eating more essential fatty acids, too. She also started cutting back on fattier cuts of meat and full-fat dairy foods. Susan had gotten used to the taste of whole milk, but she found that cutting back to 2% wasn't that bad, and soon she drank 1% effortlessly. She replaced the hamburgers she had been eating with veggie or turkey burgers and started eating the buns as well. She ate fish a few times a week for the omega-3's as well as its clean taste. By week 4, she experienced fewer mood swings and had more energy. She noticed that her workouts were feeling better, that she was stronger when she lifted weights and had more stamina on the rowing machine and stairclimber.

By week 8, Susan was noticeably less depressed and less obsessed with food. She realized she had missed carbohydrates and that they did make her feel better. Since she was more educated about her food choices, she was able to pick foods that her body really wanted. Subsequently, she got over the constipation and did not gain weight. In fact, after 8 weeks, she found that she had lost the 10 pounds she had gained since moving in with her boyfriend.

Beans. I usually count beans as a serving of protein in my daily eating plan. It's important to remember, however, that they are also an excellent source of complex carbohydrates and have a lot of soluble fiber (4 to 7 grams per half cup), which may help lower cholesterol and may prevent or control heart disease and diabetes. Studies show that ½ to 1 cup of beans eaten daily can significantly reduce blood cholesterol levels and control blood sugar in people with diabetes. Beans are a great source of vitamins including thiamin, riboflavin, niacin, and folate and minerals including calcium, iron, copper, zinc, phosphorus, potassium, and magnesium. Beans are also a great anti-cancer food because they contain phytoestrogens. Soybeans, in particular, are extremely rich in the phytoestrogen isoflavone, which may decrease the risk of certain hormone-dependent cancers like breast and prostate cancer.

In addition, beans are a good source of protein. Soybeans are unique in that they're a complete protein. To make other beans even more nutritious, eat them with (or within a few hours of) whole grains. (See page 76 for more on protein.)

If you avoid eating beans because you're afraid they're going to cause flatulence, there's a simple solution. Just add a few drops of a product called Beano to the bean dish. Beano is an enzyme that helps the body digest the sugars found in beans that lead to this problem. The way you prepare beans can also eliminate this problem. First, soak beans for 4 to 5 hours, then drain and throw out the water. Add fresh water (10 cups of water to 1 pound of beans) and boil for 10 minutes; simmer for half an hour, and throw out the water again. If the beans need more cooking, add fresh water and cook until soft. Don't worry, this cooking process won't harm the nutrients. You can also use canned or frozen beans to save time on cooking. Just rinse them well to reduce the sodium level.

Simple Carbohydrates

Simple carbohydrates are made up of short chains of only one or two sugars. They're also referred to as simple sugars and include fructose (fruit sugar), sucrose (table sugar), and lactose (milk sugar). Fresh, frozen, or dried fruit is one of the most healthful sources of simple carbohydrates.

Sucrose. Americans love their sugar, but it's a love that could lead to obesity. The consumption of sugar in our country has taken a massive leap in the past 160 years. In the 1840s, each person consumed a mere 4 teaspoons of sugar daily. Today, the average person takes in a whopping 1 cup of sugar daily.

The U.S. Department of Agriculture reported that in a large percentage of adult diets, two of the top three sources of carbohydrates are sugar and soft drinks. The average American drinks 450 glasses of soda each year. With 5 to 9 teaspoons of sugar per serving, that's 2,250 to 4,050 teaspoons of sugar from soft drinks alone! Furthermore, a recent study found that if a child increased his or her soft drink consumption by just one extra drink per day, the child was 60 percent more likely to become obese later in life. These researchers concluded that the body may have trouble adapting to intense concentrations of sugar taken in liquid form.

People are usually less concerned with the amount of sugar in their diets than the amount of fat. Just look at the boom in fat-free sweets on the market. But it's dangerous to think that sugar is innocent when it's not accompanied by lots of fat. Ironically, most fat-free foods contain more calories than regular-fat foods, because they substitute sugar for fat. Eating these products could lead to weight gain, since every 3,500 calories that go unused by the body turns into 1 pound of fat. Consuming large amounts of sugar is not only bad for your teeth, but it may well be a factor in the development and progression of obesity. Sugar is also linked to premenstrual syndrome, food cravings, fatigue, depression, and seasonal affective disorder (SAD).

Be sure to look at the Nutrition Facts label on packages of food. If sugar is one of the first three ingredients listed, the product is high in sugar and should be avoided or eaten only occasionally. (*Note:* If you have diabetes, your doctor will likely give you an eating plan that is different from the one described in this chapter.)

The U.S. Department of Agriculture recommends that you limit your added sugar intake to no more than 6 teaspoonfuls a day if you eat 1,600 calories or 12 teaspoonfuls a day if you eat 2,200 calories. What this means is that added sugar should constitute between 6 and 10 percent of your total daily calories. Currently, 16 percent of the average American's daily calories come from added sugar (with many people consuming much more than that), according to the USDA.

Lactose. For the past several years, lactose has been enmeshed in controversy. Many adults suffer dire stomach problems such as bloating, gas, diarrhea, and cramps when they consume dairy foods containing lactose. Tummy troubles arise because many adults stop producing lactase, the enzyme needed to digest lactose. While most Northern Europeans and their descendants produce lactase their entire lives, many Asians and Africans and their descendants stop producing lactase after infancy.

If you think you suffer from lactose intolerance, you can try Lactaid (a dietary supplement that helps the body process lactose), drink lactose-free milk, or substitute soy products for dairy ones. There are many soy foods available at the supermarket that resemble dairy foods and taste very much like their dairy counterparts. Try soy milk, soy yogurt, and soy cheese. Try to make sure that the soy foods have had the bone-strengthening mineral calcium sulfate added to them, so you're sure to get all the benefits you would if you had the dairy foods. If you don't think you're getting enough calcium, try a supplement. (For more information on calcium, see page 102.)

Fiber

Dietary fiber is a crucial part of our diet. It's a form of carbohydrate (often referred to as roughage) that comes from the structural part of fruits, vegetables, grains, and other plant foods. We're unable to digest dietary fiber. Most fiber travels through the gastrointestinal tract and ends up in the stool.

There are two types of dietary fiber: insoluble and soluble fiber. Most plant foods contain both types of fibers in varying amounts. Insoluble fiber doesn't dissolve in water; thus it attracts and retains water in your intestinal tract. This increases the bulk of stools and makes them softer and easier to eliminate. Insoluble fiber is found in high amounts in wheat bran and other whole grains. Soluble fiber forms a gel in water that helps to bind acids and cholesterol in the intestinal tract, preventing their reabsorption into the body. This may be why soluble fiber helps to lower cholesterol levels (and decreases the risk of heart disease) and also maintains steady blood sugar (glucose) levels. Soluble fiber is found in oats and oat bran, barley, brown rice, beans, apples, carrots, and most other fruits and vegetables.

Why Do You Need Fiber?

Even though fiber is not digested per se, it still has vital health benefits. Fiber may reduce the risk of colon cancer by either combining with, or diluting, cancer-causing agents, or altering the natural bacteria of the intestines. Fiber also speeds up the rate at which stools pass through the body, keeping the digestive tract clean and healthy and preventing constipation and hemorrhoids.

Fiber-rich foods tend to be bulky and lower in fat and calories. These foods help with weight control because they're naturally filling and they're chewy, so they take longer to eat. This will make you less likely to overeat, and you will feel fuller longer.

Complex carbohydrates are usually high in fiber and are great choices for active people needing high-endurance, long-burning foods. The carbohydrates provide the fuel needed to power the muscles used during activity. This is why low-carb diets aren't helpful. Foods with a lot of soluble fiber, such as oatmeal, lentils, and pasta, become great sources of long-term fuel because they release sugar into the bloodstream slowly. Fiber can enhance stamina during a marathon, a long bike ride, or any endurance activity.

How Much Fiber Do You Need?

For the greatest health benefits, both the Food and Drug Administration and the National Cancer Institute recommend that

High-Fiber Foods

With delicious foods like those listed below, there's no reason why getting more fiber in your diet needs to be unpleasant! All of the following are excellent sources of dietary fiber.

Cereals. Breakfast cereals are a quick and easy source of fiber. By eating a variety of grains such as wheat, corn, oats, and rice, you'll get both soluble and insoluble fiber. Mixing cereals is a way of adding a variety of tastes and fibers to your meal or snack. Try 1 cup of any of the following: Fiber One (14 grams of fiber), 100% Bran (13.5 grams), All Bran with Extra Fiber (13 grams), Kashi Go Lean (10 grams), Kashi Good Friends (8 grams), Quick Quaker Oats (8 grams), Shredded Wheat Spoon Size (5 grams), Puffed Kashi (2 grams).

Fruits. Fiber is usually concentrated in the skin and outer layer of the fruit, so opt for fruit with edible skins and seeds. Try one kiwifruit (5 grams), pear (4.5 grams), orange (4 grams), or apple (2.5 grams); 1 cup of blackberries (7 grams) or raspberries (6 grams); or two figs (4 grams).

Vegetables. Vegetables with edible skins are the best high-fiber choices, but almost every vegetable has a decent fiber content. The difference between raw and cooked is minor. Try 1 cup of winter squash (6 grams), kale (5 grams), broccoli (4 grams), spinach (4 grams), carrots (3.5 grams), cauliflower (3 grams), or green beans (3 grams).

Breads and crackers. Those with the most fiber are made from whole grain flours; check the ingredients list. Be aware that most breads contain moderate amounts of fat, so if you're following a low-fat diet, check the label and choose breads with a lower fat content. Brands of high-fiber bread to look for include The Baker (4 grams of fiber per slice), Branola (3 grams), Matthew's (2 grams), Vermont Bread Company (2 grams), and Thomas's Honey Whole Wheat or Oat Bran English Muffins (2 grams per muffin). As for crackers, I recommend Finn Crisps (3 grams per serving), Ryvita (3 grams), Wasa (3 grams), Woven Wheat (3 grams), and Kavali (2 grams).

Beans and legumes. The following are all tops in fiber (per ¼ cup, uncooked): kidney beans (10 grams), chickpeas (7 grams), lentils (4.5 grams), split peas (4.5 grams).

Snacks. Try 2 ounces of fat-free tortilla chips (8 grams), 3½ cups of air-popped popcorn (4.5 grams), or dried fruit (amount of fiber varies, but generally it's high).

adults get 25 to 30 grams of fiber each day. Most Americans consume just a third to a half of this recommended amount. It is especially important for elderly and pregnant women to get a lot of fiber because of their tendency for constipation.

It's best to increase your fiber intake gradually so that your stomach has time to adjust. Expect softer and more frequent bowel movements. You may also notice that you become a bit more gassy—this is natural and a sign that you're getting adequate fiber from your diet. Since fiber acts like a sponge and attracts water into the intestines, drinking plenty of water (at least eight 8-ounce glasses a day) is important to keep the stool soft. Too little water combined with increased fiber can result in constipation.

The best way to get the fiber you need is from foods, not from laxatives or stool softeners. The smartest way to increase your fiber is to eat a variety of fiber-rich foods including fruits, vegetables, beans, and whole grains. Try to eat these foods as close to their natural state as possible (that includes keeping skins on fruits and vegetables where possible), since a lot of fiber gets lost through processing (including juicing). Dried fruits are good because they offer concentrated fiber compared to their fresh counterparts.

Protein

Protein is an essential building block of life. It's also one of the most satisfying food groups you can eat. Most Americans get their proteins in the form of meat and dairy, but there are other, more healthful protein choices that you should try to work into your diet.

Why Do You Need Protein?

Every organism in our world—from the tiniest microbe to the largest animal—is made of protein. Protein is the primary building material for the brain, heart, muscles, blood, skin, hair, and nails, and it's essential for growth and development.

Proteins help the body to regulate water balance, aid in the formation of hormones and enzymes that control the metabolism, help maintain skin moisture levels, and regulate skin pigment. Antibodies—an important part of the immune system—also require protein to function properly.

Protein is made up of 22 different amino acids. When protein is metabolized, it gets broken back down into amino acids. Some amino acids are termed "nonessential." This doesn't mean that they aren't important; it simply means that the body can produce them from other amino acids, so they don't need to come from the diet. Other amino acids are termed "essential," which means the body can't produce them and they must come from the foods we eat.

When the body builds muscle or makes cells, it needs a variety of amino acids. If the body is chronically low in amino acids (which will happen if a diet is deficient in essential amino acids), it can't function properly. This is why it's important to consume

Kitchen CURES

Surefire Steps to Strengthen Your Nails

Have you been hiding your hands so no one sees your broken, jagged fingernails? Do you have white bands across your nails? Read on for ways to pamper your nails.

- Protein provides building material for new nails and prevents white bands across the nails, so to have good nails, you need to consume an adequate amount of protein. Be sure you're getting enough meat, eggs, soy foods, or tofu.
- Vitamin C helps prevent hangnails. Try berries, citrus fruits, broccoli, and sweet peppers.
- Vitamin A and calcium help prevent dry and brittle nails. Try eating some carrots; peaches; squash; low-fat dairy foods; dark green, leafy vegetables; and canned fish.
- The B vitamins—including folate and B_{12}—help strengthen nails and prevent ridges and dryness. Eat some asparagus, barley, bran, root veggies, sea vegetables, eggs, seafood, or soy foods.
- Zinc helps prevent white spots. Eat some lean meat, legumes, mushrooms, oysters, and whole grains.
- Essential fatty acids—found in pumpkin seeds, walnuts, flaxseed, and fish and fish oils—help to nourish the nails.

foods that contain all the essential amino acids.

Complete or Incomplete?

Proteins can be divided into two groups depending on the amino acids they contain: complete proteins or incomplete proteins. Complete proteins—also referred to as high-quality proteins—contain plenty of the essential amino acids and are found most readily in animal products like eggs, meat, poultry, fish, and dairy products; tofu and other soybean products are pretty much the only non-animal sources of complete proteins.

Incomplete proteins contain only some of the essential amino acids. Sources include beans, peas, and other legumes; grains; and leafy, green vegetables. In the past, it was thought that incomplete proteins needed to be combined with other complementary (incomplete) protein foods in the same meal to make them complete. But now we know that if you eat incomplete proteins at different meals, your body is usually able to make complete proteins using its store of bacteria found in the digestive tract. Your body will take care of the food combining it needs to do to get the maximum amount of nutrients from the food you eat.

How Much Protein Do You Need?

The risk of protein deficiency in our country is almost nonexistent. Even pregnant women and athletes are not usually at risk for protein deficiency, since a balanced food intake provides plenty of protein. Growing children, women who are breastfeeding, and people recuperating from major injury or illness typically require a little more protein, but even they can usually get it from a regular diet.

Fifteen to 20 percent of your daily calories should come from proteins. The average person really needs only 50 to 60 grams of protein per day, with 100 grams as the ceiling. In nonmetric terms, that means you need *no more* than 7 to 8 ounces of protein-rich foods a day.

Animal Protein

Meat and poultry. Our bodies absorb certain nutrients, such as iron and zinc, better when they come from meat than from plant foods. Women, in particular, tend to be low in these minerals, so eating moderate amounts of meat can be beneficial. On the other hand, diets that are very high in animal proteins tend to be lower in phytochemicals and fiber (both of which come from plant-based foods) and can lead to diet-related diseases. The bottom line? If you choose to eat meat, stick to moderate amounts. Remember that most people need no more than 8 ounces of protein-rich foods each day. Also, since meat is loaded with protein, eat it with a lot of veggies to be sure you're getting adequate amounts of phytochemicals and fiber and a wide variety of nutrients.

If you eat meat, you should look for the leanest cuts available. Chicken breast and turkey breast, both with the skin removed, are good poultry choices. Flank steak and filet mignon are my favorite lean cuts of beef.

Dairy. Dairy foods like yogurt, milk, and cheese are nutritional powerhouses. They're great sources of high-quality protein and are rich in minerals and vitamins like calcium, zinc, magnesium, phosphorus, vitamins A, D, and K, and some B vitamins. Dairy foods are very high in the amino acid lycine, which plant foods lack, so the protein in dairy complements the protein in plant-based foods like legumes and grains.

When choosing dairy foods, stick with low-fat or fat-free options. These products have as much protein and calcium as their full-fat counterparts but are, of course, much lower in saturated fats (which are directly related to higher blood cholesterol levels). I often buy organic dairy products: They're much more flavorful and "richer"-tasting than conventional dairy, and there's the added peace of mind of knowing that they're chemical-free.

Eggs. Eggs are a great source of high-quality protein and nutrients, but they are high in cholesterol. A single large egg contains 6 grams of protein, 5 grams of fat (most of it unsaturated), good amounts of vitamins B_{12} and E, riboflavin, folate, iron, and phosphorus, but two-thirds of the daily recommended amount of cholesterol. If eaten occasionally (no more than 5 a week), eggs won't raise your cholesterol levels. Egg whites, though, are fat-free and cholesterol-free and are still an excellent source of protein—so feel free to enjoy as many egg whites as you like. Just be sure that you always cook eggs (both the whites and the yolks) thoroughly before eating them.

As for egg substitutes and pasteurized bottled egg whites, they're quick and easy, but I prefer eating things closer to nature, such as fresh whole eggs or fresh egg whites. A fairly recent addition to the egg-product line is eggs enriched with omega-3 fatty acids (because the chicken feed is enriched with omega-3). They're a wise choice, so try them out if they're available in your supermarket.

Fish. Fish is an excellent source of high-quality protein, and certain varieties contain omega-3 fatty acids (a good kind of fat). Studies have shown that in countries where fish is a mainstay of the diet, people tend to be healthier and live longer. Fish is also high in water content, so it helps to flush you out, makes you feel full without feeling "stuffed," and keeps you feeling satisfied longer. Varieties of fish that are high in both protein and omega-3 fatty acids include salmon (smoked salmon is fine if there are no additives), tuna (including canned varieties packed in water), herring, sardines, mackerel, lake trout, anchovies, sablefish (a type of cod), whitefish, bluefish, and shellfish.

Plant Protein

Grains. The United States is one of the largest producers of grains in the world, but the grains harvested here contribute to only a quarter of the calories in the American diet. More than half the grains grown here are used for animal feed. In Asia, on the other hand, grains (in the form of rice) make up 65 percent of the citizens' diet, and in lesser-developed countries, grains constitute 80 to 85 percent of the diet.

Grains are a good source of low-fat protein. Amaranth, barley, quinoa, rye, triticale, whole wheat bread, buckwheat noodles, and spaghetti (made from semolina flour) are all good grain sources of protein, especially if you bulk up dishes with beans.

Beans/legumes. Beans, too, are a good

Jumping for Soy

Soybeans and foods made from soybeans are "super foods." They're the only plant-based food equivalent to animal products in terms of protein quality. Soybeans are packed with energy-producing complex carbohydrates and B vitamins, zinc, potassium, magnesium, and iron. They're also loaded with fiber—2 ounces of dried soybeans have an amazing 11 grams of fiber. Their calcium levels can hardly be beat either, with 29 milligrams of calcium per ounce (fat-free milk has 38 milligrams per ounce). They contain 9 grams of fat in a cooked half-cup serving, but it's the good, unsaturated kind.

Soy foods contain isoflavones—phytochemicals that have hormonal effects and may protect people from certain cancers. Soy also contains a huge amount of anticancer compounds called phytoestrogens (plant-based estrogens), which may raise natural estrogen levels in menopausal women and lower high estrogen levels in younger women. The high fiber in soy also may lower cancer risks. Some studies have shown that isolated soy proteins are helpful in preventing osteoporosis and heart disease and may help with symptoms of menopause.

To get the fullest benefits of soy, try to take in at least 40 to 50 grams of soy foods each day. By upping the amount of soy in your diet, you'll also increase your intake of fiber, pytochemicals, and omega-3 fatty acids (which protect against heart disease and other diseases). When you increase your soy intake, you'll likely lower your saturated fat intake because by eating more soy protein, you'll probably be eating less animal protein.

Soybeans are among the oldest cultivated crops, dating back about 10,000 years. They have

source of low-fat protein. The most filling way to enjoy them is with grains or flour products, such as rice and beans, tortillas and fat-free refried beans, or pasta and bean soup. Beans are also cholesterol-free and high in complex carbohydrates and fiber. They come in a huge variety of sizes, shapes, and colors, but most are nutritionally similar. Dried beans are often referred to as legumes (which is defined as vegetables that grow in pods) and include black beans, lima beans, chick-peas, kidney beans, split peas, and lentils.

Beans are a good source of water-soluble vitamins such as thiamin, riboflavin, niacin, and folate. These vitamins are stored in the body only for a short time and then quickly excreted through urine, so you need to take in water-soluble vitamins on a daily basis. Canned beans tend to be lower in these vitamins due to processing, but they still provide a good amount. Be sure to rinse canned beans very well (in a bowl of cold water for 3 been a staple food in Asian diets for centuries. Today, soy is available in a huge variety of forms, including tofu, miso, soy milk, soy cheese, and soy yogurt.

When the by-product of soy milk is dried, it forms the basis of mock meat products like soy burgers, soy hot dogs, and soy "chicken." When a culture is added to cooked soybeans, it binds them into solid cakes called tempeh, which can then be flavored and used like meat. Roasted soybeans are the basis of a fairly new product called soy nuts, which are a tasty nibble and have much more omega-3 than peanuts do. Soy has also recently become an important ingredient in baby foods.

A great way to get kids (or even adults) to eat their soy is with fresh soybeans called edamame. They're available whole (in their pods) or shelled frozen (boil either variety for 5 minutes). Occasionally, you can find fresh soybeans at health food stores and farmers' markets (they still require a 5-minute boil). They're a healthy, earthy-tasting snack. (They taste similar to green beans.) In their whole form, they're fun to eat since you scrape the beans out of their pods much as you would with peanuts, and kids, particularly, think this is great. But they're easier to use if you buy them already shelled.

Soy milk is a great addition to your eating plan. Soy milk is wholesome and nutritious and mixes well with other flavors—it's especially good in shakes and smoothies. Experiment with the different flavors available at the market, but make sure the brand you buy is processed with calcium sulfate, so you get all the calcium benefits you would if you used cow's milk.

to 5 minutes), which will help remove the excess salt. All beans—canned or freshly prepared—are also a very good source of minerals such as calcium, iron, copper, zinc, phosphorus, potassium, and magnesium.

Nuts and seeds. Nuts and seeds are tasty and healthful. They provide good amounts of protein, fiber, iron, potassium, calcium, magnesium, zinc, copper, selenium, vitamin E, and B vitamins. But despite their deliciousness, they are too high in fat to be a primary source of protein. When eating nuts and seeds, enjoy them sparingly—no more than a handful or so each day.

Protein Supplements

In my opinion, protein bars are expensive, glorified candy bars. I also believe that protein powders and supplements are a complete waste of money. Most Americans get more than enough protein from their regular diets and don't need extra. If you enjoy protein shakes, however, an occasional one will do no harm. Just be sure to get a soy-based one with 100 calories or fewer per scoop.

Fats

In the past 10 years, there has been a lot of noise made that people should reduce the amount of fat in their diets or eliminate it completely, since saturated fats are associated with an increased risk of heart disease. The truth is, though, that the human body requires fat to function properly. Fat acts as an intestinal lubricant and protects the internal organs. It also helps generate body heat and helps to absorb the fat-soluble vitamins A, D, E, and K—without fat, we would be deficient in these vitamins.

All cell membranes are composed of fat, as are the myelin sheaths that protect nerve fibers. Infants and children need fat for brain development, and adults need fat throughout their lives for energy and growth. In fact, fat is the most concentrated energy source available to the body.

Dietary fat makes foods taste delicious; without it, food would be less tender and flavorful, since fat is a flavor carrier. Fats also delay the emptying of the stomach, so they keep you feeling satisfied and "full" longer. Of course, excessive fat intake and eating the wrong types of fat are major factors in high cholesterol and blood pressure, obesity, heart disease, colon cancer, and diabetes.

What Kinds of Fats Are Healthiest?

Fats are made up of building blocks called fatty acids. There are three main categories of fatty acids: saturated, monounsaturated, and polyunsaturated. These classifications are based on the number of hydrogen atoms within the chemical structure of the fatty acid itself.

Saturated Fatty Acids

Saturated fats are fats that are solid at room temperature and get harder as they chill. They're usually found in animal products such as dairy foods, including whole milk, cream, butter, and cheese, and meats such as beef, lamb, and pork (the marbling of fat that makes meat so tasty is pure saturated fat). There are some plant-based saturated fats, too, notably palm kernel oil, coconut oil, and vegetable shortening.

The liver uses saturated fat to make cholesterol, so eating foods with too much saturated fat can increase cholesterol levels, especially low-density lipoproteins (LDL)—the bad cholesterol. Even more than the cholesterol content, it's important to pay close attention to the saturated fat content in food.

Not all saturated fats are alike, however. Stearic acid, a saturated fat found in both meat and chocolate, doesn't raise your LDL cholesterol but can increase the risk of blood clots. The saturated fat that does the most physical harm, myristic acid, is found in full-fat dairy products, so stick to low-fat or fat-free dairy products.

Monounsaturated Fatty Acids

Monounsaturated fats are liquid at room temperature and get more viscous when they're chilled. Good sources of monounsaturated fats include olive oil, canola oil, avocados, avocado oil, olives (be careful, though, since these can be very high in salt), and high oleic (a fatty acid that is lower in omega-6, is light tasting, and can stand up to high cooking temperatures) safflower and sunflower oils. These fats may actually help to raise levels of HDL (good cholesterol) while reducing levels of LDL (bad cholesterol). Olive oil can also help decrease the risk of blood clots because it contains squalene, a substance that has anti-clotting properties and can also lower cholesterol.

Polyunsaturated Fatty Acids

Polyunsaturated fats are liquid at room temperature and stay liquid even when chilled. Large amounts of polyunsaturated fats are found in corn oil, soybean oil, safflower oil, and sunflower oil. Polyunsaturated fats may help to lower total cholesterol, but the downside is that if you have too much of them, they may also lower your high-density lipoproteins (HDL)—the good cholesterol.

Essential fatty acids (EFAs). Polyunsaturated fatty acids can be further classified into omega-6 fatty acids and omega-3 fatty acids

(there are others as well but these are the most important). These fatty acids are called essential fatty acids (EFAs) because they are necessary for normal human growth and development, including rebuilding and producing cells. Our bodies can't produce them, so they must come from our diets.

EFAs also help reduce blood pressure, aid in the prevention of arthritis, aid in nerve impulse transmission, are needed for normal brain functioning, and are beneficial for skin and hair.

Both omega-3 and omega-6 fatty acids are converted into hormonelike substances called eicosanoids, which can profoundly affect health and well-being. Omega-3 and omega-6 produce opposite functions; this is why choosing the right fat is crucial. Eicosanoids affect blood pressure and the immune system, influence the perception of pain, and can make you more or less prone to allergies and inflammation. When you have more omega-6 in your diet than omega-3, your body produces more eicosanoids, which then increases your risk for asthma, allergies, arthritis, psoriasis, and colitis. As Americans, we eat too much omega-6 and too little omega-3, so it's important to become more aware of these fats and to find a healthier balance in consuming them. Sources of omega-6 include corn oil, safflower oil, sunflower oil, cottonseed oil, soybean oil, peanut oil, sesame oil, grapeseed oil, borage oil, and primrose oil.

Omega-3 can reduce blood pressure, may help decrease the risk of heart disease, reduces the risk of heart attacks, decreases blood clot formation, and helps to stabilize the heartbeat. Omega-3 may also decrease the incidence of depression and can lessen the severity of several inflammatory and autoimmune diseases such as asthma, allergies, arthritis, psoriasis, and colitis as well as heart disease and high blood pressure.

Fish is a primary source of omega-3. A study published in the *Journal of the American Medical Association* found that women who ate seafood two to four times a week had half the risk of strokes caused by blood clots as women who ate seafood less than once a month. The scientists concluded that the omega-3 fatty acids from the seafood appeared to protect the women against stroke.

Excellent sources of omega-3 are mackerel, herring, salmon, fresh tuna, and sardines. Good sources include trout, shellfish, flaxseed oil and flaxseed, canola oil, walnut oil, walnuts, and brazil nuts.

Trans fatty acids (TFAs). Trans fatty acids are polyunsaturated vegetable oils that have been hydrogenated to increase shelf life. Hydrogenation is a process in which oils are heated to become solid at room temperature; margarine and vegetable shortening are prime examples.

These fats are different from other polyunsaturated fats in that they act like saturated fats in the body: They increase the risk of heart disease, stroke, and diabetes by raising LDL cholesterol and decreasing HDL cholesterol. Even if you don't use margarine or shortening, you may be consuming trans fatty acids in processed foods. They're found in large amounts in foods fried in deep fat, commercial pastries, cookies, crackers, chips, and many other snack foods. Because of their health risks, you should actively try to avoid these fats in your diet. By reading food labels, you can see if products contain "partially hydrogenated oil," which is another term for trans fatty acid, and you can make a better food choice.

How Much Fat Do You Really Need?

Fats should make up 20 to 30 percent of your diet. The average person requires only one or two servings of good fatty acids per day. Most of the dietary fat we consume should come from a variety of omega-3 fatty acid sources or monounsaturated fatty acids. But remember that our bodies need fat (the good kind), so don't eliminate it from your diet.

Cholesterol

Cholesterol is a fat-like substance—called a sterol—found only in animal-based foods. Cholesterol is also naturally found in the brain, nerves, blood, and bile and is necessary for the proper functioning of the body. It's used to build membranes and produce sex hormones. The liver uses cholesterol to make bile acids, which help you digest food. Eighty percent of total body cholesterol is manufactured in the liver; the remaining 20 percent comes from the diet. While cholesterol is necessary, elevated cholesterol levels can be dangerous and can lead to plaque-filled arteries, which inhibit the flow of blood to the brain, kidneys, genitals, extremities, and heart, and can promote heart disease.

How Does Cholesterol Work?

Cholesterol travels from the liver through the bloodstream to various tissues and cells by a special class of proteins called lipoproteins. The cells take what cholesterol they need, and the remainder stays in the bloodstream until other lipoproteins pick it up and take it back to the liver.

There are two types of lipoproteins: Low-density lipoprotein (LDL), the bad form of cholesterol, and high-density lipoprotein (HDL), the good form. LDLs carry a lot of cholesterol from the liver to all the cells of the body. HDLs carry very little cholesterol, circulate in the bloodstream, and remove excess cholesterol from the blood and tissues. After HDLs travel through the bloodstream and collect the excess cholesterol, they return it to the liver, where it's incorporated into LDLs for delivery to the cells. If everything is functioning properly, this system remains in balance.

If there is too much cholesterol for the HDLs to pick up in time or if there isn't enough HDL in the body to do the job, cholesterol forms plaque that sticks to artery walls and may cause heart disease. That's why it's beneficial to have high HDL levels and low LDL levels.

Diet and Cholesterol

Since 20 percent of total body cholesterol comes from what you eat, diet and cholesterol are linked. Decreasing your intake of animal foods that contain a lot of cholesterol (and saturated fats) is important, but it's not the whole story.

It has been shown that saturated fats increase blood cholesterol even more than cholesterol does. This is because saturated fat lowers LDL receptors, so more LDL remains in the blood. So when a food product claims that it contains "no cholesterol," the product may still negatively affect your cholesterol level if it's high in saturated fats like palm oil, coconut oil, or hydrogenated oils. Sugar and uncontrolled alcohol intake may also raise the level of natural cholesterol that your body produces. Stress, too, can raise cholesterol levels.

Reducing your risk of heart disease requires reducing the amount of animal foods you eat, removing saturated fats from your diet, reducing your sugar intake, moderating your alcohol consumption (but not necessarily completely eliminating it, since drinking one 5-ounce glass of red wine a day

(continued on page 88)

LIVING A
REAL FOOD LIFE

High Cholesterol Prompted Him to Overhaul His Diet

Name: Robert
Real Food Life Issues: High cholesterol, high blood pressure

At 64, Robert was looking forward to retirement. He worked hard his whole life, he put his now-grown kids through college years ago, and now he was getting ready to travel with his wife, play golf, and do some part-time volunteer work. When I met Robert, he got practically no exercise and ate whatever he felt like, particularly fatty meats and fast foods. He especially loved doughnuts. Only when his wife forced him would he eat fresh fruit and vegetables. Here's where I found him:

July 14

I'm half inclined to check into my doctor's credentials. He looks like he graduated from medical school the same day I qualified for early retirement. I went in for a checkup and the kid told me I had to change everything—stop eating red meat, stop putting salt on my food, stop eating doughnuts. I didn't know whether to pay the bill and thank him or take the damn kid across my knee and spank him!

I guess I knew it would happen. I'm getting to that age . . . even though I'll be damned before I admit that to anyone. God knows, I don't want to give my wife any more ammunition to tell me how to eat. But I have to admit, she has been saying the same things for about 10 years. Of course, I'll never admit that to her—that would give her too much pleasure. (Just kidding.) I know the old bird has my best interests at heart—I just wish my best interests tasted a little better.

Who wants to live to be 100 if you can't eat a big slab of beef when you want to? And what's the harm in a couple of martinis in the afternoon? They don't have any of this "saturated fat" everyone seems to be terrified of. Sometimes I think it's just all a big conspiracy to drain the joy out of our best years . . .

Robert had very high cholesterol and high blood pressure along with slightly elevated blood sugar levels. His doctor told him if he couldn't change these levels through diet and exercise in a few months, he would have to be put on medication. His father died at age 65, and Robert was afraid the pattern would repeat, so that's why he came to see me.

We overhauled Robert's food life to reduce his cholesterol levels. First, he cut out almost all saturated fats and hydrogenated oils from his diet. This meant eating leaner meats, including more chicken and fish. He had lean beef only two or three times a week. He indulged in doughnuts only on rare occasions. He also added more fresh fruits and vegetables into his diet—a particularly healthy step for him because the potassium in fresh produce can help reduce blood pressure. These changes were hard at first—after all, Robert had eaten his old diet for more than half a century. But with support from his wife, his kids, his physician, and me, coupled with the memory of his own father's early death, he made an effort to make these changes.

Robert also joined his local Y and began taking exercise classes for seniors. Within a few weeks, he felt physically better and stronger than he had in years. And during his golf games, he began walking the course instead of using the cart.

Robert also began drinking 8 cups of water and 1 cup of green tea each day. I coached him on how to reduce his sodium intake by reading food labels carefully and cooking dishes without added salt; he shared these techniques with his wife as well. He began adding canned beans (no salt added and well-rinsed) to his salads and eating oatmeal for breakfast because the soluble fiber in both foods can help reduce cholesterol levels. He also took a daily B-complex vitamin to help keep his homocysteine levels down.

He started eating more foods that are high in essential fatty acids, since these acids can help reduce cholesterol. In addition to eating olive oil, flaxseed oil, and nuts and seeds, he also started eating fish three times a week. I also had him try a variety of soy-based foods to further help reduce his cholesterol. He was surprised that he actually liked edamame (cooked soy beans), flavored tofu, and soy hot dogs.

By the end of 8 weeks, Robert's blood pressure was heading toward the normal range, his cholesterol level had come down significantly, and his blood sugar level had returned to normal. Thrilled to see these improvements, his doctor held off prescribing medications and told him to continue eating this way and to continue exercising. Today, Robert continues with his new food life, is still medication-free, and is healthily and happily enjoying his retirement.

may actually raise your HDL), and reducing stress.

Reducing Cholesterol

You can lower your LDL cholesterol level by modifying your diet. Using monounsaturated fats instead of saturated ones helps to lower LDL. Physical exercise and consuming foods rich in omega-3 fatty acids will also help in this regard. A diet rich in foods that have high amounts of soluble fiber, such as barley, beans, peas, brown rice, alfalfa, fruits, and oats, can also help to decrease LDL levels.

If you have high cholesterol, you should see your doctor about changes in the recommended levels of dietary fat you should consume. According to the National Cholesterol Education Program's updated clinical guidelines, people with high cholesterol should get 25 to 35 percent of their total calories from fat. Of this number, less than 7 percent

Decoding Cholesterol

When you get your cholesterol levels checked, your doctor will draw some blood and send it to a lab for analysis. The lab will check for levels of HDL cholesterol, LDL cholesterol, total cholesterol (which includes both HDL and LDL), and triglycerides. Here's what those numbers mean.

- A normal, healthy, and safe *total cholesterol level* is less than 200 milligrams per deciliter of blood. (Milligrams per deciliter or "mg/dl" is simply the way cholesterol is measured.) A reading above 200 indicates the potential for developing heart disease. A reading of 200 to 239 is borderline dangerous, and 240 and above is considered high risk.
- If your total cholesterol is under 200 but your HDL is under 40, you are still considered at risk for heart disease. As your HDL decreases, the potential for heart disease increases, even if your total cholesterol is low.
- Normal *HDL levels* are 45 to 50 mg/dl for men and 50 to 60 mg/dl for women. Higher HDL levels (70 to 80 mg/dl) may protect against heart disease; having a lower HDL level (under 40 mg/dl) is an independent risk factor for heart disease.
- For men and women, the optimal *LDL level* is 100 mg/dl or less (the range starts at 75 mg/dl). An acceptable range is 100 to 129 mg/dl; 130 to 159 mg/dl is borderline high risk for heart disease; 160 and above is considered high risk.
- *Triglycerides* are blood fats that play a role in heart disease. They are also associated with obesity, diabetes, hypertension, and low HDL levels. A reading of 40 to 199 mg/dl is a healthy range. A reading above 200 shows a potential risk for heart disease.

should be from saturated fat, up to 10 percent should be from polyunsaturated fat, and up to 20 percent should be from monounsaturated fat. A higher intake of total fat, mostly in the form of unsaturated fat, can help to reduce triglycerides and raise HDL cholesterol in persons with high cholesterol.

The traditional advice for people with high cholesterol was to avoid shellfish because it was thought to be too high in cholesterol. This advice is outdated. The cholesterol from seafood will most likely not raise your cholesterol level. In addition, shellfish is low in fat and a great source of protein and omega-3's. In one study, volunteers ate 10 ounces of shrimp each day for 3 weeks. While their LDL did increase by 7 percent, they also had a 12 percent increase in their HDL, which more than canceled out the rise in LDL.

Finally, taking antioxidant vitamins like vitamins C, E, and beta-carotene has been shown to reduce cardiovascular risks and plaque buildup in the arteries.

Homocysteine

Several B vitamins are associated with a reduced incidence of heart disease. Vitamins B_6, B_{12}, and folate are essential in controlling a compound called homocysteine, an amino acid that can injure the walls of the coronary arteries. Levels of homocysteine rise when your diet is low in these vitamins. Higher levels of homocysteine mean an increased risk for heart disease even if your blood cholesterol levels are low. Eating plenty of fruits and vegetables daily—5 or more servings a day—will keep your homocysteine levels in line. I also recommend taking 400 micrograms of folic acid, 3 micrograms of B_{12}, and at least 2 milligrams of B_6.

4 THE ABCS OF VITAMINS AND MINERALS

Get your vitamins and minerals. It sounds like such a cliché. But for good health, you really do need to make sure you're getting enough of these powerful substances, whether you get them from the foods you eat or the supplements you take. In the following pages, I've provided sketches of several essential vitamins and minerals. You'll discover why they're necessary for good health and well-being, what can happen if you're deficient in them, what the top food sources are for each, and how much you need to be getting each day.

Vitamins are organic substances that the body needs in tiny amounts to help regulate cell functions necessary for good health. We usually get the majority of the vitamins we need through food—except for vitamin K (which the body can produce from bacteria in the intestines).

Vitamins are categorized as either fat-soluble (vitamins A, D, E, and K) or water-soluble (all the B vitamins, biotin, folic acid, and vitamin C). The body stores fat-soluble vitamins in the liver and in body fat for long periods of time; they get released and used slowly. Water-soluble vitamins are stored in tissues, stay in the body for short periods of time, and need to be replenished daily.

Minerals are inorganic basic elements from the earth's crust that are used in many bodily functions, from bone formation to the effective working of the digestive system. Minerals are also vital for the activity of enzymes (protein molecules that are necessary for almost every biochemical activity in the body). While there are more than 60 minerals in the body, only 22 are considered essential.

Both vitamins and minerals are nutrients. In 1989, the Food and Nutrition Board of the National Research Council, a government-sponsored agency, formulated Recommended Dietary Allowance (RDA) levels for most vitamins and minerals. The RDA levels are set low; they're intended to be only enough to prevent deficiency and diseases and to maintain borderline good health.

The Daily Value (DV) is a reference value for nutrients developed by the Food and Drug Administration specifically for use on food labels. The DV reflects dietary recommendations for nutrients and other dietary components that have important links to health. On food labels, you'll see "% Daily Value"; that percentage represents an estimate of how individual foods contribute to your total diet, if you're eating a 2,000-calorie diet. The precise amount of vitamins and minerals a person should get has to be adjusted to suit the individual, taking into consideration the person's age, height, weight, exercise level, stress level, diet, any illnesses, medication, smoking habit, and, if female, whether or not she's pregnant. Regardless, the USDA has found that 40 percent of Americans consume a diet that includes only 60 percent of the RDA of vitamins and minerals, the minimal amount.

In this chapter, I'll provide you with the DV for your daily needs. You can estimate how much of certain vitamins and minerals you're getting in the foods you eat by checking the Nutrition Facts label on the packages.

A Prescription for Vitamins and Minerals

The best way to get the most nutrients your body needs to maintain great health and protect and heal itself is to eat several servings of fruit and vegetables every day. But even if you eat a wholesome diet with an emphasis on fruits, vegetables, whole grains, and high-quality proteins, you may not be getting enough vitamins and minerals. So I recommend taking a multivitamin every day; it's the best way to ensure you're getting all the nutrients you need.

You may also want to take additional vitamin C and vitamin E to help boost your immune system. You can safely take up to 500 milligrams of vitamin C and 400 international units (IU) of vitamin E each day.

Most people, especially women, don't get enough calcium. While the best source of calcium is food, you may not be getting enough through your diet alone. I recommend taking a calcium supplement with added vitamin D, which helps the body absorb the additional calcium. You should try to get 1,000 milligrams a day, or 1,200 milligrams if you're age 50 or older. For best absorption, don't take more than 500 milligrams at a time.

My female clients and I take vitamin B_6 (50 to 100 milligrams) a few days before our periods and during the first few days, and then stop until the next cycle. We feel it helps with irritability and bloating.

If you plan on becoming pregnant, you should take only special prenatal multivitamins (which have higher levels of vitamins and minerals than "regular" multivitamins, and iron and folic acid). You may also want to take a B-complex vitamin that contains at least 400 to 800 micrograms of folic acid to protect against neural tube defects. It also protects against homocysteine, a protein that can cause heart disease.

Vitamins
Vitamin A and Carotenoids

Why vitamin A is important: Especially when it comes from carotenoids, vitamin A is an all-star antioxidant, which means that it helps protect cells against cancers. It is also needed for new cell growth and for the formation of teeth and bones. Vitamin A enhances the immune system, supports reproduction and growth, maintains healthy skin, and helps the body to fight infections.

In addition, it helps prevent night blindness, and it may slow down the aging process. Since vitamin A is stored in the body's fat, if it's taken in extreme quantities it can be toxic.

Carotenoids are a class of compounds related to vitamin A. There are believed to be more than 600 carotenoids in existence; 400 have been identified and named. Of those 400, 50 are precursors to vitamin A, which means the liver will convert them into vitamin A as the body needs it. After they're converted, these carotenoids perform all the functions of vitamin A, such as having antioxidant properties and disease-preventing potential.

Carotenoids taken in extreme quantities aren't believed to be toxic but may turn the skin orange. The best-known carotenoid is beta-carotene, but there are many more, including lycopene and lutein. Lycopene is a potent antioxidant that may help to prevent prostate and other cancers; it is naturally abundant in tomatoes, pink grapefruit, and watermelon. Lutein is also an antioxidant and may protect against vision disorders that can occur with age. These, and other carotenoids, are abundant in dark green, leafy vegetables (like spinach and collard greens) and dark orange fruits and vegetables (like carrots, squash, and papayas).

Symptoms of deficiency: Dry hair and skin, poor growth, and night blindness. Also

Kitchen
CURES

Find an Oasis for Dry Skin

Skin that's dry, flaky, and itchy not only is irritating but can be unsightly. Rehydrate with these all-natural remedies.

- Foods rich in beta-carotene—including yellow and orange vegetables—can help prevent and may remedy dry, flaky skin.
- Foods high in B vitamins also help relieve itchy skin. Try some fish, legumes, nuts, eggs, and whole grains—and take a B-complex supplement.
- Vitamin C helps the production of collagen and can strengthen the capillaries that feed the skin. So be sure you're getting enough dark green vegetables, sweet potatoes, berries, and oranges.
- Foods that contain sulfur can help keep skin smooth. Eat some garlic, onions, eggs, asparagus, or wheat germ at your next meal.
- Drink at least 8 glasses of water a day. Water naturally hydrates your body and skin.
- Avoid alcohol and caffeine. Both dehydrate the skin (and the body).

may lead to problems with reproduction, painful joints, insomnia, frequent colds, and skin disorders.

Symptoms of toxicity: Hair loss, skin rashes, fractures, hemorrhaging, and liver failure can all result from too much vitamin A. Women taking more than 10,000 IU daily can experience reproduction complications.

Foods rich in vitamin A: Animal and fish liver; egg yolks; milk fortified with vitamins A and D; red bell peppers; and green, yellow, and orange fruits and veggies, including apricots, asparagus, beet greens, broccoli, cantaloupe, carrots, collards, dandelion greens, kale, papayas, peaches, sweet potatoes, watercress, and yellow squash.

How much do you need a day? 5,000 IU

B-Complex Vitamins

The B-complex family of vitamins does many things. Primarily, they help to maintain the health of the nerves, skin, eyes, hair, liver, muscles, gastrointestinal tract, and brain functions. They also help prevent canker sores and other mouth sores. In addition, the Bs help produce and maintain energy, and they may help alleviate anxiety and depression. They're water-soluble vitamins, which means they need to be replenished daily.

Vitamin B_1 (Thiamin)

Why vitamin B_1 is important: It enhances circulation and assists in blood formation. It also aids in digestion, helps with brain functions, and helps the body to use carbohydrates. B_1 has positive effects on energy, growth, appetite, and learning capacity. It's also needed for muscle tone of the intestines, stomach, and heart.

Symptoms of deficiency: Constipation, edema, fatigue, forgetfulness, stomach problems, irritability, muscle atrophy, nervousness, numbness in the limbs, and general weakness.

Foods rich in vitamin B_1: Brown rice; egg yolks; fish; fortified grain products, such as bread, rice, and whole grains; legumes; oatmeal; peanuts; peas; poultry; rice bran; sunflower seeds; and wheat germ.

How much do you need a day? 1.5 milligrams

Vitamin B_2 (Riboflavin)

Why vitamin B_2 is important: It's necessary for red blood cell formation, antibody production, and cell repair and growth. Vitamin B_2 also helps in the prevention and treatment of cataracts and helps metabolize carbohydrates, fats, and protein.

Symptoms of deficiency: Sores and cracks in the corners of the mouth, eye disorders, skin lesions, skin rash, dizziness, hair loss, insomnia, light sensitivity, and slowed growth and mental response.

Foods rich in vitamin B_2: Cheese, egg yolks, fish, legumes, meat, milk, poultry, sardines, spinach, whole grains, and yogurt.

How much do you need a day? 1.7 milligrams

Vitamin B_3 (Niacin)

Why vitamin B_3 is important: It's necessary for good circulation and healthy skin. It also helps the nervous and digestive systems function properly, and helps to metabolize carbohydrates, fats, and protein. Plus, it can be used to lower LDL (bad) cholesterol—under the supervision of your doctor—and may help to enhance memory.

Symptoms of deficiency: Canker sores, depression, diarrhea, halitosis, indigestion, insomnia, weakness, and skin bumps and inflammation.

Symptoms of toxicity: Niacin flush—a burning, tingling, and itching sensation. Diarrhea, heartburn, nausea, ulcer, vomiting, and headache.

Foods rich in vitamin B_3: Broccoli, carrots, cheese, chicken breasts, corn flour, dandelion greens, dates, eggs, fish, milk, oatmeal, peanuts, potatoes, tomatoes, tuna, turkey, wheat germ, and whole wheat products.

How much do you need a day? 20 milligrams

Vitamin B₅ (Pantothenic Acid)

Why vitamin B₅ is important: Known as the anti-stress vitamin, vitamin B₅ is needed to form antibodies and for the proper functioning of the gastrointestinal tract. It helps the body use other vitamins and helps to convert fats, proteins, and carbohydrates into energy. It also enhances stamina, helps to prevent certain forms of anemia, and is proving helpful in treating depression and anxiety.

Symptoms of deficiency: Fatigue, headache, and nausea.

Foods rich in vitamin B₅: Avocados, beef, eggs, fish, legumes, mushrooms, nuts, poultry, saltwater fish, and whole grains including whole rye flour and whole wheat.

How much do you need a day? 10 milligrams

Vitamin B₆ (Pyridoxine)

Why vitamin B₆ is important: This vitamin is involved with more bodily functions than almost any other single nutrient. It helps produce serotonin and other neurotransmitters (brain chemicals that are important for good mental balance). It also helps protect against heart disease by reducing the level of homocysteine (a protein that can injure the walls of the coronary arteries) in the blood. It helps to maintain the balance of sodium and potassium and helps the production and digestion of fats and proteins. It also promotes the formation of red blood cells and the production of antibodies. It is needed for proper functioning of the brain, nervous system, and immune system and helps to prevent kidney stones. B₆ is also a mild diuretic, so it is great for relieving water retention and may help with symptoms of PMS.

Symptoms of deficiency: Anemia, convulsions, headaches, nausea, acne, depression, fatigue, irritability, inflammation of the mouth, smooth tongue, and hair loss.

Symptoms of toxicity: Bloating, fatigue, headaches, and bone pain.

Foods rich in vitamin B₆: Avocados, bananas, carrots, chicken, eggs, liver, nuts, peas, pork, potatoes, salmon, spinach, sunflower seeds, tuna, walnuts, and wheat germ.

How much do you need a day? 2 milligrams

Vitamin B₁₂ (Cyanocobalamin)

Why vitamin B₁₂ is important: B₁₂ will prevent anemia and nerve damage, and it works with folic acid to regulate red blood cell formation. It helps the body to use iron, protein, carbohydrates, and fat and aids in digestion. It also will promote growth, helps to maintain fertility, and may help with memory and learning.

Symptoms of deficiency: Anemia, constipation, depression, problems with digestion, drowsiness, fatigue, eye disorders, moodiness, and heart palpitations.

Foods rich in vitamin B₁₂: Dairy products, eggs, fortified soybeans and soy products, herring, mackerel, meats, milk, seafood, and sea vegetables (including dulse, kelp, kombu, and nori).

Kitchen CURES

Curb the Symptoms of PMS

Just because you're going to be getting your period soon doesn't mean that you have to feel bloated, irritable, and crampy. The following remedies will gently soothe the symptoms of PMS.

- A daily B-complex vitamin supplement can help relieve irritability, moodiness, swelling, and bloating.
- Calcium can help decrease bloating and irritability, muscle cramps, pelvic pain, and nervousness. Take a 500-milligram supplement twice a day, and be sure to eat at least two or three calcium-rich foods a day. Good options include low-fat yogurt, fat-free milk, and canned sardines or salmon.
- Magnesium helps with cravings, mood swings, bloating, and breast tenderness. Zinc helps with headaches, irritability, depression, and cramps. Try eating foods rich in both minerals, including whole grains; soy beans; nuts and seeds; and dark green, leafy vegetables.
- Exercise helps with cramping and helps your system to flow properly.
- Iron prevents fatigue and anemia, so eat some eggs, fish, meat, poultry, beans, legumes, or dried fruit to prevent iron-poor blood.
- If you slightly increase your protein intake and slightly decrease your carbohydrate intake, you can reduce that bloated feeling often associated with PMS.
- If you have sweet cravings that you just can't ignore, eat a frozen fudge bar or hard candy in small portions.
- Don't forget: Stay away from salty processed foods because they make your body retain more fluid and therefore increase PMS symptoms.

How much do you need a day? 6 micrograms (Vegetarians—especially vegetarian women who are breastfeeding—need to be sure they get this daily requirement, usually from a multivitamin.)

Folate

Why folate is important: This vitamin is crucial for women who are or plan on becoming pregnant. They should start getting at least 400 micrograms of folate (or a folic acid sup-

(continued on page 100)

LIVING A
REAL FOOD LIFE

A Diet Packed with Vitamins and Minerals—Instead of Take-Out—Turned Her Life Around

Name: Julia

Real Food Life Issue: social isolation, using food for comfort/activity, frequent colds, and depression

When I met Julia, she was a college student living away from home for the first time. She was depressed because she missed her family terribly, she was overweight, and she caught colds all the time. Plus, she felt isolated because she didn't live on campus near the few friends she had met at school. She used food as a source of comfort and for company—especially when she was bored and lonely. At that point, Julia's days pretty much entailed going to class, eating, coming home, eating, studying, eating, and sleeping. Here's where I found her:

October 10

The days are getting darker earlier now. I can't wait to get home in the after-noons—I just want to be inside all the time. I've gotten into kind of a ritual lately: I get off the bus from school, head straight to my apartment, turn on the TV, and check my messages (usually empty). Then I grab the phone, stick my hand in the top kitchen drawer, and pull out a take-out menu at random. Sometimes I spend the bus trip thinking about what's going to come out of the drawer that night.

I have a favorite meal at each place: cheeseburger and fries, pizza and moz-zarella sticks, cheese steak and fried onion rings. Everyone delivers around here, even the convenience store! Dessert is the thing that never changes: chocolate chip cookie dough ice cream. I know all the delivery guys by name, and I think they like me—probably because I tip them well. They always say hi, but I just throw the money at them and grab the bag out of their hands. Then I settle in front of the TV—although these days, I have to limit my TV because school is gearing up for midterms. I let myself watch only while I eat. I'll dawdle over dessert, because I know as soon as I'm done, the TV goes off and the books get opened.

Most days, I feel like I'm on autopilot. I wonder what would happen if I just stopped going to class. I'm terrified I'm going to fail...

At her off-campus apartment, Julia ordered in most of her meals. Her tastes ran to foods that are very high in saturated fat, such as pizza and cheeseburgers. She would also have a pint of ice cream almost every night. She ate no fruits, vegetables, whole grains, or foods high in essential fatty acids, such as fish and nuts. Her depression made her not care about what she ate or looked like, and that made her even more depressed.

Our first plan of action was to go grocery shopping. I showed Julia how to stock up on healthy foods for quick and nourishing meals and snacks. We bought a variety of whole grains (crackers, quick brown rice, cereals), high-quality proteins (veggie burgers, frozen shrimp, canned beans), essential fatty acids (olive oil, nuts, and seeds), and some fresh and dried fruits and frozen and fresh vegetables. We even got her some treats.

I started her on vitamin supplements, including a B-complex to help with her depression and vitamins C and E to help her immune system. I also recommended—and she embraced—eating fish three times a week (usually grilled salmon or canned tuna). She also started eating salads daily, topped with a few walnuts and dressed with olive oil and lemon.

We pored over all of her delivery menus, and I pointed out delicious and wholesome choices in each one; I also showed her which dishes she'd do best to avoid. Julia soon replaced her nightly pint of ice cream with an ounce of high-quality dark chocolate or a chocolate sorbet pop, and she came to realize that sometimes she didn't even need her nighttime sweet. By week 4, she was drinking 8 cups of water a day, and her colds had cleared up.

Instead of rushing home to study and mope and eat, she also started going to the gym on campus. She began taking a few exercise classes there each week, which allowed her to start feeling better about her body and meet more people at the same time. She also began volunteering at the nearby soup kitchen once a week, helping to serve the needy. This really improved her self-esteem because she was doing something for someone other than herself, and making a small contribution to bettering her new community (and she met even more new people).

By the end of 8 weeks, Julia's depression had improved tremendously. Between her involvement at the soup kitchen and her newfound workout schedule, her energy increased significantly and she felt much better about herself and her situation. Even her grades improved. And much to her pleasure and surprise, she lost a little weight, even though that was not her main goal.

plement) before conception and then take 600 micrograms when they become pregnant. Why? Because folate protects against neural tube defects such as spina bifida and anencephaly, and it may also help prevent premature birth. Folate is also needed for healthy cell division and replication, energy, and the formation of red blood cells. It can strengthen the immune system and may help alleviate depression and anxiety. It may protect against colon and lung cancer, and it decreases homocysteine (a protein that causes heart disease).

Symptoms of deficiency: Anemia, apathy, gastrointestinal disturbances, fatigue, growth impairment, memory problems, general weakness, and birth defects.

Foods rich in folate: Asparagus; barley; bran; brown rice; cheese; chicken; chicory; dates; green, leafy veggies; lamb; legumes; lentils; milk; mushrooms; oatmeal; oranges; root veggies; salmon; seaweed; split peas; sunflower seeds; tuna; wheat germ; and whole grains and whole wheat.

How much do you need a day? 400 micrograms

Vitamin C

Why vitamin C is important: This may be the most well-known of all the vitamins, due to its ability to strengthen the immune system (which is why it's often taken just before or during a cold) and the fact that it's a powerful antioxidant that helps rid the body of free radicals. Needed for tissue growth and repair,

vitamin C is also necessary for proper functioning of the adrenal glands (which regulate hormones) and for healthy gums. It protects against damage from pollution, cancer, and infections. Essential for the formation and repair of collagen (which gives skin its suppleness and strengthens bones and blood vessels), it promotes the healing of wounds and burns. It also increases absorption of iron and reinforces and strengthens vitamin E's antioxidant properties. Vitamin C also helps to reduce LDL (bad) cholesterol and high blood pressure, and may prevent osteoporosis.

Symptoms of deficiency: Scurvy (symptoms include soft and spongy, bleeding gums and loose teeth), edema, bleeding gums, increased susceptibility to infections, slower wound healing, lack of energy, poor digestion, bruises, and tooth loss.

Symptoms of toxicity: Nausea, abdominal cramps, and diarrhea.

Foods rich in vitamin C: Asparagus; avocados; beet greens; berries; broccoli; Brussels sprouts; cantaloupe; citrus fruits; green, leafy vegetables; mangoes; papayas; potatoes; red and green bell peppers; spinach; and tomatoes.

How much do you need a day? 60 milligrams (Look for a buffered variety if you're taking a supplement, since it's easier on the stomach.)

Vitamin D

Why vitamin D is important: It helps the body absorb—and efficiently use—calcium and phosphorus and is necessary for growth, particularly of children's teeth and bones. Vitamin D also strengthens muscles, enhances immunity and thyroid functions, regulates the heartbeat, and prevents and may remedy osteoporosis. Vitamin D is stored in the body's fat.

Symptoms of deficiency: Bone disorders, diarrhea, and insomnia.

Symptoms of toxicity: Kidney stones, hardening of blood vessels, nausea, vomiting, and loss of appetite.

Foods rich in vitamin D: Sunlight helps convert vitamin D to its active form, so if you're outside for just 10 to 15 minutes of midday sun 2 or 3 times a week, you get all the D you need. During the winter months, you'll need a supplement if you live in cold climates or are homebound. Vitamin D is also found in dairy foods, eggs, and fatty saltwater fish like salmon, mackerel, and tuna.

How much do you need a day? 400 IU (*Note:* If you drink at least 2 glasses of milk per day, you don't need a vitamin D supplement.)

Vitamin E

Why vitamin E is important: It promotes healthy skin, hair, nerves, and muscles. It also stabilizes cell membranes, enhances the immune system, and may help to prevent certain cancers and heart disease. Vital for healing, vitamin E repairs tissues, clots blood, heals wounds, and reduces scarring. It slows tumor growth, decreases blood pressure, and strengthens coronary arteries to repair the effects of heart disease. This vitamin also helps relieve leg cramps, and helps treat PMS, hot flashes, and breast tenderness. Plus, it's an important antioxidant.

Symptoms of deficiency: Potential nerve and red blood cell damage, infertility, menstrual problems, miscarriage, and heart disease.

Foods rich in vitamin E: Avocados; brown rice; canola oil; cereals and breads made with 100 percent whole grain; eggs; extra-virgin olive oil; green, leafy vegetables; legumes; milk; nuts; oatmeal; seeds; soybeans; and wheat germ.

How much do you need a day? 30 IU (Buy vitamin E labeled "d-alpha tocopherol," which is the best source of natural vitamin E. Avoid vitamin E labeled "DL," which is synthetically derived and not as good.)

Vitamin K

Why vitamin K is important: Necessary for proper blood clotting and bone formation and repair, vitamin K is also used by our bodies for making bone protein, which helps prevent osteoporosis. It also helps to increase our resistance to infection, particularly in children. Like vitamins A and D, K is fat-soluble.

Symptoms of deficiency: Abnormal and/or internal bleeding.

Foods rich in vitamin K: Asparagus; broccoli; Brussels sprouts; cabbage; cauliflower; dark green, leafy vegetables including kale, spinach, and Swiss Chard; eggs; oatmeal; oats; onions; rye; soybeans; and wheat. Green tea has some, too.

How much do you need a day? 80 micrograms

Coenzyme Q$_{10}$

Why coenzyme Q$_{10}$ is important: Coenzyme Q$_{10}$ isn't an actual vitamin. Rather, it's a vitamin-like substance that resembles vitamin E. It's a powerful antioxidant that has enormous anti-aging properties. For this reason, it's often used in skin creams. It also is critical for energy production, aids in circulation, stimulates the immune system, and alleviates allergies, asthma, and respiratory diseases. Finally, coenzyme Q$_{10}$ is used in the treatment of some cancers and heart disease (because it helps strengthen the heart muscle).

Foods rich in coenzyme Q$_{10}$: Beef, mackerel, peanuts, salmon, sardines, and spinach.

How much do you need a day? No DV

Minerals
Calcium

Why calcium is important: Ninety-nine percent of your body's calcium is found in your bones and teeth, so it's no wonder that this mineral is vital for forming and growing strong bones and teeth. Calcium also helps to maintain healthy gums and a regular heartbeat. Plus, it aids in neuromuscular activity, helps keep skin healthy, protects against preeclampsia, and can help with symptoms of PMS. Calcium is needed for blood clotting and may help to protect against colon cancer, prevent heart disease, prevent muscle cramps, and lower both blood pressure and cholesterol levels. Because of its bone mass–building properties, it's also beneficial in the prevention of osteoporosis.

Symptoms of deficiency: Aching joints, osteoporosis, brittle nails, high blood cholesterol, eczema, heart palpitations, high blood pressure, insomnia, muscle cramps, nervousness, pasty complexion, and depression.

Symptoms of toxicity: Constipation, interference with aborption of other minerals, urinary stone formation, and kidney dysfunction.

Foods rich in calcium: Low-fat or fat-free yogurt, milk, and cheese ("reduced-fat" and "part-skim" cheeses can be almost as high in fat and calories as regular cheese, so stick with low-fat or fat-free varieties). Other good sources include almonds; asparagus; broccoli; cabbage; calcium-fortified orange juice; cereals; figs; goat's milk; green, leafy vegetables; oats; prunes; sardines and salmon (canned); seafood; sesame seeds; and soy products including soy milk, soy yogurt, soy cheese, and tofu processed with calcium sulfate.

How much do you need a day? 1,000 milligrams if you're under the age of 50; 1,200 milligrams if you're 50 or older

Chromium

Why chromium is important: Chromium helps metabolize glucose (blood sugar), which

Top 10 Ways to Boost Your Calcium Intake

Having trouble getting enough calcium in your diet? Check out these simple—and delicious—strategies for boosting your daily calcium consumption.

1. Eat more yogurt. (Eight ounces of yogurt has 100 milligrams more calcium than the same amount of milk.)
2. Have cereal with milk.
3. Cook oatmeal in fat-free milk instead of water.
4. Choose calcium-fortified orange juice.
5. Have a big serving of broccoli.
6. Add fat-free powdered milk to mashed potatoes, casseroles, sauces, and soups.
7. Add fresh or frozen kale or chard to soups or pasta sauce.
8. Add calcium-fortified tofu to smoothies, sauces, soups, salads, and chili.
9. Snack on fat-free tortilla chips with melted fat-free cheese.
10. Treat yourself to a glass of fat-free milk with fat-free chocolate sauce.

gives us energy. It's also vital for burning fats and proteins, and the body needs it to use insulin properly and to maintain stable blood sugar levels. Without chromium, insulin can't make glucose available to cells. Chromium can be especially helpful for people with diabetes and hypoglycemia.

Symptoms of deficiency: Anxiety, fatigue, and insulin resistance (when the body doesn't use glucose as it should), particularly in people with diabetes. May lead to arteriosclerosis (hardening of the arteries). A diet high in processed foods can decrease the chromium levels in the blood and wreak havoc with blood sugar levels. This is another reason to limit the amount of processed foods you eat.

Foods rich in chromium: Brown rice, cheese, eggs, meat, seafood, and whole grains.

How much do you need a day? 120 micrograms

Copper

Why copper is important: Copper aids in bone and red blood cell formation and has anti-inflammatory properties. It plays a role in the healing process, energy production, the sense of taste, and hair and skin pigmentation. It also increases the strength of collagen, a protein that gives strength and elasticity to skin and connective tissues.

In the body, the levels of copper are directly related to the levels of vitamin C and zinc. If too much vitamin C or zinc is consumed, copper levels will drop; if copper levels are too high, vitamin C and zinc levels will drop, so it's important not to take too much of either supplement.

Symptoms of deficiency: Osteoporosis, anemia, diarrhea, impaired respiratory functions, and sores.

Foods rich in copper: Almonds, avocados, barley, beans, beets, broccoli, garlic, lentils, mushrooms, oats, oranges, oysters, pecans, sardines, and sunflower seeds.

How much do you need a day? 2 milligrams

Iodine

Why iodine is important: It's vital for maintaining healthy thyroid glands (which control metabolism and growth), and it prevents goiter (enlargement of the thyroid caused by lack of iodine). Iodine is important for mental and physical development in children. It's also essential for the absorption of carbohydrates and necessary for reproduction.

Foods rich in iodine: Dairy foods, iodized salt, kelp, saltwater fish, and seafood.

How much do you need a day? 150 micrograms

Iron

Why iron is important: An essential part of hemoglobin (a protein that gives blood its red color and carries oxygen to all the cells), iron is also part of myoglobin (which stores oxygen in the muscles to provide energy for muscle contractions). Iron is important for growth, a healthy immune system, and energy production.

There are two kinds of iron, heme and nonheme. Heme is found mostly in animal-based foods and is absorbed much more efficiently than nonheme; nonheme is found mostly in plant-based foods and is poorly absorbed by the body. Vitamin C increases nonheme iron absorption by up to 30 percent. For this reason, it's best to eat foods that are high in vitamin C along with iron-rich foods to increase iron's absorption. For example, drink orange juice along with your tofu or rice and beans. You might also cook acidic foods such as tomatoes in cast-iron pans because the iron leaches into the food.

Symptoms of deficiency: Anemia, brittle hair, digestive problems, inflammation of the mouth tissues, nervousness, slowed mental reactions, intestinal bleeding, weakness, and fatigue. Too much phosphorus in the diet, poor digestion, eating too many antacids, or drinking too much coffee or tea could prevent you from getting enough iron. A deficiency in vitamins B_6 or B_{12} could also cause iron deficiency. Strenuous exercise and heavy perspiration also deplete iron.

Symptoms of toxicity: Upset stomach, diarrhea, constipation, fatigue, hemosiderosis—a genetic disorder that enhances iron absorption—and possibly kidney damage. Excessive iron may also lead to heart disease and cancer.

Foods rich in iron: Beans and legumes, cream of wheat (fortified); dried fruit; eggs; fish; green, leafy vegetables; liver; poultry; red meat; seeds; tofu; and whole grains.

How much do you need a day? 18 milligrams

Magnesium

Why magnesium is important: The main function of magnesium is energy production. Magnesium is a major component of bones and teeth and helps to regulate heart rhythm and calcium and potassium metabolism. In addition, it enhances the immune system and may help to increase HDL (good) cholesterol and prevent cardiovascular disease and osteoporosis. It also helps ensure good sleep. Magnesium can help prevent depression, PMS, dizziness, muscle weakness and twitching, and premature labor and convulsions in pregnant women.

Symptoms of deficiency: Too little magnesium could interfere with the transmission of nerve and muscle impulses and cause irritability, tiredness, and nervousness. Too little of this mineral could also result in loss of appetite, cramps, abnormal heart rhythms, and feelings of "weakness."

Foods rich in magnesium: Apples; apricots; avocados; bananas; Brazil nuts; brown rice; cantaloupe; dairy products (fat-free or low-fat), figs; fish; garlic; grapefruit; green, leafy vegetables; hazelnuts; lemons; lima beans; meat; nuts; pumpkin seeds; salmon; sardines; seafood; sesame seeds; soybeans; sunflower seeds; tofu; watercress; and whole wheat and whole grains including quinoa and amaranth.

How much do you need a day? 400 milligrams

Manganese

Why manganese is important: Manganese metabolizes protein and fat, and it is also needed for healthy nerves, a strong immune system, and the regulation of blood sugar. It's required for reproduction and for normal bone growth, and for the formation of cartilage and synovial (lubricating) joint fluids. Women need manganese for the production of breast milk. When taken with B-complex vitamins, manganese helps to give an overall sense of well-being.

Symptoms of deficiency: Hardening of the arteries, confusion, eye problems, hearing problems, high cholesterol, high blood pressure, memory loss, profuse sweating, rapid pulse, and teeth grinding.

Foods rich in manganese: Avocados; blueberries; dried peas; egg yolks; green, leafy vegetables; legumes; nuts and seeds; pineapples; seaweed; and whole grains.

How much do you need a day? 2 milligrams

Phosphorus

Why phosphorus is important: It's needed for bone and tooth formation, cell growth, heart contractions, and proper kidney functioning.

BESTBITES

Foods to Keep You Loving All Night Long

Choosing the right foods can enhance all aspects of your life—including your love life! Before a night of romance, take a peek at the following tips.

- Carbohydrates provide energy and stamina, so try some sexy fruits such as pomegranates, cherries, passion fruit, blood oranges, mangoes, papayas, and figs.
- Zinc is great for sex hormones. Indulge in some shellfish (especially oysters), lean beef, whole grains, wheat germ, beans, cashews, chicken, or turkey.
- Essential fatty acids help regulate hormones—including the sex hormones. To get more of these good fats in your diet, sprinkle walnuts or pumpkin seeds on a salad and drizzle with olive oil.
- Vitamin C helps with sperm production. So try some melons, berries, sweet potatoes, red and green peppers, and citrus fruit (and be careful).
- Avoid gas-producing foods like beans and legumes.
- Hot peppers help with circulation. Spice up your meals with cayenne or other hot peppers.
- Ginger tea also helps with blood circulation.
- Dark chocolate is a good source of antioxidants and is just plain sensual—especially when melted on strawberries!

Phosphorus also assists in the utilization of vitamins and helps convert food to energy.

A proper balance of magnesium, calcium, and phosphorus needs to be maintained at all times. If the body has too much or too little of one of these minerals, it won't function properly.

Symptoms of deficiency: Since phosphorus is found in most foods, deficiency is very rare, but prolonged use of antacids can cause it.

Symptoms of toxicity: Interferes with calcium and iron uptake. Excessive phosphorus may be a problem for people who drink more than 32 ounces of soft drinks a day.

Foods rich in phosphorus: Most foods contain some phosphorus. The following foods, however, are top sources: asparagus; bran; corn; dairy products; eggs; fish; fruit (dried); garlic; legumes; meats; nuts; poultry; pumpkin, sesame, and sunflower seeds; salmon; and whole grains.

How much do you need a day? 1,000 milligrams

Potassium

Why potassium is important: Vital for a healthy nervous system, potassium also regulates the heartbeat, prevents strokes, aids in muscle contractions, maintains stable blood pressure, and works with sodium to control the body's water balance.

Symptoms of deficiency: Critically dry skin, acne, chills, constipation, diarrhea, erratic heartbeat, and depression.

Foods rich in potassium: Apricots, avocados, bananas, brown rice, dairy foods, dates, figs, fish, fruit (including dried), garlic, legumes, meat, oats, potatoes, poultry, raisins, vegetables, wheat bran, whole grains, winter squash, and yams.

How much do you need a day? No DV, but try for 3,500 milligrams from food only.

Selenium

Why selenium is important: Selenium and vitamin E work together to help produce antibodies and maintain a healthy heart and liver. Alone, selenium enhances the immune system and has antiviral and anti-inflammatory properties and is necessary for both pancreatic functioning and tissue elasticity. It also has antioxidant properties, which means that it helps to prevent the formation of free radicals that can damage the body.

Symptoms of deficiency: Exhaustion, high cholesterol, and infections. Also linked to cancer and heart disease.

Symptoms of toxicity: Arthritis, brittle nails, stomach upset, hair loss, irritability, and skin problems.

Foods rich in selenium: One Brazil nut gives you as much selenium as you need in a day. Other sources include broccoli, brown rice, chicken, dairy foods, garlic, and salmon.

How much do you need a day? 70 micrograms

Sodium

Why sodium is important: Sodium is necessary for maintaining proper water balance and proper pH levels. It's also needed for stomach, nerve, and muscle functions. The proper balance of sodium and potassium is vital for good health; an imbalance could lead to heart disease.

Symptoms of deficiency: It's rare to have a sodium deficiency, but it can happen if someone has a kidney disorder, perspires excessively, or takes too many diuretics.

Symptoms of toxicity: Water retention, high blood pressure, potassium deficiency, and liver and kidney disease.

Foods rich in sodium: Sodium is found in virtually all foods, and most people have adequate—or excessive—amounts of sodium in their bodies.

How much do you need a day? No more

Kitchen CURES

A Natural Prescription to Soothe Acne

Whether you're a teenager or an adult, there's *never* a good time for a case of acne. Soothe your skin with the power of the following herbs and foods.

- Zinc helps prevent scarring and is necessary for oil-producing skin glands and tissue repair. So eat some zinc-rich foods, including shellfish, soybeans, whole grains, sunflower seeds, and nuts.
- Use tea tree oil, a natural antibiotic and antiseptic. Dab a little oil on a cotton swab and apply to affected areas up to three times a day.
- Beta-carotene helps heal and construct new skin. Have some dark green vegetables and orange fruit.
- Chamomile tea helps to nourish the skin, so be sure to have a cup or two each day.
- Add flaxseeds or flaxseed oil to your diet. Flax helps heal skin disorders, keeps the skin smooth and soft, and repairs damaged skin cells.
- Try to keep your stress levels low, since stress may cause skin flare-ups.

than 2,400 milligrams (this is equivalent to 1 teaspoon of table salt).

Zinc

Why zinc is important: Needed for healing wounds, growth, and bone formation, zinc also enhances the immune system and is a natural anti-inflammatory. It helps the prostate gland function properly and aids in the development of reproductive organs. Zinc also facilitates the senses of taste and smell. It may help prevent acne and regulate the activity of oil glands.

Symptoms of deficiency: Loss of taste and smell; fingernails can become thin and peel and develop white spots. Wound healing slows. Zinc deficiency may also lead to a recurrence of colds, impaired night vision, infertility, and hair loss.

Foods rich in zinc: Egg yolks, fish and shellfish, lamb and other meats, legumes, lima beans, mushrooms, oysters, pecans, poultry, pumpkin seeds, soybeans, sunflower seeds, and whole grains.

How much do you need a day? 15 milligrams

5 HUNGER AND METABOLISM

You get hungry, so you eat. Simple, right?

Not quite. There are two kinds of hunger: physical hunger and emotional, or "head," hunger. In this chapter, you'll learn to distinguish between the two. You'll also learn about the role metabolism plays in your food life. And, best of all, you'll discover a fool-proof way to boost your metabolism, regardless of the genes you were born with.

How Do You Know You're Hungry?

Hunger is the body's mechanism to remind us to fuel it. The body needs food just as a car needs gasoline—without it neither could operate. While most people won't ignore their gas gauge when it hovers at empty, many don't pay attention to their body's hunger signals. But ignoring hunger signals can confuse the body's natural chemicals that activate the appetite and hunger.

Hunger more or less originates in the hypothalamus, an area in the brain partly responsible for eating behavior. The hypothalamus sends signals to other areas of the brain, which then emit chemicals called neurotransmitters that help regulate how much we eat and what we eat.

When the body's levels of blood sugar and glycogen (the store of carbohydrates) are low, a neurotransmitter called neuropeptide Y (also known as NPY) is released from the hypothalamus. As NPY levels increase, so does the body's urge for sweet and starchy foods (carbohydrates).

For example, while you sleep, your glycogen and blood sugar levels naturally drop and then signal your brain to release NPY; that's why people naturally crave carbohydrates like breads, cereals, bagels, and fruit for breakfast. If you don't eat breakfast, NPY levels will keep going up all day and eventually set you up for a carb-binge in the late afternoon. So, sometimes carb cravings and binges are not because you "lack control"; rather, they're a natural function of your body's own chemistry. Not only does eating carbohydrates turn off the flow of NPY, but it also releases serotonin, a neurotransmitter that produces a feeling of satisfaction with your food and an overall sense of well-being.

Why Low-Calorie Diets Don't Work

Another chemical important to hunger is cholecystokinin (CCK). CCK is a neurotransmitter whose function is to send signals to stop eating, to switch off the appetite, and to activate feelings of fullness.

Some researchers believe that certain conditions, such as existing on very low calorie diets, may cause CCK to become "numbed." As a result, the dieter is no longer able to recognize the signal to stop eating. Because very restrictive diets don't supply enough nutrients to the body and the body constantly wants to fuel up on nutrients, the "stop eating" signal from the brain gets mixed messages and then fails to function properly. For this reason, this dieting strategy will

never be successful in the long term. Fortunately, when the person resumes eating a normal diet, CCK functions also return to normal.

Studies also show that those who engage in these extreme dieting practices lose their ability to recognize their natural hunger signals. Since these people have denied their hunger signals for so long, when they do eat, they're at risk of overeating because they can no longer register what "fullness" feels like and they don't know when to stop.

Learning to Listen

The bottom line when it comes to hunger? Learn to listen to your body's hunger signals, eat, and then acknowledge your body's feelings of fullness and satisfaction (rather than continuing to eat until you feel stuffed and uncomfortable). Check out the following strategies, which will help you to tune in to your body's signals.

Get off the clock. Many people eat because of external circumstances, not because their bodies are telling them to eat. It could be the time of day ("It's noon, so I must have lunch") or certain beliefs ("I have to finish this pizza because I don't want to be wasteful") that lead to this sort of eating. These habits—especially when coupled with large portion sizes—contribute to people's food lives spinning out of control. Instead, opt for flexible meal times, and eat when your body

Blood Sugar and Hypoglycemia

When people speak of blood sugar level, they're referring to the measure of the concentration of glucose in the bloodstream. (Glucose is the main source of energy for all bodily functions and comes from carbohydrates.) It's important to keep your blood sugar level stable, because if it gets out of balance, you won't feel your best. Also called hypoglycemia, low blood sugar, in particular, is blamed for many conditions—from lack of energy to psychiatric disorders.

Hypoglycemia is not a disease; rather, it's a set of symptoms that indicate blood sugar levels aren't normal. Symptoms may include one, some, or many of the following: fatigue, irritability, lack of concentration, rapid heart rate, anxiety, hunger, shakiness, and headaches. The only way to determine if you're actually hypoglycemic is to get a blood sugar test.

Each individual has a different response to blood sugar levels. Some people may feel hypoglycemic even when their blood sugar levels are in the normal range; others may not feel any symptoms even if their blood sugar levels have dipped into the clinically hypoglycemic range. If you feel that you suffer from hypoglycemia (and some of my clients do), you need to get your blood sugar levels tested by your doctor.

An acute episode of hypoglycemia requires immediate treatment. If your blood glucose level is anywhere between 20 to 60 mg/dL, you should receive treatment. People with levels between 40 to 60 mg/dL should eat crackers or drink milk, while those with the lower end of 20 to 40 mg/dL should eat 2 to 3 teaspoons of simple sugar, such as honey or table sugar, followed by a well-balanced meal in 10 to 15 minutes.

tells you to, not when the clock does.

Slow down. After you've eaten, it takes the brain about 20 minutes to register that you're full. If you slow down while you eat, your body will have time to recognize that it's being fed and satisfied. Put your fork down between bites, chew your food longer, and drink plenty of water throughout the meal. All of these will force you to slow down while eating.

Eat when you're hungry, not starving. Don't allow yourself to get to the point of starving before you eat. If you eat when you feel famished, you are much more likely to overeat or binge than if you eat when you're moderately hungry.

Recognize your thirst. It's easy to confuse your body's thirst signals with a desire for food. As a result, you may think you're hungry when you're actually thirsty. Instead of automatically reaching for food, first have a large glass of water to see if that's what your body really needs.

(continued on page 114)

LIVING A REAL FOOD LIFE

Mini-Bar Raids Are a Thing of the Past for This Healthy Traveler

Name: Ted
Real Food Life Issues: overweight, travels for work, human garbage pail

Ted is in his early forties. He's married with three kids ranging in age from 7 to 12. His demanding job in construction requires long hours at work and about 2 weeks of business travel each month. When we met, he was in a constant state of anxiety and felt so tightly wound that his stomach was chronically upset and he was able to sleep only 4 hours a night. Regularly traveling to different time zones didn't help matters. Here's where I found him:

June 5

Can't write much today—taking off for Houston tonight. Or Tulsa. Always get those confused because the hotels' mini-bars are exactly the same—on the small side, plenty of chips and sodas, not too many chocolate bars. Not like Denver—those people know how to treat me right! Chocolate bars and a nice cheese danish. My kind of people.

Eating dinner tomorrow night with the head of construction on a major project. Last time we met, I hadn't eaten since 2 that afternoon and I nearly ate the centerpiece off the table. He said, "You gotta respect a guy who relishes his dinner." He offered me the rest of his steak—nice guy. Or at least I thought so. This time he wants to go for sushi . . .

One constant in Ted's life was his food. He always felt hungry and was afraid of food deprivation (even though he was never poor and was financially successful), so he always cleaned his plate because he never wanted to get hungry and be unable to feed himself. Not only did he always finish his own food, but he also finished all of his children's leftovers. They had nicknamed him "the Human Garbage Pail."

His whole life, Ted was overweight. But he had become so big over the past few years that he barely recognized himself anymore. The stress of balancing his family and his career, and the regular business traveling, caused him to overeat even more than he previously had. Even though he was an experienced traveler, he felt that he never knew what to eat when he was away from home, and he'd soothe his travel nerves with food. When he checked into his hotel, he would inevitably inhale the entire contents of the mini-bar. Plus, he had a particular weakness for fried chicken sandwiches, candy, and sweet rolls—cravings that were easy to satisfy on his many trips to various airports.

The way for Ted to get a Real Food Life was to set him up on an eating plan that he could easily follow when traveling. The first was to make sure he didn't go to the airport hungry. If he was hungry before he left, he ate a nourishing snack or meal. If he wasn't hungry before he left, he brought along some good snacks such as yogurt, low-fat cheese sandwiches, or dried fruit and nuts—that way, he was prepared when hunger did strike. He also made sure to prearrange low-fat meals for his flights. To put an end to his mini-bar raids at the hotel, he always called ahead and made the hotel empty the mini-bar before he even arrived so he couldn't be tempted.

Ted started eating fish four times a week with a salad or a cooked vegetable; this was easily achieved on business dinners. In the early years of his marriage, he used to do all the cooking, so he was fairly comfortable in the kitchen. When he was around on weekends, he cooked dinner for the whole family and made dishes to freeze for future meals.

Whether at home or traveling, Ted started drinking much more water. It surprised him that water helped to boost his energy, calm his stomach, and quiet his hunger. He also started drinking a few daily cups of ginger or chamomile tea to soothe his stomach. In an effort to slow his pace, he tried to get at least 6 to 7 hours of sleep each night. A month into his new way with food, he felt much less anxious and much more energized.

Ted gave serious thought to his compulsive need to finish all food in sight. We talked about hunger levels, and I coached him to slow down while eating. At first, this was pretty hard for him. When he made a conscious effort, he slowed down, recognized how quickly he got full, and eventually even learned to leave his kids' leftovers alone. He either saved them for another meal or threw them away (which made him crazy, but he knew he was doing his body a favor).

By the end of 8 weeks, Ted had lost 20 pounds. He also felt stronger, was sharper at work, had more energy, and had greater patience with his kids—and more balance in his life.

Buy small. Resist the come-ons from food manufacturers who want you to buy giant packages of their products. If you buy only small packages of foods you love and crave (like cookies, chips, or candy), you will eat less. Research has shown that people eat less of a food when it's in a small package than when it's in a larger package.

Eat often. Eating small but frequent meals throughout the day will keep your blood sugar levels more stable than if you eat three large meals. And stable blood sugar levels could mean fewer and less severe mood swings, fewer cravings, and greater energy. Further, eating regular meals and snacks throughout the day will help you get in touch with your true, biological hunger levels. If you retrain yourself to recognize feelings of hunger, you can acknowledge them and eat only when you're truly hungry.

Cravings

"Craving" is just another word for emotional hunger. When you're biologically hungry, many different kinds of food can quell your hunger and fill you up. But if you have a craving, you have an overwhelming desire for a very specific taste, and only by eating that thing will you get satisfaction. If you're craving a candy bar, tuna won't satisfy you.

Ninety-seven percent of all women and 68 percent of all men experience cravings at some point. More women have cravings be-cause hormones released during the men-strual cycle and pregnancy promote cravings. For most people, cravings hit the hardest between 3:00 and 6:00 P.M. and after 8:00 P.M.

On the other hand, perpetual dieters have cravings around the clock. Studies have shown that people who go on and off short-term, highly restrictive fad diets (with mo-notonous eating plans and many "forbidden" foods) usually have intense cravings. They es-pecially crave foods they aren't "allowed" to eat—and end up thinking about them all day and ultimately becoming obsessed with them. Conversely, people who go on long-term eating plans tend to have fewer cravings. They have cravings less frequently because their diets are not only more sensible than re-strictive ones, but these diets also tend to pro-vide a wide variety of food options so they don't foster feelings of starvation or promote emotional eating.

If you are having a food craving, don't ig-nore it: Acknowledge it and find a way to sat-isfy it. The more you fight a craving, the more it will become an issue. To move past your craving, you have to give yourself permission to satisfy it and enjoy the food you're craving—but do so in smaller quantities. Try eating a small portion of the food you crave and then end it. Stop eating, and move on. After you've fed your craving, try not to focus on it anymore. Recognize that you've in-dulged it and that you're satisfied, and con-tinue on with the rest of your day.

Metabolism

While hunger is our bodies' way of telling us that we need fuel, metabolism is the engine that burns and uses that fuel. We all need a minimum number of calories to keep our bodies operational and to maintain basic vital functions, including heartbeat, liver func- tions, and breathing. The minimum number of calories required is measured by the Basal Metabolic Rate (BMR). This is what people are referring to when they talk about the "base" metabolism or metabolism at complete rest. Body shape and size as well as activity levels also help to determine the amount of calories a person needs for her

Restrictive Diets: Enemy Number One to Metabolism and Hunger

If you're on a restrictive diet and eat fewer than 1,000 calories a day, your metabolism will slow down and adjust itself to conserve energy and preserve bodily functions.

Why? When you restrict your calories, your body doesn't know it's dieting; it thinks it's starving because of famine. Your body will slow down all its basic physiological functions because it doesn't know when it will be fed again. First, your heart rate slows down. Next, your body temperature drops and your energy levels decrease. Then your metabolism slows down, causing you to become cranky and sluggish. Your body does this to conserve energy and calories so that it can maintain basic body functions.

In one study, participants were placed on severe diets that would cause them to lose 25 percent of their body weight (basically, it starved them). During this diet, the subjects became totally obsessed with food. They collected recipes and hung pictures of food on their walls; they also became irritable, cranky, upset, and lethargic. When they were allowed to put the weight back on, they binged and felt out of control with their eating, and still the food obsessions lingered. Chronic dieters may be at risk of developing these same traits.

Another study weighed a group of chronic dieters and a group of nondieters. The researchers told half the subjects they weighed 5 pounds less than they actually did and told the other half they weighed 5 pounds more. Both the dieters and nondieters who were told they weighed 5 pounds less were unaffected by what the researchers told them. However, unlike the nondieters, the *dieters* who were told they weighed 5 pounds more had a big drop in self-esteem, experienced bad mood swings, and binged excessively on food, despite the hunger signals their bodies gave them. You don't need to be a scientist to analyze this data: Chronic dieting is bad for your mind and body.

day. Simply put, some people need a lot of fuel to keep them going, while others don't need as much, depending on their genes and activity level.

Lean muscle mass has a higher metabolism (that is, it burns more calories at rest) than fat does. So if you are more muscular, your metabolism will be higher than that of someone who has less muscle and more fat. Since a man has 10 to 20 percent more muscle than a comparably sized and aged woman, and since muscle burns more calories than fat does, men's metabolisms tend to be higher than women's. As a result, men can eat 5 to 10 percent more than women without gaining an ounce.

The BMR accounts for 60 percent of your total daily energy needs, but it can go up to 75 percent if you increase your muscle mass through resistance exercises like lifting weights, running, and dancing. Since muscles are the body's calorie-burning furnace, when you build muscle, your metabolism will rise, which can cause even more calories to be burned both during and after exercise.

The metabolism, like many bodily attributes, is an inherited genetic trait—and it's hard to change biological destiny. Genetics can explain why a woman who is the same size and has the same activity level as her friend may be able to eat a lot more than her friend and still not gain any weight. But don't despair if your genes have dealt you a sluggish metabolism. You can increase your lean muscle mass and shrink your stores of body fat and, in so doing, boost your metabolism if you regularly lift weights and do a variety of weight-bearing exercises.

Maintaining Your Metabolism

Your calorie needs peak at age 25. After that, they start to decline by 2 percent every 10 years. This happens because as you age, the amount of lean muscle tissue you have usually decreases while your fat stores increase. If you remain active and exercise regularly, however, your metabolism can remain strong your entire life. Remember: It doesn't matter at what age you begin exercising, because at any age, exercise will increase your metabolic rate.

Measure Your Metabolism: A Ballpark Estimate

To get an absolutely accurate measurement of your BMR, you would need to go to a medical facility (usually a hospital) where they specialize in weight management and metabolism. There they would use very high tech machinery and methods, and the work would be very expensive. Fortunately, most people don't need to get that kind of precise measurement. Instead, you can measure your BMR yourself. While it won't be as accurate, it is free.

A crude way to approximate your BMR is to multiply your current weight by 10 if you're a woman or 11 if you're a man. The body needs 10 to 11 calories for each pound it weighs to meet its very basic functional needs. So, a 140-pound woman needs no less than 1,400 calories a day, and a 180-pound man needs at least 1,980 calories a day. You should add 500 to that number, since the figure is based on a resting body, not an active one, and is really the fewest number of calories needed.

As I mentioned earlier, a person's calorie needs can go up or down, based on his or her individual activity levels and body shape and size. Unless you are a tiny woman, you will need at least 1,500 calories a day. If you're a taller woman, you probably need about 2,000 calories a day; if you're a man, you need about 2,500 to 3,500 calories each day, depending on your size.

If you take in more calories than you expend, it will result in your body storing fat—and you gaining weight. To gain a pound of fat, you have to take in 3,500 calories more than you're using.

Note: This BMR formula is intended to give you a rough idea of how many calories you burn daily. I don't ever want you to count calories in your daily life, however. My clients don't count them, and you shouldn't either. Base your eating plan on how your body feels, not on what your calculator tells you.

6 HEALING FOODS AND HERBS

As you're developing your Real Food Life, you may want to add some healing foods or herbs to your diet to boost your energy level, help maintain overall good health, or occasionally help fight a cold. In this chapter, I'll discuss the varieties available and explain how to incorporate them smartly and safely into your Real Food Life.

Personally, I have found herbs to be helpful because they make me feel good and make me feel that I'm doing something extra to enhance my health. I don't use them daily, just when I need a boost. I also eat plenty of fruits and vegetables every day to ensure I get the medicinal properties they contain in a pure and natural form. For example, I regularly eat dandelion greens and fresh garlic to help control my blood pressure. When I feel a cold coming on, I use echinacea and drink fresh ginger tea. I love chamomile tea because it helps me relax after a long day. I also try to drink at least a cup of green tea daily because I love that it's loaded with antioxidants.

While this chapter includes foods and herbs I've used myself and recommended, to good effect, to my clients, they are not intended as a cure for any health condition you may be experiencing. Rather, they should be used to enhance your health now and in the future.

Using Herbs and Other Natural Supplements

Natural food supplements and herb-based remedies have been around for centuries. Records indicate that many ancient cultures, including the Chinese, Indians, Romans, and Native Americans, used a variety of herbs, plants, and foods to cure illnesses. Modern medicine is rooted in herbal medicine; in fact, today at least 25 percent of pharmaceutical prescription drugs are derived from plants.

Herbs can play many roles. Certain ones, like parsley and basil, are most commonly used in cooking to enhance the taste of foods. But medicinal herbs—including the roots, bark, and leaves—can be used to treat ailments or diseases and maintain good health. Natural food remedies are foods that, when eaten, have particular healthful attributes.

Medicinal herbs were once considered "folk" or "alternative" medicine, but they have become increasingly popular in recent years and have now started to enter the mainstream. This is a result of several factors, such as an increased awareness of the benefits of keeping fit and maintaining overall wellness, an awareness of the benefits of eating "natural" foods, and more widespread knowledge about disease prevention. Between the rising cost of and safety concerns about conventional medicines and a noted increase in the prevalence of chronic diseases, many people

are turning to a natural way to maintain or improve overall health.

Many herbs have chemical properties that, when the herb is used correctly, can help protect and heal the body. But herbs always need to be used with caution. Most people in the United States self-medicate with herbs because medical doctors don't usually prescribe them. (In many other countries, particularly throughout Europe and Asia, doctors regularly prescribe herbs to their patients.) If you decide to use herbs, you need to be aware that some herbs may have negative interactions with prescription and nonprescription drugs. Natural doesn't always mean safe. If you're concerned about negative reactions, or you want to learn more about herbs, you may want to talk with a qualified herbalist. Look for an M.D. with special training in herbs, a naturopathic (N.D.) or Chinese medicine doctor (O.M.D.), or a certified herbal practitioner through the American Herbalist Guild (AHG) or other reputable organization.

If you're currently taking prescription drugs, please talk with your doctor before trying any of the herbs and supplements listed below. Some of the drugs they are known to interact with are named, but not all of them.

Since the U.S. government and FDA have not officially approved herbs for medicinal use, they neither govern herb manufacturers nor protect consumers by requiring warnings on the labels about contraindications, adverse reactions, or doses that may be toxic. So you need to be careful about what you buy. Just because a label says the product contains an herb doesn't guarantee the herb is actually in the product. Further, you need to be aware of the form of the herb and the concentration level that is most effective. A qualified herbalist can help you with this. Some health food stores have someone on staff who is qualified to help you.

My preferred brands, in alphabetical order, are:

▶ Eclectic Institute: (888) 799-4372

▶ Enzymatic Therapy/Phytopharmic (European formulas): (800) 558-7372

▶ Frontier Organic: (800) 786-1388

▶ Gaia Herbs (organic): (800) 831-7780

▶ Herbalist and Alchemist (organic): (800) 611-8235

▶ Herb Pharm (organic whole herbs): (800) 348-4372

▶ Nature's Way: (800) 962-8873

▶ Warner Lambert (European formulas): (877) 782-6837

▶ Whitehall-Robins (Centrum brand): (877) 236-8786

For more information, I recommend logging on to www.consumerlab.com. This is a nonprofit organization that tests for purity, strength, and quality control of herbs, vitamins, and minerals.

Natural Food Supplements and Herbs

Ready to be introduced to some of the most effective healing foods and herbs? Read on.

Cayenne (Also Known as Capsicum, Hot Pepper, or Red Pepper)

What cayenne does: Cayenne aids digestion and improves circulation. It alleviates ulcers and helps to ward off colds, sinus infections, and sore throats. It's good for the heart, lungs, kidneys, and stomach.

Dosage: Sprinkle on foods throughout the day.

Chamomile

What chamomile does: Chamomile may help promote sleep and alleviate stress and anxiety. It also acts as an anti-inflammatory for the digestive system.

Dosage: One cup of tea. Pour 10 ounces of boiling water over 1 heaping teaspoon of dried flower heads (or use a tea ball) and let steep, covered, for 5 to 10 minutes; strain and serve. If you can't find dried flower heads, use a good-quality tea bag such as Pompadour or Twinings.

Cinnamon

What cinnamon does: Cinnamon relieves diarrhea and nausea and enhances digestion. It also helps to decongest nasal passages.

Dosage: Sprinkle on food.

Kitchen CURES

Powerful Pointers for Boosting Your Immune System

Every day, your immune system defends you from invading marauders such as viruses and bacteria. Sometimes, though, it can use a boost. If you've noticed that you've been sick a lot lately, help your immune system out with the following natural strategies.

- Vitamins C and E are both powerful antioxidants that increase resistance to infection and enhance the immune system. Be sure to get 60 milligrams of vitamin C and 30 IU of vitamin E each day.
- Try eating several antioxidant-rich foods each day. Good choices include tomatoes; sweet potatoes; carrots; bell peppers; broccoli; leafy, dark green vegetables; apricots; melons; citrus fruit; strawberries; wheat germ; cold-pressed vegetable oils; and nuts and seeds.
- Garlic is a great antioxidant and antibiotic that can protect against infection. It also contains phytochemicals that stop bacterial growth and may help stimulate the immune system. Be sure to eat a few cloves of raw or lightly cooked garlic regularly.
- Omega-3 fatty acids can help reduce chronic inflammation that stems from a hyperactive immune system. They also help strengthen cell membranes, which are our bodies' first defense against infection. Eat fish, nuts, and seeds several times a week.
- Laughter, getting 8 hours of sleep each night, exercise, and having strong emotional connections with others can help keep you healthy.

Dandelion Greens

What dandelion greens do: Dandelion greens work as a diuretic (helping to release retained water) and relieve bloating. They're also loaded with B vitamins.

Dosage: Steam dandelion greens until soft, let cool, and then add a squeeze of fresh lemon and a drizzle of extra-virgin olive oil. Toss well before eating.

Garlic

What garlic does: Garlic has anti-inflammatory, antioxidant, and anti-yeast properties. It helps heal gastric ulcers, enhances the immune system, and may help prevent cancers. It also may lower blood pressure, LDL (bad) cholesterol, and triglycerides, and may raise HDL (good) cholesterol. The allicin in garlic gives its characteristic odor and taste and is where most of the medicinal properties are found.

Dosage: 1 clove of fresh garlic a day (if you choose to cook it, limit the cooking time to no more than 15 minutes or the allicin becomes inactive).

Ginger

What ginger does: A powerful antioxidant and effective antimicrobial agent, ginger is useful for treating bowel disorders, circulatory problems, motion sickness, indigestion, nausea, vomiting, and morning sickness. It contains shogaols, which are natural anti-inflammatory agents.

Dosage: 1 inch square of candied, crystallized, or fresh ginger; or one cup of ginger tea (1 to 2 tablespoons of peeled, chopped fresh ginger simmered in 10 ounces of water for about 15 minutes); or one or two 500-milligram capsules daily.

Caution: Avoid ginger supplements if you're taking anticoagulant or blood-thinning medications.

Green Tea

What green tea does: Green tea contains an antioxidant that is 100 times more effective than vitamin C and 25 times more effective than vitamin E in protecting against cancers including esophageal, stomach, lung, bladder, pancreatic, and colon. It also promotes healthy teeth and contains polyphenols that increase HDL (good) cholesterol and de-

crease LDL (bad) cholesterol and can protect against heart disease. Green tea is made from unfermented dried tea leaves, usually grown in India or Asia. It contains about a quarter of the caffeine of coffee and half the caffeine of regular tea; feel free to drink decaffeinated green tea if you're affected by caffeine. (*Note:* Milk deactivates the antioxidant properties of any tea.)

Dosage: One cup or more a day. Steep 1 teaspoon of tea leaves (use a tea ball, if you have one) in 1 cup hot (just under boiling) water for 1 to 3 minutes, strain, and drink.

Peppermint

What peppermint does: Peppermint enhances digestion and stimulates the appetite. It also alleviates chills, colic, diarrhea, headache, and indigestion.

Dosage: One cup of tea as needed. Pour 10 ounces of boiling water over 1 heaping teaspoon of dried leaves (or use a tea ball) and let steep, covered, for 5 to 10 minutes; strain and serve.

Caution: If you have gastroesophageal problems, such as acid reflux, do not use peppermint.

Yogurt

What yogurt does: Yogurt contains bacteria (*L. acidophilus*) that can help maintain the gastrointestinal tract. It also maintains the vaginal canal and reduces the incidence of candidal vaginitis (candida yeast).

Kitchen CURES

Get Relief When You're Feeling Bloated and Gassy

If you're so bloated that you're wondering how your ring *ever* fit on your finger, sample the following suggestions. They're guaranteed to relieve that bloated, gassy feeling.

- Avoid salty foods, which can cause you to retain water and make you feel and look puffy.
- If you're eating a lot of gas-promoting foods, such as fiber-rich beans, try cutting down on your portions. Also add a few drops of Beano (an enzyme that helps digest gas-causing sugars) to your gas-producing food. Beano is available in most supermarkets and health food stores.
- Lack of vitamin E causes fluid retention as well as cramps and breast tenderness. You can increase the amount of vitamin E you get by adding some extra-virgin olive oil, nuts, seeds, brown rice, or legumes to your diet. Also, take a 400 IU supplement.
- Too little protein in your diet can also cause fluid retention. Be sure to have some fish, tofu, chicken, or lean meat each day.
- Acidophilus can help with gas. Eat all-natural yogurt made with active cultures or take an acidophilus supplement daily.
- Fresh pineapple contains an enzyme that helps with gas and soothes the stomach.
- Fresh papaya contains enzymes that aid digestion, as does mint. Try a papaya and mint salad.
- Anise seeds or fennel seeds can help soothe your belly, decrease gas, and aid digestion. Add some to your food or chew on a teaspoonful after eating.
- Drink ginger or chamomile tea. Both are age-old remedies known to help calm the stomach.
- If you get gas after eating dairy products, you may be sensitive to dairy or lactose intolerant. Try Lactaid with your milk—it's an over-the-counter lactose digestion aid.

Dosage: Eat 1 cup of low-fat plain yogurt daily.

The following herbs are ingested either in pill form (like traditional medicine or vitamins) or liquid form (you place drops on or under your tongue) or applied as a topical lotion, liquid, or oil. You can purchase these herbs in health food stores and better drug stores. You can also order them by calling the manufacturers listed on page 121.

Echinacea

What echinacea does: Echinacea decreases the severity of cold symptoms and may lower your chance of catching the common cold. It's been approved in Germany for treating colds, influenza, and upper respiratory infections. When applied topically, it enhances wound healing.

Dosage: No more than nine 300- to 400-milligram capsules per day. It's most effective when taken at the first sign of a cold or infection; take for 8 to 10 days, then stop.

Caution: Do not use echinacea if you're allergic to closely related plants such as ragweed, asters, and chrysanthemums. Do not use if you have tuberculosis or an autoimmune condition because echinacea stimulates the immune system. Avoid this herb if you're pregnant.

Ginkgo Biloba

What ginkgo biloba does: Used to treat lack of concentration, lack of energy, dizziness, absentmindedness, and confusion, ginkgo biloba increases cerebral bloodflow. It may help with tinnitus (ringing in the ear) and may improve hearing.

Dosage: 3 capsules of 40-milligram standardized extract a day. It takes 6 to 8 weeks before results are evident. Look for Ginkgold, which is a good brand.

Caution: Do not use with antidepressant MAO inhibitor drugs, aspirin, or other non-steroidal anti-inflammatory medications, or blood-thinning medications such as warfarin (Coumadin). Do not use if you're being treated for infertility.

Kava Kava

What kava kava does: This herb helps relieve anxiety and insomnia without morning grogginess. It also relieves menopausal anxiety and may help with hot flashes. Kava kava has been used for hundreds of years by native South Pacific Islanders as a calming drink.

Dosage: No more than six 400- to 500-milligram capsules a day.

Caution: Do not take more than the recommended dose on the package. Do not take with alcohol or barbiturates. Use with caution when driving since it is a muscle relaxant. Do not use if you're taking drugs for depression. Do not take it for more than 3 months, because you can become dependent on it. Do not use if you're pregnant or lactating.

Saw Palmetto

What saw palmetto does: This herb improves urine flow, reduces prostate swelling, and prevents further progression of an enlarged prostate gland. It can help boost the immune system and can alleviate cystitis.

Dosage: Six 500-milligram capsules a day.

Caution: Consult your doctor for proper diagnosis and monitoring before using saw palmetto to treat an enlarged prostate.

Valerian Root

What valerian root does: It improves sleep without daytime drowsiness. Valerian root has been used for hundreds of years throughout Europe as a sedative, to relieve insomnia, anxiety, and muscle spasms.

Dosage: For sleep only: 300 to 400 milligrams 1 hour before bed.

Caution: Do not use with sleep or mood medications because it may intensify their effects. Sensitive individuals may experience heart palpitations and nervousness; if you experience these symptoms, discontinue use.

Supplements Especially for Women

Many herbs and natural foods are particularly useful in treating women's health problems. Below I've noted a few that I've found especially beneficial.

Black Cohosh

What black cohosh does: Black cohosh controls the changes associated with menopause. It reduces the number and severity of hot flashes and increases the strength of pelvic floor muscles. Black cohosh also reduces depression, irritability, fatigue, headache, and vaginal dryness and promotes sleep. It has been used in Germany since the 1950s for menopausal symptoms.

Dosage: Three 500- to 600-milligram capsules a day of the dried root (often marketed under the name Remifemin).

Dong Quai

What dong quai does: Dong quai is helpful for relieving urinary tract infections, PMS symptoms, and irregular and difficult menses. It's used with vitex or black cohosh for menstrual and menopausal symptoms.

Dosage: Up to six 500- to 600-milligram capsules a day.

Caution: Do not use for more than 6 months. Do not use with blood-thinning or anti-platelet drugs.

Flaxseed

What flaxseed does: A stool softener and a great source of fiber, flaxseed is a natural laxative. It's an antioxidant that can protect against breast, ovarian, and prostate cancers. It's also high in omega-3 fatty acids, which may reduce LDL (bad) cholesterol. It also reduces symptoms of PMS and menopause. One of the world's oldest cultivated plants, flaxseed is currently grown for fiber (linen), seed oil (linseed oil), and seeds.

Dosage: 1 teaspoon freshly crushed seeds

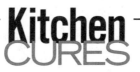

Say Goodbye to Constipation

Don't be embarrassed by a case of constipation. Cure it with one of the following home remedies.

- Increase your fiber intake. Slowly start to include more fruits, vegetables, and whole grains in your eating plan each day.
- Brown rice; dark green, leafy vegetables (such as collards, kale, cabbage, and Brussels spouts); beans; asparagus; figs; prunes; nuts and seeds; toasted wheat germ; and berries will help fill you, flush you, and give you needed fiber.
- Rhubarb is a natural laxative. Don't eat the leaves—they're poisonous. But do cut the stalks into inch-long pieces, add sugar or honey to taste, and cook over medium heat for about 10 minutes. Add a pint of hulled strawberries, raspberries, blackberries, or blueberries (frozen are fine) and cook for another minute or so, and you have a fresh, sweet-and-sour dessert that will make you "regular."
- Freshly ground flaxseed is a great natural laxative. Add a tablespoon or two to your cereal or salads.
- Essential fatty acids help lubricate the intestines, so add some olive oil or walnut oil to your next salad or steamed vegetable dish.
- Pour yourself a bowl of high-fiber cereal, such as Kashi Go Lean, which contains 10 grams of fiber—that's one-third of your recommended daily fiber intake!
- Water is a great lubricant for your system. Drink at least eight 8-ounce glasses a day.

twice a day (sprinkled on food). Grind flaxseeds in a coffee grinder (seeds need to be crushed and eaten within 20 minutes or the medicinal properties will be destroyed). Or take 1 to 4 tablespoons of flaxseed oil a day. Four tablespoons a day can increase HDL

(good) cholesterol and decrease LDL (bad) cholesterol and triglycerides.

Caution: Do not take if you have a bowel obstruction. Take with at least 8 ounces of water. Do not use if you have intestinal or esophageal problems.

Phytoestrogens

What phytoestrogens do: These are estrogen-like substances found in plants. Before the onset of menopause, they can protect against estrogen-related cancers; after menopause occurs, they rebuild depleted levels of "good" estrogens.

Phytoestrogens that can help with symptoms of menopause include alfalfa, aniseed, basil, beans, caraway, chervil, fennel, hops, licorice, parsley, sage, and especially soy foods like tofu (try to purchase organic soy food products).

Dosage: Try to have at least one good source of phytoestrogen-rich food daily. For example, try half a cup of beans, an herb salad, 1 cup of edamame, or 4 ounces of tofu. Also, cook with liberal amounts of herbs.

Vitex

What vitex does: This herb alleviates menstrual cramps and breast tenderness and regulates irregular menstrual cycles. It relieves PMS anxiety and other PMS symptoms including migraines, cramps, bloating, and constipation. It stimulates milk production in lactating women. Vitex is also used to treat premenopausal symptoms including hot flashes and vaginal dryness. It has been used to treat women's health problems for more than 2,000 years. It's best used in conjunction with black cohosh, dong quai, and omega-3 fatty acids.

Dosage: Three 650-milligram capsules a day.

Caution: May counteract the effectiveness of birth control pills.

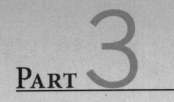

PART 3

The 8-Week Food Life

MAKEOVER PLAN

Welcome to the 8-Week Makeover Plan

Let's get started!

You are literally holding, in your very own hands, the power to develop your Real Food Life. I've developed this program over years of working with all kinds of clients, from a young teen who struggled with body consciousness to a retiree who needed to let go of his high-fat diet in order to save his own life. While everyone's individual circumstances are different, we all go through the same process in adopting the changes of our Real Food Lives. During these 8 weeks, you'll learn all the skills you need to define, em-brace, and rejoice in your very own Real Food Life.

A big part of developing your own Real Food Life is evaluating where you are now, targeting your most limiting old food life habits, sweeping them out of your life, and filling in the space that remains with new, healthy, invigorating food choices. Although I can't be with you while you move through these next 2 months, I'll do my best to answer each of your questions as they arise.

In week 1, you'll become a student of your own habits, thinking about the larger issues that may have shaped your current food life. You'll set your ultimate goal and answer the question, "What will my Real Food Life look like and how will I know when I get there?"

You'll don a spiffy doctor's coat in week 2 to study your results and give yourself a food life diagnosis—what kind of eater are you? You'll also begin setting weekly mini-goals that will guide your choices during the week, and you'll check your progress at the end with your weekly Get Real Check-In.

Week 3 is a fun one—I'll have you do a Kitchen Makeover. We take a good, hard look at the food you've been surrounding yourself with, evaluating each item to determine if it has what it takes to remain a part of your Real Food Life. Then we'll take your show on the road, hitting the supermarket to map out a strategy for the fastest, highest-value shopping trips.

Cooking is a big part of taking responsibility for your Real Food Life, and in week 4, you'll draw on everything you've learned before to enjoy the power of cooking your first Real Food Life meal.

In week 5, I'll give you fun and interesting ways to tackle the nuts and bolts of any Real Food Life week: eating a healthy, satisfying lunch and fitting in energizing exercise.

By this point in your program, you'll have made some enormous changes. During week 6, we'll take a moment to study your progress, savor your accomplishments, and chart a course for the remaining 3 weeks. I've also anticipated many of your most challenging food moments, from the holiday dinner at Mom's to the vacation buffet brunch, and given you specific methods to deal with each one.

During week 7, we go back to the scene of your most common food life crimes—the restaurant. I'll give you targeted strategies to zoom in on the best choices on any menu, so you can relish dining out without sabotaging your Real Food Life.

Triumphant and buzzing with new possibilities, we'll launch week 8 with a talk about some hurdles that may still be holding you back (or may pop up in the future). Armed with the strength of these suggestions, you'll give any resistance to your Real Food Life the one-two punch!

In each week, I'll introduce new tasks for you to continue working on as the plan progresses. Each week builds on the next, and while I might not remind you of certain ongoing tasks in the main part of the week's chapter, I've provided a handy reminder at the beginning of the week (in the checklist) and at the end of the week (in the Get Real Check-In). Along the way, I'll share shopping lists, mental strategies, Instant Makeovers—all the powerful tools in my bag of tricks—to catapult you into your new, rich, rewarding Real Food Life. With my help and your hard work, you are about to be reborn!

Week One:
KICK-STARTING YOUR REAL FOOD LIFE

During this week, you will:

- Accomplish Instant Makeover #1: Replace two sugared drinks per day with two glasses of water
- Schedule an appointment with your doctor for a checkup
- Buy a kicky notepad or journal
- Fill out a quick questionnaire on the broad aspects of your food life
- Choose one or two ultimate goals for your plan
- Begin keeping your personalized food journal
- Complete week 1 of your Get Real Check-In

Are those trumpets I hear? Well, if they're not playing for you, they should be. You've made a big first step—you've decided you want to get a Real Food Life. Congratulations and welcome. Now let's get started!

Just like most of the long-lasting changes we make in our lives, your Real Food Life is built of small steps that add up to big payoffs. Each week, I'll guide you through a series of very doable, very *satisfying* tasks that help you reach your ultimate goals. The work you do in week 1 will be the first small steps on the road to achieving significant positive changes in your food life.

Though this plan covers the span of

Instant Makeover #1:

Replace Two Sugared Drinks with Two Extra Glasses of Water

This week, I won't be asking you to make a single change in the way you eat, but I do want you to replace two glasses of flavored or sugar-added drinks (such as soda and coffee) with two glasses of water every day. Now, I ask you—isn't that a pretty low-stress way to kick-start your Real Food Life?

As the first of eight bad habits you'll cleanse yourself of over these weeks, re-placing two sugared or flavored drinks with water is the primary one for good reason. Water plays a key role in nearly every func-tion of our bodies, including digestion, waste control, circulation, and body temper-ature maintenance. In addition, water fills you up, so you tend to eat less. And water is instant energy when you're feeling tired. (In fact, tiredness is one of the most common signs of dehydration.) Because dehydration can leave you feeling mentally fuzzy, drinking more water can help you to think more clearly.

Now, if for some reason you never drink any sweetened drinks (coffee included), just add two glasses of water. Unless you're al-ready downing at least ten 8-ounce glasses of water a day, you could always use a little extra.

2 months, there's no need to feel nervous about it. Your biggest task this week is pretty simple—just be you.

Imagine that you're taking a long road trip. The first thing you'd probably do is buy a big map that will give you detailed informa-tion about the best roads to take. But you can't chart out your course on a map without knowing where you're starting from!

Likewise, when you begin your Real Food Life journey, you first need a plan that will "map out" the best strategies to follow. In Week 1, I'll guide you through a process that will give you an accurate view of the place you come from, food-wise. Once you estab-lish a starting point, you can confidently point yourself toward your goal, and nothing will stand between you and your Real Food Life. As you go along, these first 8 weeks will allow you to get rid of unhealthy food habits and replace them with positive, health-en-hancing ones.

1. Schedule a Visit with Your Doctor

Okay, so let's say your road trip is a cross-country move—you're starting a new life in a whole new state. Would you just jump in your car and head out for the hills? You'd probably want to make sure your car is up to the challenge—you'd take it to the garage, have the mechanic check under the hood, fill the tires, change the oil.

Think of your doctor as the mechanic who can pronounce your vehicle sound for the journey. Before you start your Real Food Life, I strongly recommend making an appointment with your doctor for a checkup. If you're taking any medications, your doctor can advise you on any precautions you should take with your diet, or if you have any medical conditions that might limit your ability to exercise. Chances are, she'll be thrilled with the positive changes you plan to make.

2. Purchase a Notepad or Journal

Phobic about school supplies? Just know I'm not going to ask you to do any homework. Your food journal is more like the notes you used to pass to your best friend in class: detailed, confessional, and *very* educational.

Your food journal will be your constant companion, developing into a comprehensive information bank about *you*. In it, you'll record your goals, your emotions, and everything you put in your mouth for the next 56 days.

Oh, and your bathroom habits. Can't forget that.

You're going to carry it around for a while, so take some time to think about what type of journal will make you feel good to write in. If you get into this kind of thing, think about color, paper texture, size. Where will you put it—in your purse? Hip pocket? Briefcase? Do you prefer the flexibility and convenience of spiral bound, or the soul-soothing solidity of a cloth-covered diary? Remember, you'll be looking at it every day for the next 8 weeks, so try to love it a little. Shoot for at least 100 pages. Slap on an inspirational bumper sticker. Break out the glitter pen. Go crazy.

3. Look at the Big Picture

I've designed the questionnaire on page 136 to help you get started thinking about your current food life. Take some time to work through it now. Answer as truthfully as possible—the outcome will help you analyze the broader issues at work in your current food life and help you develop your ultimate Real Food Life goal. (If you prefer not to write in this book, you can jot down your answers in your newly purchased journal.)

4. Determine Your Real Food Life Ultimate Goals

Now that you've thought about the big picture, it's time to hone in on your ultimate goal for the next 8 weeks. Perhaps even be-

(continued on page 140)

Your Real Food Life Starting Point: The Questionnaire

Food touches every part of your life—and you're about to find out if that touch is a tickle or a sucker punch. These questions, grouped by general category, cover many of the basic issues that affect how—and what—you eat. I tried to make this fun, but underneath the jokes, these are real questions. Circle the letter of the answer that most closely describes how you feel.

Food Likes and Dislikes

1. Fruits and veggies factor into my eating with
   a. two kinds at every meal and one at every snack
   b. a salad with lunch and boiled carrots with dinner
   c. an extra scoop of ketchup on my nearly daily fries

2. You will see me in the kitchen
   a. wielding zucchini and a chopping knife (I cook for myself at least 5 nights a week)
   b. tearing open a Lean Cuisine (I eat at home about 3 times a week)
   c. when hell freezes over (I never eat at home)

3. The colors of my diet
   a. look like a rainbow (with a variety of phytochemical-rich foods)
   b. look like a stoplight (two or three favorite foods)
   c. look like a 1970s beige living room (lots of refined carbs)

4. The last time I was at a fast-food restaurant
   a. I ordered a happy meal and played on the jungle gym (haven't eaten it for years)
   b. I gave into a craving, but felt a little sick afterward (eat it less than monthly)
   c. the counter guy greeted me with "your standard order, miss/sir?" (eat it at least once a week)

5. If I'm really honest, I'd say fish is
   a. nature's irresistible power food (eat it 2+ times a week)
   b. tolerable when I'm in the mood (eat it monthly)
   c. best served crunchy (eaten deep-fried only)

Diet Mentality

1. When a new diet comes out, I
   a. don't consider following it for a minute
   b. read up on it, try it for a couple of days, then revert to my old ways
   c. make it my religion

2. If I made a chart of my weight over the past few years, it would look like
   a. a Kansas horizon line (very stable)
   b. the rolling hills of Tuscany (repeatedly lost and gained the same 5 to 10 pounds)
   c. the Himalayas (repeatedly lost and gained 10 percent of my body weight)

3. "Bad" foods
   a. don't exist
   b. can feel so good
   c. make the best friends

4. I think about food
   a. when I'm hungry
   b. when I'm bored
   c. when I'm breathing

5. If I eat well during the week, by the weekend
   a. I restock fresh foods from the grocery store
   b. I reward myself with Friday night pizza and beer
   c. I backslide into a blur of brunch buffets and Biggie Fries

Work Issues

1. Working through lunch usually means
   a. unwrapping a homemade low-fat turkey or smoked tofu sandwich on whole grain bread
   b. taking a stab at whatever "diet" dish the cafeteria is serving
   c. ordering in a cheese steak and fries—and a couple of Cokes to get me through the midafternoon slump

2. When I'm feeling overwhelmed at work
   a. I strap on my sneakers and take a walk around the building until my head clears
   b. I scavenge some nuts and low-fat crackers from the bottom drawer of my desk
   c. I use up a roll of quarters in the vending machine

3. On the extremely rare slow day at work
   a. I catch up on paperwork and take an extra-long walk at lunchtime
   b. I linger over lunch, adding dessert and coffee to my normal meal
   c. I find myself irresistibly drawn to the receptionist's bowl of M&M's

(continued)

Your Real Food Life Starting Point: The Questionnaire (cont.)

4. When I'm mad at my boss
   a. I take a walk to clear my head and sort out my feelings
   b. I vent to my friends over lunch at the steakhouse
   c. I dive into a bag of chips and pretend I'm crushing his head with every crunch

Home Life

1. My partner and I
   a. eat together every night, at the table
   b. eat together four times a week, twice at our favorite Chinese place
   c. eat together every night, side-by-side on the couch

2. If I were honest about my relationship, I'd say
   a. my partner supports my efforts, often offering to make the changes along with me
   b. my partner is okay with any changes I make, as long as I don't ask him or her to change!
   c. my partner criticizes my efforts and is convinced I'll fail

3. Since we got together, my weight
   a. has stayed the same
   b. has gone up or down more than 10 percent
   c. has yo-yoed depending on life stresses

4. I love eating alone because
   a. I cook to my taste and don't have anyone to please but myself
   b. my dinner routine is comfortable—me, the cat, and the TV
   c. the drive-thru bills are always under $10!

5. My roommate and I
   a. share cooking and shopping duties and like preparing meals together
   b. bond over bags of cookies
   c. size each other up and compete about everything

Family and Friends

1. Growing up, my mom and dad
   a. didn't get stressed about what or how much I ate

  b. made comments, but backed off when I gave them The Look

  c. hovered to the point of blocking airspace

2. When I go home for the holidays, I

  a. bring my own cereal, for clutch situations

  b. look forward to my favorite home-baked cookies, but they lose their charm after the first dozen

  c. resist reacting to criticism by keeping my mouth full—the whole visit

3. When I was growing up

  a. all food was fair game, but there wasn't that much junk in the house

  b. Mom limited me to three sodas a day

  c. I spent my allowance on economy packs of forbidden Hostess snacks

4. A standard evening with my best friends includes

  a. dinner and a movie

  b. dinner and a movie and a regular box of Milk Duds

  c. dinner and a movie, a tub of popcorn, and a soda so large you need two hands to hold it

5. For me, standard bar fare is:

  a. a glass (or two) of wine, interspersed with club soda

  b. a few handfuls of bar nuts washed down with a Rum and coke

  c. as many turbo hot wings as the beer special can extinguish

Emotions

1. When I'm feeling lonely or bored, I

  a. borrow a neighbor's dog and head for the park

  b. park myself on the couch with a trashy novel and a low-fat snack

  c. commune with my good buddies Ben and Jerry

2. When I'm angry or frustrated, I

  a. take a moment to breathe, then write in my journal about what's upsetting me

  b. call my girlfriend for an emergency meeting over double lattes

  c. take the phone off the hook and work my way through the Girl Scout cookies that were stashed in the back of the cupboard

(continued)

Your Real Food Life Starting Point: The Questionnaire (cont.)

3. After I order a big, rich piece of cheesecake, I
   a. split it with my dinner mate and savor every bite
   b. regret it, chastise myself, and resolve to eat more healthfully at my next meal
   c. order a coffee drink with whipped cream—when I blow it, I go big!

4. My food philosophy is
   a. eat to live
   b. eat now, repent later
   c. live to eat

5. When it comes to counting calories or grams of fat, I
   a. focus my efforts on checking food labels and portion sizes
   b. look only at grams of fat—calories aren't important
   c. methodically track each calorie and gram of fat as if dieting were quantum physics

Health

1. When I run to get the phone, I
   a. answer it on the first ring
   b. take a second to catch my breath and gasp out my hello
   c. why run? Screening is so much less effort

2. At 2:00 in the afternoon, you're most likely to find me
   a. happily plugging away at work
   b. working steadily, but starting to think about dinner
   c. slumped at my desk, mumbling, "must . . . stay . . . awake . . ."

fore you started the questionnaire, you knew that you wanted to lose weight, gain more energy, or get your heart running more efficiently. All of those are excellent goals. While you were taking the quiz, maybe you noticed that your diet could use some more fruits and veggies, or perhaps your trips to the bathroom have been few and far between—in which case, fiber will be your new best friend.

Remember: As you develop possible goals, make sure each one is realistic. A goal of losing 50 pounds in 8 weeks is unrealistic and bound to set you up for disappointment. Reducing the amount of unhealthy foods you eat, increasing your energy level, trimming your waistline by a couple of

3. When my doctor tests my blood pressure, she
   a. puts a gold star on my chart (120/80)
   b. says it's passable, but she's not turning cartwheels (130/85)
   c. rolls in the crash cart just to be safe (140/90)

4. When it comes to my bathroom business, I
   a. am so regular, you could set a watch by me
   b. am more or less regular, but sometimes need a little laxative help
   c. could write a novel in the time I spend in there

5. When I look at the hours adding up in my "sleep bank"
   a. I feel like Rockefeller (average 8+ per night)
   b. I'm living paycheck to paycheck (6 to 8 per night)
   c. I'm staring foreclosure in the face (less than 6 per night)

Now go back and count up the number of *c* answers you've circled in each category. As you may have guessed, a *c* indicates you may be struggling with that particular food life issue. Do you notice any patterns in the way you responded? Does a particular category seem to be of special concern?

On the following lines, write down the top two categories that seem to be the biggest challenges for you.

_____

_____

inches—these goals are not only achievable, they're probable! Getting a Real Food Life means starting a wholesome eating program that you can live with for the rest of your life.

For now, narrow your ultimate goals to one or two—these are your compass for the weeks ahead. Don't worry about how you're going to accomplish them just yet—we'll get to that in week 2, when we develop mini-goals, specific steps that will steadily get you toward your ultimate goal. (For instance, if your ultimate goal is to gain more energy, your mini-goals might include drinking 64 ounces of water a day and replacing refined carbohydrates, such as white bread and bagels, with complex carbs, such as whole grain bread and fruits and vegetables.) Your ultimate goal is the destination; your mini-goals are the highways and byways that will get you there.

Keep in mind that if at any time you want to change your goals or add to them, you can. For example, if you've met your ultimate goal by week 4, look back to your quiz answers and see if there's another issue you're grappling with in your food life—but first give yourself a pat on the back for achieving your first goal!

Take a look at the following list of common goals clients have shared with me over the years.

> *I want more energy!* Do you need stamina? Do you want to find foods that make you feel revved up and keep illness at bay?

> *I want to reeducate myself about food!* Do you want to become your own nutritionist so you can better understand food and make smart food choices?

> *I want to lose weight!* Do you want to find an eating plan loaded with foods lower in calories and fat that satisfy you and fill you up?

> *I simply want to find foods I like that are good for me!* Do you want to find an eating plan that you can live with, that's enjoyable, tasty, and easy, with a variety of foods that are emotionally and physically satisfying?

> *I want to eat healthier!* Do you want to find foods that lower your cholesterol and re-duce your risk of heart disease, diabetes, and cancers?

> *I want to drop the food obsessions once and for all!* Do you want to find a place with your food where you simply feel calmer and more relaxed?

Open your journal and write your ultimate goals on the first page. The physical act of putting them on paper will strengthen your resolve and help solidify them in your mind. Then flip to the last page and write down an ultimate reward you'll give yourself when you complete the plan. Sure, the achievement of your goal is a tremendous gift in and of itself, but how will you mark the occasion of your success—with a new dress? A fancy night out on the town with just the two of you? That new cappuccino maker you've had your eye on? Make it something you'd consider too extravagant for everyday—you really want this to feel like getting a gold medal.

Once you've made this contract with yourself, you have your destination. Now you just have to gather information for the journey.

5. Start Your Food Journal

Now that you've set your ultimate goals, the next step in getting a Real Food Life is to start keeping a food journal. I have all my clients do it, and you need to do it, too. It may seem

WEEK: _____ DAY: _____		
Time	**Food** (include amount)	**Comments** (include the situation or activity, how you felt before and after eating, etc.)

like a drag at first, but in fact it's the most valuable tool you have. Keeping a food journal not only makes you accountable for what you eat, but it will help you to see your eating patterns and understand just how much (or how little) you eat, when you eat, and why you eat.

Start your food journal on the next blank page of your notebook. Check out the template above. I recommend copying this simple chart into your notebook. It will help you to remember to include all the informa-

tion that will be so vital when you begin your analysis of your journal. After noting that this is week 1, day 1, use the journal to record absolutely everything you eat and drink during the day. (This may seem daunting at first, but once it becomes a habit, my clients tell me it keeps them accountable for what they eat, is very gratifying, and helps them feel in control.)

The first column will not only help you to keep track of the times when you ate but also how frequently you ate (perhaps you'll

(continued on page 146)

LIVING A REAL FOOD LIFE

Her New Food Life Has Her Sailing through Menopause

Name: Nancy
Real Food Life Issues: experiencing symptoms of menopause, craving carbohydrates

When I met Nancy, she was a 51-year-old grade school teacher and mother of three (two at college and one teenager still at home). She was going through menopause and had many common symptoms, including hot flashes, weight gain around her waist, mild depression, and exhaustion. She had never before had a sweet tooth, but for the first time in her life, she craved (and indulged in) cookies and candy. On top of this, she always felt bloated—like she was retaining water all the time. Here's where I found her:

November 3

Stevie Johnson busted me today. I was reaching into my desk, trying to get a piece of candy while the kids had their heads down. I almost had the candy all the way unwrapped, inwardly cursing the loud plastic crinkling, when I nearly jumped out of my skin. Stevie yelled, "Mrs. M, how come you're allowed to eat candy and we're not?"

Instantly, every kid's head shot up and they all started half-whimpering about how "it's not fair" and "teachers are always...." It was humiliating. I had to stand up and eat some ceremonial crow, which was not the flavor I was craving. I told Stevie he was right. I even apologized. I took the bag of candy out of my drawer and very dramatically dumped it in the trash can.

Of course, I fished it out at recess.

In analyzing Nancy's food journal, I saw that she ate a lot of high-sugar foods and very little protein. The first thing I asked her to do was cut back on those high-sugar foods. This would help stabilize her mood, reduce her depression, and cut down on the hot flashes. I also had her significantly cut her intake of refined carbohydrates, such as wheat pastas like macaroni and spaghetti, and replace them with whole grains including quinoa and brown rice for lunches and dinners and high-fiber cereal for breakfasts and snacks.

Nancy had avoided protein because she thought it was too "fatty" and would contribute to her weight gain. I explained that the body needs protein to release water and repair muscles. I also noted that it would improve her concentration and would help curb her sweet cravings. She gradually added some to her eating plan. She especially liked fish and began eating it several times a week. Not only was it a great source of low-fat protein, but it was also a great source of omega-3 fatty acids. To get even more healthy essential fatty acids, she added pumpkin seeds to her salads and dressed her vegetables with olive oil. On my recommendation, she also started to take the nutritional herb black cohosh each day to help with her hot flashes.

For years, Nancy had avoided breakfast. She thought it took too much time, and she didn't feel hungry in the morning. But this neglect caused her to have severe blood sugar swings and contributed to her afternoon candy binges. Together, we found quick and light breakfasts she could enjoy. Fruit smoothies were a good choice for her. When she felt a little more hungry, she would opt for a hard-boiled egg with whole wheat toast and a piece of fruit. She quickly realized that eating breakfast gave her the energy she needed to last until lunch.

Nancy also began taking lunch with her to school, instead of foraging around the cafeteria or grabbing something quick, and usually nutritionally unsound, at a fast-food restaurant near the school. Her brown-bag lunches now always included some high-quality protein, such as a grilled chicken breast or boiled shrimp, along with a lot of vegetables and some whole grain leftovers like brown rice or barley. Nancy recognized that having a hearty lunch really helped her to maintain her energy level through the afternoon—and almost completely squashed her desire for a 3:00 candy fix. We made sure, however, that she had a snack if she wanted it, but instead of a bag of cookies, she would reach for a soy yogurt with wheat germ and walnuts or an apple with a little bit of peanut butter.

By the end of 8 weeks, Nancy was pleased to find that she had lost 10 pounds. Her body had released the excess water that made her feel puffy. Nancy was finally able to put on her rings and take them off easily, and that was a boost to her mood. She was excited that her new food life fit into her lifestyle with little effort. She was especially excited that the hot flashes had virtually disappeared and her cravings for sweets were no longer a constant issue. Overall, Nancy felt happier and more energized than she had since the onset of her menopause.

discover that you feel best when you're grazing on mini-meals throughout the day, for example). In the second column, be sure to record the approximate amount of food you ate. In the final column, write down all other relevant information, including what you were doing before eating; whether or not you were alone or with others; and how you felt both physically and emotionally before, during, and after eating.

Finally, in a tiny, discreet area, reserve a bit of space in your journal to record your bathroom visits. You could use a personalized system, but why not go for the old standards #1 and #2? While this may feel slightly gross at first, I assure you that this will help you to monitor how your system is functioning. If you have a bowel movement only every 2 days, that's an indication that you aren't eating enough fruits, vegetables, and whole grain, fiber-rich foods (and maybe one of your goals should be to get regular!).

Don't forget to include a weekend in your food journal, so it reflects 7 consecutive days. After all, everyone knows weekend eating is an entirely different animal than the regimen of weekday meals. Remember: The only difference in what goes into your mouth this week is more water. Don't change a thing about the way you eat this week. We need this time to see patterns in the way you eat and to identify the areas of your food life that need to change. For ex-

ample, maybe you'll discover that you eat differently on weekends, that family dynamics trigger "food reactions" in you, that boredom causes you to eat a lot at night, or that damaging thoughts about yourself influence what you eat.

The cardinal rule of getting a Real Food Life: Be honest. About what you eat, how much, how often, and, most important, how it feels. If you aren't honest, this whole process will be an exercise in futility. There's a compelling reason you picked up this book, and being honest is how you'll find out what's behind it. This isn't a diet. There is no such thing as "cheating" or "being bad." By honestly and accurately recording what you eat, you'll give yourself the information you need to make positive changes and ultimately feel better about yourself in relation to food.

To get started, look at some sample entries from a few of my clients. Because they included detailed information about their motives for eating, how they were feeling at the time, and the activities they were doing prior to eating, they were able to gain important insights into their eating patterns.

Your food journal is a powerful magnifying glass; with it, you'll get a much clearer picture of what you put into your body and how it makes you feel. Busy lives and a lack of basic knowledge about eating well have caused many of us to block the signals that pass between our bodies and minds. We don't

Time	Food	Comments
1:00 P.M.	1 chicken roll	Feeling like I totally messed up lunch. It was late and I was starving. Went to see a movie with the kids and HAD to get something before then. Had the chicken roll from a pizzeria next door instead of having popcorn, but it wasn't great.

Time	Food	Comments
3:00pm	Small Crab salad w/ touch of mayo, lettuce, and tomato.	Was in the fridge. I really wasn't hungry but it was there... I was helping my husband put away groceries

Time	Food	Comments
Around 10:30 P.M.	Handful of M&M's two handfuls of potato chips	Had a craving for chocolate, which I haven't eaten in a long time. Had some M&M's while I watched TV, but then I craved salt, so I had chips.

know how to acknowledge different levels of hunger or to recognize if we're eating to fill emotional hunger or actual physical hunger. As you work to develop a Real Food Life, you will start eating mindfully; you will recognize true hunger signals; and you will start hearing what your body really needs and wants and know how to satisfy it.

Finally, take special note of meals that are dominated by carbohydrates or protein. Then, note how you feel just before you eat your next meal. Say, for example, you eat some black bean soup for lunch, which is high in fiber and protein. Then, you notice that it's 6:00 before you're even thinking about food

again, and you've skipped your typical 3:00 trip to the vending machine (which was one of your goals!). You need to record that you had a positive response to proteins. Conversely, maybe you had a muffin for breakfast, which is mainly carbs, and you notice that you're ready for lunch at 11:00 A.M. instead of 1:00, which is when you usually start considering lunch. Note then that pure carbs don't sustain you as long as other foods (in fact, they're quickly emptied from the stomach when eaten alone). This awareness of how your body responds to different food groups will help you in the weeks to come and aid you in sculpting your Real Food Life.

6. Complete Your First Get Real Check-In

When you're on a road trip, doesn't it feel good to occasionally stop and check the map to reassure yourself you're on the right path? At the end of your Real Food week, maybe on a Sunday afternoon, take your food journal to your favorite chair, settle in with a cup of ginger or green tea, and assess your progress.

Checking off the boxes in your Get Real Check-In will give you a well-deserved sense of accomplishment. Take time to record your feelings in your journal. Consider them notes to the new you, the one who will exist in the future, after you've achieved your goals.

When you look back, you'll see how far you've come and how much you have to be proud of.

You'll notice that there's also a checkbox for a weekly reward. This might be a quick lunch-hour manicure, a longer-than-average soak in the tub, a CD you've had your eye on. Too many of us rush by our smaller successes, keeping our eyes on the big prize—losing 20 pounds, cutting 50 points off our cholesterol, exercising four times a week. But each completed step is its own finish line and deserves to be heralded as the victory it is—after all, you're not just drinking more water or becoming aware of what you're putting in your mouth, you are taking control of your food life.

Get Real Check-In

Assess your progress by checking off each of the following items you achieved during week 1.

❏ Instant Makeover #1: I replaced 2 sugared drinks with 2 glasses of water.

❏ I scheduled a checkup with my doctor, to tell her of my plans for a new food life.

❏ I purchased a notebook or journal and personalized it.

❏ I completed the "Real Food Life Starting Point" questionnaire and thought about the broad aspects of my food life.

❏ I selected one or two ultimate goals for the next 7 weeks.

❏ I kept my food journal each day.

❏ I rewarded myself for my intentions and my efforts.

Weekly Words: On a blank page in your journal, write a couple of paragraphs about what it feels like to keep your food journal. Has it been empowering? Annoying? Educational? Discuss how you think keeping a food journal will help you reach your goal.

Week Two:

8 Analyzing Your Current Food Life

How do your arms feel right now? They should feel good and stretched out from all the pats on the back you should be giving yourself! By completing week 1, you've taken a very important step in beginning your Real Food Life.

Put on your lab coat—it's time to get down to some serious analysis. All the great research you did in week 1 feeds directly into week 2's main purpose: to analyze your current food life and create a new eating plan that will be the core of your Real Food Life. The work you do now will benefit you forever. Don't worry—I'll take you through it step-by-step.

Instant Makeover #2:

Replace Your Current Breakfast with a High-Fiber Cereal

First off, know that if you don't currently eat breakfast, this is like a double whammy to your Real Food Life. The body needs breakfast to kick its metabolism into gear for the day— if you don't eat breakfast, you could be slowing your metabolism down by up to 5 percent. Further, by not eating in the morning, you set yourself up for energy drain, mental fuzziness, and lunchtime bingeing.

Fiber is a key to your Real Food Life for so many reasons: It fills you up, keeps your blood sugar stable, helps relieve constipation, and helps cut down on how much fat you eat. Fiber itself has no calories and is found only in plant-based foods, so when you're eating a high-fiber meal, you're automatically increasing your intake of the healthiest stuff.

High-fiber cereal sticks with you, digesting more slowly than a bagel, to keep you satisfied longer. And never fear, today's high-fiber cereals are not the prunes-and-wheat-germ fare of our parents' generation—many are so tasty you'll find yourself looking forward to your morning meal.

1. Do a Complete Analysis of Your Week 1 Food Journal

When I work with clients, I have them submit their food journals to me after 7 days and I analyze what they've written. By studying their journals, I'll see their main source of calories and fats and note their nutritional deficiencies. The timing of their food choices is amazingly telling—I can immediately recognize when they eat mindlessly and when they're actually hungry. I notice what foods they like and eat all the time and the foods they don't include. Since I can't be with you in person, I'll show you how to analyze your journal for yourself.

Nutritional Analysis

Take your food journal from week 1 and count the number of servings of foods and food groups you ate from throughout each day. Using the Food Journal Analysis Chart (see page 154), tally up your portions. You might want to make several photocopies of this chart or duplicate it in your journal so you can use it not only for this week, but for the weeks to come as well.

In part 2 of this book, I discussed in detail the food components of a Real Food Life. As you work through the following journal analysis, flip back to the previous section whenever you feel you need a refresher on this information.

After you've filled out the chart, turn to a fresh page in your journal to answer the questions below. The Real Food Life Targets that appear after each section will help you see where you need to increase certain food intakes and decrease others.

Carbohydrates

▶ Complex carbohydrates are found in foods such as breads, grains, and cereals. How many servings of complex carbs did you have this week?

▶ Where are your complex carbohydrates coming from?

▶ Is your total number of servings more or less than you thought?

▶ Are the carbs you eat mostly in the form of refined white flour such as bagels, white bread, and white rice? These refined carbohydrates are probably responsible for a great deal of your hunger after meals. Replace refined carbs with complex, and you'll definitely feel a difference.

▶ Are you eating any whole grains or whole grain products? Whole grains provide extra fiber and balance blood sugar.

Real Food Life Target: You need 3 to 10 servings of complex carbohydrates each day (where you fall in the range depends on your individual penchant for carbohydrates).

Fruit and Vegetables

▶ Fruit is nature's healthful snack, providing antioxidants, phytochemicals, and fiber. How many servings of fruit did you have this week?

▶ What kinds of fruit did you choose?

▶ Is your total number of servings more or less than you thought?

▶ As much as we might wish for it, apple pie, blueberry cobbler, and fruit roll-ups *do not* count as fruit servings. If you drink 100 percent pure fruit juice, count one 8-ounce glass as only half a serving of fruit when it comes to health benefits since fruit juice has none of the fiber and only some of the phytochemicals of whole fruit. Further, fruit juice has a lot more calories than whole fruit.

▶ Vegetables will soon become the foundation of your Real Food Life. How many servings of vegetables did you have this week?

▶ What kinds of vegetables did you choose?

▶ Is your total number of servings more or less than you thought?

▶ Are you counting white potatoes—especially when french-fried—as a vegetable? While that may technically be true, that bland monotone white translates to very little nutritional value and tons of carbs. Try eating sweet potatoes instead, a power food packed with phytochemicals.

▶ Do you eat any dark-colored vegetables such as broccoli, spinach, bell peppers, asparagus, sweet potatoes, carrots, collard greens,

(continued on page 156)

The Food Journal Analysis Chart

For each of the 7 days that you kept your food journal last week, record the number of servings that you ate of each of the following foods. Then tally up the number of servings that you ate from each group, such as carbohydrates, fruit, vegetables, and so on.

Servings

Food	Day 1	Day 2	Day 3	Day 4	Day 5	Day 6	Day 7
CARBOHYDRATES							
White bread							
Whole wheat bread							
Muffins							
Bagels							
White rice							
Brown rice							
Grains							
Whole grains							
Cereal							
Whole grain cereal							
Pasta							
Other							
TOTAL							
FRUIT							
Fresh, canned, or frozen fruit							
100 percent fruit juice							
Dried fruit							
TOTAL							
VEGETABLES							
Fresh vegetables							
Cooked vegetables							
TOTAL							
PROTEINS							
Chicken (without skin)							
Chicken (with skin)							
Eggs							

Servings

Food	Day 1	Day 2	Day 3	Day 4	Day 5	Day 6	Day 7
Turkey (without skin)							
Turkey (with skin)							
Fish							
Beef (lean)							
Beef (fatty)							
Pork							
Lamb							
Lunchmeats							
Sausage							
Beans/legumes							
Soy food							
Other							
TOTAL							
DAIRY FOODS							
Whole milk							
Low-fat milk							
Fat-free milk							
Full-fat cheese							
Reduced-fat cheese							
Yogurt							
Other							
TOTAL							
FATS							
Butter							
Margarine							
Shortening							
Peanut or coconut oil							
Lard							
Corn oil							
Bacon							
Other							
TOTAL SATURATED/ HYDROGENATED FAT							

(continued)

The Food Journal Analysis Chart (cont.)

Servings

Food	Day 1	Day 2	Day 3	Day 4	Day 5	Day 6	Day 7
Avocados							
Nuts and seeds							
Olive oil							
Canola, sunflower, or safflower oil							
Other							
TOTAL MONOUNSAT- URATED OR POLY- UNSATURATED FATS							
BEVERAGES Water							
Green tea							
TOTAL WATER							
Soda							
Diet soda							
Fruit juice drink							
Coffee (hot or iced)							
Black tea (hot or iced)							
Herbal tea							
Other							
TOTAL SOFT DRINKS/ JUICE/COFFEE/TEA							

or kale? Expand your veggie repertoire to include a wide spectrum of colors. Check out my recipes beginning on page 259 for some ideas, then try one new recipe every week to expand your vegetable diet.

Real Food Life Target: You should eat at least 4 servings of vegetables and 3 to 4 servings of fruit each day. Filled with vitamins, minerals, phytochemicals, and fiber, vegetables and fruit are crucial to a Real Food Life.

Protein

❱ Protein builds muscle and helps our brains function well—it's also one of the most satisfying food groups we can eat. How many

Servings

Food	Day 1	Day 2	Day 3	Day 4	Day 5	Day 6	Day 7
Beer							
Wine							
Coolers							
Mixed drinks							
Other							
TOTAL ALCOHOLIC BEVERAGES							
SNACK FOODS/ FAST FOODS							
Cake							
Cookies							
Candy							
Chips							
Pretzels							
Ice cream							
Pizza							
Burgers							
French fries							
Fried chicken (or fried chicken sandwich)							
Other							
TOTAL							

servings of protein did you have this week?

▶ What kinds of protein did you choose?

▶ Is your total number of servings more or less than you thought?

▶ Is your protein mainly from animals or plants? If it's mainly from meat, are you making lean choices (chicken, turkey, fish, or lean beef) or fatty ones (ground meats, fried foods, lunchmeats, hot dogs)? The saturated fats in the second group are deadly business.

▶ Are you eating any protein from soy foods such as soy beans, soy nuts, or tofu? The grocery store is full of tasty options.

▶ Do you get most of your protein from processed meat such as bacon, baloney, salami, corned beef, pastrami, and ham?

What's a Serving?

This handy chart shows you at a glance what constitutes a serving of each type of food.

Complex carbohydrates: One slice of bread; an ounce of ready-to-eat cereal; ½ cup cooked cereal, rice, or pasta; or one medium sweet or regular potato

Fruit: A medium apple, banana, or orange; ½ cup of cooked or canned fruit, chopped; ½ cup of berries; ¾ cup fruit juice; or ¼ cup dried fruit

Vegetables: 1 cup of raw leafy greens; ½ cup of other types of veggies that are cooked or raw and chopped; ¾ cup low-sodium vegetable juice; or 7 to 8 carrot sticks

Protein: 2 to 3 ounces of cooked lean meat, fish, poultry, or tofu; 1 egg; or ½ cup of cooked dry beans

Dairy: 1 cup of cow's milk, soy milk, or yogurt; 2 ounces of processed cheese or soy cheese; or 1½ ounces of natural cheese

Fats: 1 tablespoon of olive or canola oils; 1 tablespoon of butter; 2 tablespoons of low-fat mayonnaise or 1 tablespoon mayonnaise-like salad dressing; 2 tablespoons of sunflower or pumpkin seeds; 4 to 6 walnuts; 1 tablespoon of nut butter; 3 to 4 tablespoons of hummus; or one-quarter of an avocado

Water: 8 ounces

Processed foods add high levels of sodium that can aggravate high blood pressure.

▶ Are you incorporating beans and legumes into your diet, or do you avoid them because they upset your stomach? Beano can help digest fiber-rich foods such as beans and other vegetables. You can purchase Beano at most supermarkets and health food stores.

▶ Is there any fish in your diet? You should eat fish at least twice a week; more often is even better because fish is so rich in omega-3 fatty acids, which can reduce your risk of heart disease.

▶ How often do you eat eggs? Eggs are a good source of high-quality protein; just

make sure they are prepared with a minimum of butter and other fats. If you have diabetes or high cholesterol or are overweight, you can eat up to four eggs a week. Otherwise, you can eat up to seven a week.

Real Food Life Target: You should eat between 6 and 8 ounces of lean protein daily.

Dairy

▶ Calcium is essential to everyone's diet, to keep bones strong and cells functioning well. How many servings of calcium-rich foods did you have this week?

▶ What kinds of calcium-rich foods did you choose?

▶ Is your total number of servings more or less than you thought?

▶ Are you lactose-intolerant and avoid milk because of discomfort? If so, try the lactose-free options, or even calcium-fortified soy milk—many of my clients like vanilla flavored. You can also try Lactaid when you eat dairy foods. It's an over-the-counter product that helps you digest lactose.

▶ Do you eat yogurt on a regular basis? One cup of plain yogurt can give you about 30 percent of your daily requirement for calcium and a solid boost of protein—try it with berries, cereal, or even in dips.

Real Food Life Target: You should be taking in at least 1,000 milligrams of calcium each day. If you're 50 or older, you should get 1,200 milligrams a day, which amounts to three servings of calcium-rich foods daily.

Fat

▶ Believe me, not all fats are bad—the brain and hormones require fat to operate effectively. How many kinds of foods with fat did you have this week?

▶ What kinds of fat did you choose?

▶ Is your total number of servings more or less than you thought?

▶ Do you know where your fat is coming from? Is it saturated or unsaturated? Read food labels to see what kinds of fats you're

consuming (see page 48 for a primer on deciphering food labels). Most of your dietary fat should come from a variety of omega-3 fatty acids or monounsaturated fatty acids.

▶ Are you eating any foods that contain omega-3 fatty acids (such as enriched eggs, cold-water fish, walnuts, Brazil nuts, flaxseeds or flaxseed oil, canola oil, sunflower seeds, or pumpkin seeds)? Are you eating any monounsaturated fats (such as avocados, olive oil, olives, high oleic sunflower and safflower oils, and almonds)? If you answered no to these questions, try to gradually change your fat sources to those listed, which are good fats.

▶ Are you using margarine or butter in your cooking? Do you eat out at fast-food restaurants a few times a week? Do you try to eat fat-free? Do you eat a very low fat diet all day but then binge on ice cream or baked goods at night? Do you use full-fat salad dressing? If any of these pertain to you, you are probably not getting enough essential fatty acids and may be getting too much saturated and hydrogenated fats.

Real Food Life Target: You need 1 to 2 servings total of essential fatty acids and monounsaturated fats each day. Always avoid saturated and hydrogenated fats.

Beverages

▶ Remember, water is essential to a Real Food Life. It helps in every aspect, from keeping food moving through your system to helping you determine if you're hungry or not. How many beverage servings did you have this week?

▶ What kinds of drinks did you choose?

▶ Is your total number of servings more or less than you thought?

▶ Have you noticed how much water you drink each day? This includes seltzer water, mineral water, and tap water. Try to drink at least eight 8-ounce glasses of water each day.

▶ Take note of the number of caffeinated drinks you consume each day. Are you drinking mostly sodas? Is coffee your idea of water? Do you crave sugary sodas to keep you going? If you answered yes to any of these questions, revisit your Instant Makeover from week 1 and replace two flavored drinks with water.

▶ Have you included green tea? How about peppermint or ginger tea? Green tea contains antioxidants and may protect against cancers and high cholesterol. Ginger and peppermint teas aid digestion and are available in the supermarket or your local coffee house. Don't drink peppermint tea if you have problems with acid reflux, however.

▶ Do you drink a number of glasses of beer, wine, or other alcoholic drinks each day? Alcohol is a diuretic, so for every alcoholic beverage you consume, you should drink a comparable amount of water. Alcohol is also very high in calories.

▶ Is your urine darker than straw? Do you need to urinate only a few times a day? If so, you need to drink more fluids. Your extra bathroom breaks will be balanced out with more energy and less snacking.

Real Food Life Target: You should drink at least eight 8-ounce glasses of water each day, and even more if you drink coffee or other caffeinated beverages.

Physical Analysis

Now that you know exactly what you ate last week and have analyzed the nutritional value of the foods you consumed, take a minute to figure out how your body felt about those foods. We are all individuals—everyone's body reacts in its own way to different meals. Once you make the connections between your foods and feelings, you'll automatically start choosing food that makes you feel healthy, energized, balanced, and satisfied but not stuffed.

In week 1's quiz, "Your Real Food Life Starting Point," you looked at the big picture of your body's reactions to foods. Now we're getting down to the nitty-gritty. To assess your physical reactions to food, turn to the next page in your journal and write down your answers to the following questions.

Energy: Did some meals give you a lot of quick energy but then make you crash? Did some meals give you energy for hours?

From your week 1 food journal, take note of which foods caused you to get energized and stay that way. Those foods—which are different for everyone—should become the mainstay of your new food life. As often as you can, avoid foods that make you crash and burn.

Bathroom business: Are your bowel movements regular? Do you suffer from constipation? You should have at least one bowel movement a day. If you "go" less than once a day, chances are you're suffering from constipation. Drink more water and eat more high-fiber foods including fruit, vegetables, and whole grains.

Bloat factor: After you eat a salty dinner, do your face and hands swell the next day and do you feel uncomfortable and puffy? If so, you're probably sensitive to sodium and need to cut back on your salt intake. Don't add salt when you cook—most foods contain ample amounts of natural sodium. When you eat out, don't hesitate to request that your meal be prepared with very little added salt. If you can't avoid eating a salty meal, drink lots of water both during and after the meal. And the next day, eat plenty of foods that have a high water content, such as fruits and vegetables, to flush out your system. (See "High-Water Foods" on page 66 for a list of specific foods.)

Sugar cravings: When you have a craving for sweets, do you eat an entire box of cookies in a sitting? And then do you feel really guilty for eating all of them? Refer to the lists of snacks on pages 23, 25, and 30, and choose two that appeal to your taste-buds. Have the first when you're craving something sweet. If that doesn't do the trick, have the second snack. By sticking to healthy snacks like these, you'll be able to get through your craving without the guilt.

Some of the following foods are notoriously troublesome among my clients—how about you?

Complex carbohydrates: How did you feel after eating a meal high in complex carbohydrates (such as pasta or pizza)? Did you get sleepy or more energetic?

▶ If you got sleepy, then you should eat this type of meal less often or only at night. Or have just a small portion along with some lean protein.

▶ If you felt energized, you'll probably want to keep that meal as part of your Real Food Life.

Meat: Do you like the taste of meat, or do you avoid it because you think it's too fatty and unhealthful?

▶ If you like the taste of meat, you can dine on it, but stick to small portions of leaner cuts, which are kinder on your system and won't make you feel as sluggish. Lean meats, like roasted turkey, are a great source of high-quality protein, vitamins, and minerals.

▶ If you're vegetarian or don't have a taste for meat, you can get high-quality protein and nutrients from other sources such as soy foods, seafood, and beans and legumes.

Dairy: How did you feel after you ate a meal with a lot of dairy? Some people's bodies can tolerate dairy foods; other people's bodies can't digest it at all.

▶ If you have no problem eating dairy foods, great! They're a great source of calcium and protein—feel free to enjoy two or three servings daily.

▶ If you don't feel well after consuming dairy, avoid it, but make sure you're getting your calcium from other sources, such as leafy green vegetables, canned sardines, and a supplement.

You may never have noticed that feeling bloated or sluggish is a result of the foods you eat until you started keeping your food journal. If a food makes you feel bad, you should probably avoid it. But beware—eliminating an entire food group from your diet will lead to food obsessions and can also lead to nutritional deficiencies. If you love a food and absolutely must have it, eat it only occasionally, realizing you'll have to deal with the consequences. You may notice that when you cut back on foods like this, you actually love them less when you do have them. You may also discover new favorites to substitute that actually make you feel fantastic.

Emotional Analysis

We eat for many reasons—physical hunger, emotional pain, chronic stress. (Sometimes we're more likely *not* to eat when we're under stress.) Part of discovering your eating patterns and adjusting them, if necessary, requires you to examine all the emotional components of your eating patterns.

After keeping your food journal and analyzing it, you will likely notice that emotions affect your eating patterns. We touched on

some of these issues in week 1's quiz, but here are a few more targeted questions.

▶ When you've had a particularly tough day, do you find yourself eating a large meal, then lying on the couch to unwind?

▶ After a confrontation with your boss, coworker, friend, spouse, or child, do you find solace in whatever food makes you "happy"?

▶ Do you find that binge-eating when you're frustrated or upset gives you comfort and relief (at least until reality sets in)?

▶ When you've finally accomplished a long, hard project, do you treat yourself by buying favorite foods and then eating until you fall into a food coma?

▶ When you're alone at night, do you find yourself eating uncontrollably?

▶ Do you feel guilty after having a large dinner complete with a rich dessert?

▶ Does drinking too much coffee or cola make you feel jittery and cranky?

▶ When you eat a fast-food meal, do you feel sluggish and depressed?

▶ Does eating a big dinner prevent you from sleeping well, and then the lack of sleep affects your whole next day?

All of the above are examples of emotional eating. While there's no way to completely separate food from feelings, you need to recognize your emotional reactions to food and minimize their significance. Refer to chapter 2 for strategies for handling specific food/emotion issues. It's critical to remember that food's purpose is to nourish your body and make you feel good, not torture you or make you feel guilty. Learning what your emotional eating triggers are and how to master them is a cornerstone of a Real Food Life.

2. Diagnose Your Type: Protein-Based or Carbohydrate-Based Eater?

In my practice, I've found that I can group people's eating habits and tendencies into two basic categories, either protein-based or carb-based. If you find you respond well to either carbs or protein, you will want to make sure you include a serving of your favored nutrient in each of your meals. Also, protein- or carb-rich snacks will be more satisfying to you. Using your food journal and the descriptions below, discover which group you best fit into.

Protein-Based Eater

Many of my clients find that protein keeps them more satisfied, more energetic, and less hungry all day long. Does this sound like you?

When you eat more protein, you seem to think about food less often and don't feel the need to constantly forage for other foods to satisfy you. You find that eating a decent portion of protein, such as lean meat, fish, soy foods, dairy, or even beans, with each meal and snack helps prevent mood swings while helping to curb cravings—especially sugar

cravings. You feel "bloated" when you eat a lot of carbs at one time. (Note: *Even if you're a vegetarian, you could be a protein-based eater if you find you feel best when you've eaten veggie-based protein like soy foods and beans.*)

Here's the key: Just because you might feel better eating a protein-based plan doesn't mean you don't still need your fruits, vegetables, and complex carbohydrates every day. The fiber, nutrients, and energy-power of carb-based foods are an integral part of a Real Food Life.

Carbohydrate-Based Eater

On the flip side, many others among my clients prefer a carbohydrate-rich diet. Are you like them?

Carbs fill you up without making you feel overstuffed. You love the way carbohydrates give you stamina that lasts all day. You feel that eating more carbs helps you to think better and helps stabilize your mood—with carbs, you feel calmer, more relaxed, and less cranky. For you, eating carb-rich foods with every meal and snack helps curb your "sweet/salty/junk food tooth" in the afternoon. You don't feel your meal is "complete" unless you have a nice serving of pasta, rice, potatoes, or whole wheat bread. If you're more athletic, you particularly like to eat carbs before and after your workouts because you find it improves your strength during the workouts and helps refuel your body afterward. If you're vegetarian, you find this option easy to adopt, as carbohydrates come mainly from plant-based foods.

One thing to keep in mind if you determine that you are a carb-based eater is that eating a little bit of protein is necessary. Protein not only helps repair muscles and is necessary for the good functioning of the body, but eating a little protein with each meal will keep cravings, hunger, and binges at bay.

3. Diagnose Your Style: Are You a Grazer or a Traditional Three-Squares Eater?

Once you figure out whether you tend toward eating protein-based foods or carbohydrate-based foods, another focus of your eating plan is whether to graze or eat more structured meals. Some people prefer grazing, eating five to six small, light "meals" throughout the day; others prefer to eat more conventionally, with three "big" meals and a light snack or two. Again, your body will tell you what's right for you—you just have to listen!

Grazing

Your parents were probably always after you with admonitions like, "Don't eat that! You'll spoil your appetite!" Well, this time mom was wrong—as long as you don't eat more calories than you would with three regular meals.

Many of my clients love grazing—eating up to six small, low-calorie, balanced meals each day—because it makes them feel like they're eating all day long. Grazing greatly reduces cravings and helps you feel in control of your food life because *you* decide when it's time to eat, not the clock. By eating every 2 to 3 hours, you never get too hungry, so you're less likely to binge. You may also find that you're good at listening to your body and can tell when your appetite first gears up, signaling that you should eat. If you've experienced this sensation, you're probably a grazer.

Biologically, grazing helps to maintain blood sugar levels, which prevents mood swings and that "starving" feeling that comes from low blood sugar. Small meals tell the body to release less of the hormone insulin, so more calories are burned.

Personally, I love grazing. It helps me keep my Food Life in check. When I eat six small meals a day, I feel really good, energetic, and balanced all day long.

Three-Squares Eating Style

Still, some of my clients prefer eating in a more conventional structure of three main meals. Eating three squares with a light snack or two fits into their lifestyle better than planning several mini-meals. You may find that grazing feels a little out of control, because you may *think* you're eating too often.

You can get a Real Food Life and still enjoy bigger meals—the two are not mutually exclusive. If you choose to eat larger meals, however, I still recommend eating a light snack, such as a yogurt and fruit, between meals to maintain blood sugar levels, prevent "crashing," and prevent that starving feeling that often leads to overeating at subsequent meals.

BEST BITES

Top 5 Foods to Eat for Energy before the Big Meeting

Before your next big meeting, snack on one of the foods below. Then go into your meeting with confidence, knowing that you'll still have plenty of energy when the last agenda item is wrapped up.

- 1 or 2 slices of whole wheat bread with nut butter and jam or low-fat cheese
- Large mixed fruit salad with low-fat regular or soy yogurt and wheat germ
- Chopped salad with olive oil and lemon and grilled chicken or smoked tofu with a small whole wheat roll
- A bowl of high-fiber cereal (such as Kashi Go Lean or Good Friends) with fat-free or soy milk, a banana, and a small handful of chopped walnuts
- 1 whole egg and 3 egg whites, scrambled, with whole wheat bread and a piece of fruit

Once you know your basic eating style, we'll move on to creating your eating plan.

4. Experiment with Sample Menus

The best thing about getting a Real Food Life is that you get to make it your very own. In the upcoming weeks, you will be changing and fine-tuning your plan, and you'll definitely notice a change in how you feel.

To get you started, I've designed the sample eating plans beginning on page 166. Focus your food life around these kinds of foods—I've included options that will give you a maximum amount of energy. Use these sample menus as a guideline in designing your own perfect meals and snacks. Whether you select a protein-based or carbohydrate-based, grazing or meal-oriented plan, feel free to sample from any of the other plans. Just cut your portions at mealtimes if you're a grazer. If you're going the meal-eating route, be sure to have much smaller snacks.

Notice that many of the sample meals are vegetarian—proof positive that you can still get a Real Food Life despite any special dietary concerns you might have.

If you start out on one plan—say, for example, the protein-based sample menus—but aren't satisfied after a few days, tinker and tweak. Maybe you want protein in the morning and carbs in the afternoon, or vice versa. Remember, it's *your* plan. Having a Real Food Life is all about balance, variety, feeling good, and finding out what works for you.

Protein-Based Sample Menus

Breakfast

1 cup water

Three-Squares Style

A. Tomato and Cheese Omelette: 1 whole egg and 4 egg whites, 2 teaspoons grated Parmesan cheese or 2 tablespoons reduced-fat Cheddar cheese, 1 sliced tomato, and 1 teaspoon olive oil (to coat the pan)

1 cup melon

B. Protein Smoothie: 1 cup fat-free plain or soy yogurt, 1 cup ice cubes, 1 cup blueberries (or other fruit), 1 teaspoon vanilla (optional), and 2 ounces plain tofu (optional) mixed in a blender

C. 2 slices low-fat cheese or low-fat soy cheese (2 ounces)

1 or 2 soy breakfast links or soy hot dogs

1 leftover Baked Apple (see page 321) topped with 2 tablespoons chopped walnuts or pumpkin seeds, or 1 raw apple

Grazing Style

A. Egg, Cheese, and Veggie Scramble: 1 scrambled egg (use an egg enriched with omega-3, if your store carries them), 1 ounce grated low-fat cheese,

> *Protein-based daily food intake at a glance:*
> - 2 to 4 servings carbohydrates
> - 8 ounces protein
> - 3 servings fruit
> - 4 to 6 servings vegetables
> - 2 to 4 servings fat
> - 2 to 3 servings calcium-rich food

1 sliced tomato, 1 green onion, 1 tablespoon parsley or basil, and 1 teaspoon olive oil to coat pan

B. ½ cup Kashi Go Lean Cereal (or other high-fiber, low-sugar, low-salt cereal)

4 walnuts, crushed

1 cup fat-free milk or low-fat soy milk

½ banana or ½ cup blueberries

C. 1 cup low-fat yogurt

1 boiled egg

1 ounce cheese

Midmorning snack

1 cup green tea and 1 cup water

Three-Squares Style

A. 2 whole wheat crackers with 2 slices (2 ounces) roast turkey breast and mustard

B. 2 whole grain crackers with ½ cup whipped cottage cheese and 2 tablespoons salsa

C. 1 bowl (8 to 10 ounces) Creamy Carrot Soup (see page 277) and 1 piece fruit

Grazing Style

A. 10 baked tortilla chips

½ cup low-fat bean dip

Unlimited baby carrots

B. 1 small apple

1 tablespoon all-natural nut butter (peanut, almond, or walnut) or a small handful of nuts or seeds

C. 1 low-fat fruit yogurt or low-fat soy yogurt

2 tablespoons wheat germ and 4 crushed walnuts

Lunch

2 cups water

Three-Squares Style

A. 1 or 2 Turkey Burgers (see page 297), each with 1 small whole wheat pita, lettuce and sliced tomato, 2 teaspoons ketchup, and 1 tablespoon low-fat mayonnaise or low-fat canola mayonnaise

1 serving (4 ounces) Eggplant Caponata (see page 270)

B. Tossed salad: 2 cups lettuce (salad in a bag), unlimited tomatoes and carrots, 3 ounces sliced roast turkey breast, ½ cup canned beans (rinsed well), 1 slice (1 ounce) low-fat soy cheese, ¼ avo-

cado, 1 tablespoon extra-virgin olive oil, and unlimited vinegar or lemon juice

C. Chopped vegetable salad: 2 cups vegetables (carrots, tomatoes, peppers, red onions, broccoli, and cauliflower), 1 small can (3 ounces) drained tuna, 1 hard-boiled egg (enriched with omega-3, if possible), ½ cup edamame, and 2 tablespoons Blue Cheese Dressing (see page 263)

Grazing Style

A. Mixed salad: 3 cups salad, 2 tablespoons Caesar dressing (see page 262), 3 ounces lean roast beef, and ½ cup cooked beans

B. 1 bowl (8 to 10 ounces) Chicken Soup (see page 275)

2 to 3 whole wheat crackers

C. 2 Boca or veggie burgers, each with 1 slice whole wheat bread, 1 slice (1 ounce) low-fat soy cheese, 2 teaspoons ketchup, and 1 tablespoon low-fat mayonnaise or low-fat canola mayonnaise

1 pear

D. 1 cup Lentil Salad with Lemon and Feta (see page 284)

1 small whole wheat pita

3 ounces smoked tofu

1 grapefruit

Afternoon snack

1 cup water

Three-Squares Style

A. 1 slice (1-ounce) low-fat soy cheese

1 piece fruit

B. 3 tablespoons Lemony Hummus (see page 284)

Unlimited baby carrots

C. ½ cup edamame

1 small handful nuts or seeds

Grazing Style

A. ½ raw apple

2 tablespoons low-fat vanilla yogurt or soy yogurt

1 tablespoon chopped nuts or seeds

B. 2 ounces leftover meat, fish, chicken, or tofu

1 cup Roasted Vegetables (see page 267)

C. 2 whole grain crackers topped with ½ cup whipped low-fat cottage cheese and either a chopped pear or 1 teaspoon mango chutney

Dinner

2 cups water

Three-Squares Style

A. 4 ounces Tuna with Green-Herb Pesto (see page 308)

1½ cups sautéed mixed vegetables (spinach, mushrooms, and broccoli cooked in 1 teaspoon sesame oil and 2 teaspoons olive oil, with 2 teaspoons of low-sodium soy sauce)

1 sliced beefsteak tomato with 1 tablespoon Caesar Dressing (see page 262)

B. 1 bowl (8 to 10 ounces) French Onion Soup (see page 274)

4 ounces Filet Mignon with Mushrooms (see page 316)

1 small baked sweet potato or ½ cup Pureed Sweet Potatoes (see page 271)

2 cups mixed salad with 1 tablespoon extra-virgin olive oil and unlimited balsamic vinegar or lemon juice

C. 1 slice (5 ounces) Mama's Meat Loaf (see page 309)

1 serving Herbed Tomato Salad (see page 260)

1 serving Layered Potato and Zucchini Pie (see page 268)

Grazing Style

A. Chinese takeout: steamed mixed vegetables (unlimited); 4 ounces steamed chicken, tofu, or shrimp; ½ cup brown rice; and 2 tablespoons brown, black bean, or garlic sauce

B. 1 piece (4 ounces) Oven-Baked Crispy Sole (see page 307)

2 cups Sautéed Broccoli and Garlic (see page 272)

1 small baked sweet potato

C. 1 can Health Valley Chili

½ cup brown rice

2 cups broccoli and zucchini sautéed in 2 teaspoons olive oil and 1 teaspoon sesame oil, with 2 teaspoons low-sodium soy sauce, 1 clove crushed garlic, lemon, and ½ teaspoon sesame seeds

D. Unlimited Roasted Vegetables (see page 267)

½ cup Quinoa with Fried Onions (see page 290) mixed with 1 cup canned and rinsed kidney beans and 1 tablespoon grated Parmesan cheese

Nighttime snack

1 cup water

Three-Squares Style

A. 1 slice (2 ounces) Very Creamy Cheesecake (see page 325)

1 cup chamomile tea

Grazing Style

A. 1 cup vanilla yogurt with 5 crushed almonds and a sprinkle of cinnamon

Carbohydrate-Based Sample Menus

Breakfast

1 cup water

Three-Squares Style

A. 2 Van's brand whole wheat waffles

1 tablespoon low-fat cream cheese

1 tablespoon jam or all-fruit spread

1 medium banana

B. 1 Muffin Galore (see page 319)

2 teaspoons nut butter

2 teaspoons jam or all-fruit spread

1 Baked Apple (see page 321)

C. 1 cup Kashi Go Lean

Carbohydrate-based daily food intake at a glance:

- 6 to 10 servings carbohydrates
- 6 ounces protein
- 3 to 4 servings fruit
- 4 to 6 servings vegetables
- 2 to 4 servings fat
- 2 to 3 servings calcium-rich food

1 cup fat-free milk or 1 cup soy milk

1 cup berries or 1 medium banana

2 tablespoons chopped walnuts or pumpkin seeds

Grazing Style

A. 1 honey whole wheat or oat bran English muffin

1 tablespoon nut butter

1 tablespoon jam or all-fruit spread

B. ¾ cup high-fiber cereal

½ cup low-fat or soy yogurt

½ cup berries

C. 1 cup cooked oatmeal (½ cup uncooked), made with 1 cup fat-free milk or soy milk

1 small box (1 ounce) raisins

Sprinkle of cinnamon

1 piece fresh fruit (optional)

D. 1 or 2 Van's brand whole wheat waffles

2 teaspoons all-natural peanut butter or 1 tablespoon low-fat cream cheese

2 teaspoons jam or all-fruit spread

1 cup fruit salad or 1 piece fruit

Midmorning snack

1 cup green tea or ginger tea and 1 cup water

Three-Squares Style

A. 2 whole wheat crackers

1 slice low-fat cheese

B. 1 slice whole wheat bread

2 tablespoons Lemony Hummus (see page 284)

Grazing Style

A. 1 cup mixed fruit

1 tablespoon toasted wheat germ

2 tablespoons low-fat whipped cottage cheese

B. 2 whole wheat crackers

2 tablespoons Roasted Garlic and White Bean Spread (see page 283)

C. 4 whole wheat crackers

2 tablespoons Lemony Hummus (see page 284)

1 sliced tomato

Lunch

2 cups water

Three-Squares Style

A. 2 rolls sushi (tuna, salmon, yellowtail, crab, shrimp—your choice)

2 cups green salad with 1 tablespoon Japanese dressing

½ cup edamame

B. 1 cup Middle Eastern Tabbouleh Salad (see page 291)

1 small (3 ounces) can tuna or salmon

2 tablespoons low-fat mayonnaise or canola mayonnaise

1 medium whole wheat roll

C. 1½ cups Pasta Primavera (see page 295)

4 tablespoons Roasted Garlic

and White Bean Spread (see page 283)

4 whole wheat crackers

Grazing Style

A. 1 Vegetarian Asian Tofu Sandwich (see page 299)

1 cup salad with 2 teaspoons olive oil and lemon

B. 2 slices whole wheat bread with ½ avocado, mashed; 1 slice (1 ounce) low-fat cheese; sliced tomatoes and lettuce; and 1 tablespoon low-fat mayonnaise or low-fat canola mayonnaise

1 apple

Afternoon snack

1 cup water

Three-Squares Style

A. 1 tablespoon all-natural peanut butter

1 slice whole wheat bread

1 apple

B. 1 cup low-fat fruit yogurt or low-fat fruit soy yogurt

1 chopped pear

½ cup high-fiber cereal

Grazing Style

A. Unlimited fresh vegetables

2 tablespoons Blue Cheese Dressing (see page 263)

1 piece fruit

B. Fruit Smoothie: 1 cup fat-free plain yogurt, 1 cup frozen blueberries, 2 tablespoons wheat germ, and 1 cup crushed ice

C. 1 small low-fat bran muffin

2 teaspoons all-natural peanut butter

D. 1 can Health Valley vegetable soup or 1 bowl (8 to 10 ounces) Chunky Mixed Vegetable Soup (see page 281)

E. 1-ounce bag Robert's American Gourmet Pirate Booty and 1 piece fruit

Dinner

2 cups water

Three-Squares Style

A. 1 cup Texas Black Bean Soup (see page 279)

1 serving Mac and Cheese (see page 294)

2 cups cooked spinach (sautéed in 1 tablespoon extra-virgin olive oil with 1 clove chopped garlic)

B. 1 can Health Valley vegetarian chili

1 medium baked sweet potato

2 to 3 cups salad with ¼ avocado, 1 tablespoon olive oil, and lemon juice or vinegar

C. 4 ounces Salmon Teriyaki (see page 306)

1½ cups Mexican Rice and Beans (see page 286)

2 cups mixed vegetables or broccoli sautéed with chopped garlic, 1 teaspoon sesame oil, 2 teaspoons canola oil, and 2 teaspoons low-sodium soy sauce

Grazing Style

A. 1 serving (4 to 5 ounces) Eggplant Parmesan (see page 303)

3 cups mixed salad with 1 tablespoon olive oil and lemon

1 whole Incredibly Tasty Mediterranean Roasted Pepper (see page 265)

B. 1 serving Spinach and Cheese Pie (see page 305)

1 cup cooked brown rice

2 cups mixed vegetables sautéed in 1 tablespoon olive oil

2 cups mixed salad with 1 tablespoon olive oil and lemon

Nighttime snack

1 cup water

Three-Squares Style

A. 1 slice (2 ounces) Banana-Date Cake (see page 323)

1 cup ginger tea

Grazing Style

A. 1 piece fruit

1 slice (2 inches wide) Blueberry Angel Food Cake (see page 322)

B. 1 piece fruit

½ ounce dark chocolate

5. Set Mini-Goals

You've already taken great leaps and bounds in your Real Food Life—so why shouldn't you give yourself credit for them? Mini-goals are a fun, easy way to stay on course to achieve your ultimate goal, but they also give you something to celebrate in the here and now. Achieving mini-goals is a great way to boost your motivation every day.

You've done a lot of investigative work this week. Look back over the week's findings and see where you'd like to make changes, then turn to the first page of your journal and just meditate on your ultimate goal for a second. What changes could you make that would make your ultimate goal a reality? Don't forget to think about your bigger-picture issues from week 1's quiz.

When setting mini-goals, think "quantifiable, measurable, and achievable." For example, "I will eat one serving of green vegetables (quantifiable) six times (measurable) this week (achievable)."

Shoot for at least one nutritional goal and one emotional goal for each week. To remind yourself, note them at the top of your food diary page every morning.

Though I won't discuss your mini-goals in detail within each of the next 6 weeks, I'll remind you to set them in the checklist that begins each chapter—and to congratulate yourself on achieving them in the Get Real Check-In at the end of each chapter.

Get Real Check-In

Assess your progress by checking off each of the following items you achieved during week 2.

❏ Instant Makeover #2: I replaced a low-fiber breakfast with a high-fiber cereal.

❏ I added an extra glass of water. I'm now drinking at least six glasses per day.

❏ I did a complete analysis of my findings from week 1.

❏ I determined whether I am a protein-based or carb-based eater.

❏ I determined if I'm a grazer or a traditional meal eater.

❏ I tried at least one sample menu.

❏ I set week 3 mini-goals that will help me achieve my ultimate goals.

❏ I kept my food journal each day.

❏ I rewarded myself for my intentions and my efforts.

Weekly Words: Write a couple of paragraphs in your journal about the biggest surprise you felt when you looked at your food analysis. Discuss the way you think your mini-goals will help you achieve your ultimate goal.

Week Three:

DOING THE REAL FOOD LIFE KITCHEN MAKEOVER

During this week, you will:

▶ Accomplish Instant Makeover #3: Replace a half-hour of TV-watching with sleep

▶ Add one extra glass of water (shoot for at least 7)

▶ Follow your week 3 mini-goals

▶ Keep week 3 of your food journal

▶ Give your kitchen a Real Food Life Makeover

▶ Go grocery shopping

▶ Complete week 3 of your Get Real Check-In

Your Real Food Life is about to hit home—your home. Week 3 of the Food Life Makeover Plan is all about remaking your home and your shopping habits so they'll support you, not sabotage you.

First, you'll do the Real Food Life Kitchen Makeover. You'll sweep out those items that can hamstring your efforts, clearing the way for the nutrition-packed all-stars that will easily, seamlessly take their place. While this makeover won't feature a manicure or a foot massage,

Instant Makeover #3:

Replace the Nightly News with Some Extra Snooze Time

While sleep and food don't appear to go hand in hand, getting more Zzzs is a major step toward a healthier lifestyle. I regularly see that sleep deprivation exacerbates many of my clients' food issues. When you are overtired, you may have noticed feeling hungrier—that's because your body is crying out for more energy! Still, you have to get through the day, and as your energy plummets, so does your mood— another prime risk factor for snacking and bingeing.

Instead of staying up late watching an extra half-hour of primetime shows or news that probably has little impact on your life, get some extra sleep. When you wake up feeling refreshed, you will be better-equipped to make good food choices and resist the temptations that would sound so appealing to a sleep-deprived mind. You won't be groggy in the afternoon—and you won't need a sugar-loaded snack or soda for a lift. Plus, you'll feel more in tune with your body and what it really needs—often just a tall drink of water!—instead of just quickly turning to food to fill all of your needs.

I promise it will be equally invigorating!

Then we'll take our show on the road and hit the supermarket, where you'll learn how to size up the store at a glance and devise a strategy to get the best foods in the least amount of time. The skills you learn now will help you automatically gravitate toward the best foods for you, so you can restock with solid nutritional staples every time you go shopping.

1. Give Your Kitchen a Real Food Life Makeover

When you tried out your tailor-made menu plan in week 2, did you need to make a spe-cial trip to the grocery store? Part of the idea behind the Kitchen Makeover is to ensure that you'll have smart, nourishing choices on hand all the time.

Try to schedule your Kitchen Makeover for a time when you have several hours to spend. Or, if you're in a crunch week at work and can't carve out a block of time, split up the following tasks over a series of nights. Monday, the cupboards. Tuesday, the refrigerator. And so on. Each segment of the makeover should take less than 30 minutes. If you're really in a time bind, try the 10-Step Kitchen Makeover (see page 180), distilled down to the most powerful changes.

Kitchen CURES

Simple Ways to Improve Your Slumber

Having trouble getting your Zzzs? Sleep tight tonight with these slumber-inducing strategies.

- Avoid spicy or fatty dinners, both of which can cause indigestion that may keep you awake at night.
- People who eat too few calories during the day often wake up hungry during the night or very early in the morning, so be sure to get enough food. It's a good idea to eat some protein with your dinner. Because it stays in your stomach longer than some other foods, it will keep you from awakening because of hunger.
- Watch what you're eating: Gassy foods such as cabbage, broccoli, peppers, and cauliflower can cause bloating and may cause restless nights.
- Munch on a carbohydrate-rich snack after dinner. Carbs help release serotonin, a brain chemical that makes you feel calm and relaxed. A few whole wheat crackers with a teaspoon of nut butter might do the trick.
- Cut down on or completely eliminate caffeine. This includes coffee, black tea, cola, and chocolate. (It's best to do this gradually, since cutting caffeine out of your diet quickly can lead to headaches and fatigue.) Though it contains much less than black tea or coffee, green tea does have some caffeine, so drink it only before 2:00 P.M. if caffeine affects your sleep. Another option is to buy decaffeinated green tea.

The kitchen makeover is one of my favorite things to do with clients because it's so liberating! You make a fresh start, physically removing the vestiges of your old food life to reinforce the positive choices you've made for your Real Food Life. Whether you cook a lot or rarely, filling your kitchen with a variety of fresh fruits and vegetables, healthy choices for snacks and quick meals, and even no-fuss frozen and convenience foods will keep you and your Food Life on track.

These five suggestions will help you make a smooth start.

1. Tackle the cupboards/pantry and the refrigerator/freezer separately.
2. Systematically read the ingredient label of

every product you have, keeping this question in mind: "Will this food be part of my Real Food Life?"

3. Keep a pad of paper and a pen nearby, so you can keep a running shopping list of new foods you will need.

4. Keep garbage bags handy. They will be used to hold the food you will throw away or give away.

5. Be patient. Your Kitchen Makeover may take an investment of time, but the dividends are worth it!

Cupboards

Start your kitchen makeover with your cupboards. Take everything out of your cupboards and place it on your kitchen table. If you have too much stuff to stack there at one time, work in segments: above the stove, below the counter, and so on. As you read the label to evaluate each food product, ask yourself, "Does this help or hinder my progress to my Real Food Life ultimate goal?" (See page 48 for information on how to read labels.) Put the "no's" immediately to the side to be thrown away. If you're on the fence about an item, remember my motto: When in doubt, throw it out.

Some of my clients feel wasteful throwing "perfectly good" food away. My answer? I would not ask you to throw "perfectly good" food away. I'm asking you to release the burden of food that does not support your goals. If being "wasteful" still makes you un-

comfortable, pack up unopened boxes and cans to donate to a food shelter or give away at work. Then, toss anything already opened that directly sabotages your goals for getting a Real Food Life. Keeping items around that aren't good for you isn't doing yourself any favors.

The foods below often pop up in my new clients' homes. I'll suggest certain items to add or subtract from your cupboards, but remember—the choice is always yours. This is *your* new food life.

High-sugar cereals. Do you have several boxes of sugary cereals? Do you have any whole grain, low-sugar, and low-salt cereals (hot or cold)?

Consider throwing away any cereals that contain 12 grams of sugar or more per serving. If you really love sugary cereal as an occasional treat for you or your kids, consider buying the small snack packs—you'll get variety and controlled portions. Otherwise, get rid of it. If you don't have any whole grain cereal, add it to your shopping list.

Processed foods. Do you have a lot of canned or packaged foods that are high in sodium, saturated fat, hydrogenated oils, and preservatives?

Take these foods to a local food bank, give them to a friend, or throw them out. If you're afraid your family will feel deprived without these foods they love, know this— there is no upside to these foods. By getting rid of processed foods, you are saving your family's health.

Vegetable oils. Is most of the oil in your cupboard sunflower or corn oil? Do you have vegetable shortening? Do you have olive oil?

Throw out shortening immediately—it's cement for your arteries. You should also toss the regular sunflower and corn oil. Replace them with olive oil and canola oil (also available in cooking sprays). Consider trying walnut oil, flaxseed oil, or high oleic sunflower oil.

Refined grain products. Are the only grains you have egg noodles and white rice? Do you have any semolina or whole wheat pasta? Do you have any grains such as quinoa, barley, buckwheat, bulgur wheat, or brown rice?

Whole grains and whole wheat pastas are a must—add them to your shopping list. Save the white rice and egg noodles for occasional use.

Canned goods. Do you have cans of processed meat like deviled ham or corned beef hash? Pork and beans? Refried beans with lard? Tuna packed in oil? Any sardines? Are your soups creamy chowders and high-fat instant noodle soups, or are they low-fat, high-fiber, and filled with vegetables? Do you have plain canned beans and stewed tomatoes?

The tinned meat, pork and beans, full-fat refried beans, and vegetable oil–packed tuna should be donated to a food bank. Keep tuna packed in olive oil. If you have none on hand, add low-fat canned soups and tuna packed in water to your shopping list. Canned beans, canned salmon, and stewed tomatoes make excellent, versatile staples.

Snack foods. Do you have boxes or bags of candy or cookies that contain "partially hydrogenated oil" as one of the first three ingredients? What about crackers—do they contain any fiber at all? Do you have potato chips, corn crisps, or tortilla chips? Are they in big bags that make it difficult to stop eating?

Toss the cookies and candy bars, and replace them with high-quality dark chocolate and dried fruit (such as raisins and apricots), which will satisfy the sweet cravings. Get rid of the white-flour, no-fiber crackers and add whole grain crackers to your list. Low-fat bean dip and fat-free salsa can make an excellent addition, if they sound good to you. (Try them with baby carrots instead of chips.) Low-fat tortilla chips can stay, if you can limit yourself. If you can't resist them, toss them.

Root vegetables. Do you have 10-pound bags of white potatoes? A net bag of white or red onions? Fresh garlic or ginger?

Unless you have a large family, get in the habit of buying potatoes in smaller bags, or even individually, so you're more conscious of how often you eat them. Consider acquiring a taste for sweet potatoes—they're more nutritious than white. Buy only as much garlic as you need for each week, thereby ensuring

The 10-Step Kitchen Makeover

The last thing I want is for the time commitment required for the Kitchen Makeover to be an obstacle that hinders you from getting a Real Food Life. If time's short but your intentions are good, these 10 easy switches will get you a lot closer to your goals.

1. Replace vegetable shortening with olive oil.
2. Replace "marshmallowy" refined white bread with whole wheat bread.
3. Replace fatty cold cuts with canned tuna or sliced turkey breast or lean roast beef.
4. Replace processed peanut butter, which contains hydrogenated oil and added sugar, with natural nut butter (such as peanut, almond, walnut, or soy).
5. Replace full-fat mayonnaise with low-fat mayo.
6. Replace whole milk with fat-free milk or low-fat soy milk.
7. Replace potato chips with nuts and seeds.
8. Replace cola and coffee with water and green or herbal tea.
9. Replace instant, dehydrated soups with good-quality, organic canned soups.
10. Replace sweetened sugary cereals with whole grain cereals.

freshness. On the flip side, buy onions in bulk and use them often. Store fresh ginger and garlic in the fridge after you cut it.

Breads. What variety of breads do you have? Do you have any dark or whole wheat breads?

Toss the marshmallowy white bread to make room for whole wheat breads—they're more filling, satisfying, and fiber-filled than white breads.

Tea and coffee. Do you have cans of coffee and only black (regular) tea? Do you have any herbal tea at all? Any green tea?

If you don't have any, add herbal tea and green tea to your shopping list. You might also want to try Caffix, a chicory-based bev-erage. Coffee and black tea are fine in moderation, but a great habit to get into is drinking more green and herbal tea.

Cooking staples. Do you have any flour other than bleached, like whole wheat? What about sugar? Honey? Saccharine or aspartame? Hot sauces? Spices and herbs?

Whole wheat flour can be a satisfying supplement to your white flour. (In baking, substitute up to half of the amount of white flour called for with whole wheat flour for very satisfactory results.) Use sugar and honey sparingly, but throw away all products containing saccharine or aspartame. (They promote a "sugar tooth," the bane of many food lives. And we still have little definitive proof of their long-term effects.) As for the herbs, spices, and hot sauces, use them to your heart's content.

Refrigerator

When you go through your refrigerator, go through a shelf at a time. Ask yourself the same question as you did when you went through your cupboards: Will this item help me toward my goals or keep me from achieving them? The goal is to make room for lots of fresh vegetables, fruits, and refreshing waters.

Water. Do you have bottles of water, a container, or a filter jug? Do you keep seltzer or mineral water on hand? What about sodas?

The top shelf of your fridge should be dominated by water in any and all forms. Keep your water jug or bottle toward the front, and pour a glass whenever you open the fridge. Seltzer counts. Soda doesn't. Soda should be a special-treat beverage, not a staple. If you simply can't resist the daily soda, you should get rid of it.

Fruit. How many pieces of fruit are in your fridge, if any? What about fresh vegetables?

You should have enough fruit and veggies to last you at least a few days or the entire week (depending on how often you market). Opening the door to your fridge should reveal a rainbow of color—prepared salad greens, carrots, roasted red peppers, spinach, broccoli, dandelion greens, asparagus, celery, carrots, squash, peas.

Dairy. Do you have any full-fat dairy

products? Any low-fat yogurts, milk, and cheeses?

Many people lose their taste for full-fat milk when they transition down to 2%, then 1%—even if you don't like fat-free milk, these modest changes can make a big difference. Stock up with other low-fat dairy items like low-fat cottage cheese and yogurt.

Processed meats. Do you have sandwich meat? Meat and breakfast meat products? Do you have any soy food products in your fridge?

Throw away baloney, salami, bacon, sausage, and other processed meats. Replace them with fresh turkey breast and lean roast beef. All-natural chicken sausage or soy hot dogs can be used instead of pork sausage. If you haven't already, consider buying soy foods such as smoked tofu (it tastes like smoked cheese), Veggie Singles (pre-sliced soy cheese that tastes like dairy cheese singles), or regular tofu (which comes in a variety of flavors); all of these are great as part of a snack or meal.

Eggs. Do you have eggs? Are they enriched with omega-3?

Keep the eggs (check their expiration date), since they're a fast and nourishing meal or snack. Consider hard-boiling a few for quick, convenient snacks.

Fats. Do you have any margarine or butter? What about nut butters and nuts and seeds?

Throw out the overprocessed margarine, but keep the butter to use in very small amounts. (I like mashed avocado as a bread-

(continued on page 184)

LIVING A
REAL FOOD LIFE

A Kitchen Makeover Got This
Stay-at-Home Mom Back On Track

Name: Nadine
Real Food Life Issues: overstressed, fast-food diet, no time to cook

Nadine is a busy stay-at-home mother of two small children. When she left the workforce to take care of her first baby 6 years ago, she was excited to have more time to make a nice home, raise her child, and even have some time for herself. But several years and another child later, she still didn't have the time to keep her house as nice as she wanted. And forget about exercise or quality time for herself. Time was always about the children, and Nadine felt worn out, stressed out, bloated, and blah. Here's where I found her:

> *May 20*
>
> *Right after breakfast this morning, Ethan started screaming about getting one of those action figure dolls at the fast-food place. I'd been up all night with Samantha's croup, and my last nerve was shot by 10 A.M. That kid can really belt out the whines when he wants something! Finally, I gave in and we all piled into the car. He got the toy and went to play on the jungle gym, and I finally had peace. I savored the moment with a milk shake and large fries. I was actually starting to feel human again when I saw that busybody PTA lady. I swear she gave my sweats and stained T-shirt the once over before she put on a fake smile and asked me to make cookies for the bake sale. I said yes, of course, while inwardly seething. I probably would've decked her if I could have summoned the energy to make a fist! Yeah, right, Nadine, you big baby. . . .*

After I analyzed her first week's food journal, I saw lots of nutritional black holes. Nadine ate hardly any fruits, vegetables, fish, or whole grains, so it was no wonder to me that she felt bloated much of the time. The majority of her diet was refined carbohydrates in the form of muffins, bagels, and pastries, and very high saturated fat and high-sodium fast food.

I wasn't surprised that she had been unsuccessful in her efforts to lose the 35 pounds she gained during her second pregnancy.

Before long, I got Nadine to break the fast-food habit (the kids came later). When I explained that the only good thing about this food is that it is fast—and that's no reason to eat it—and that it's almost completely devoid of any vitamins and minerals, Nadine reevaluated its convenience. I also explained that her diet of refined carbs and fast food contributed not only to her inability to lose weight, but more important, to her feelings of being worn out, stressed out, and bloated. Together, we created a wholesome eating plan she could stick with, filled with foods she liked and could prepare quickly and with minimal fuss. I also had her start drinking at least 4 cups of water a day, which quickly turned into 8 cups a day.

Next up, Nadine and I gave her kitchen a makeover. I showed her how to read food labels and explained what to look for—and avoid—in packaged foods. We tossed out most of the unhealthful foods in her larder, especially those with hydrogenated fats, refined white flour, and too much sugar. We then went grocery shopping and stocked her cabinets, refrigerator, and freezer with an assortment of healthful and fast foods including soy foods, frozen and fresh vegetables, dried and fresh fruit, nuts and seeds, olive oil, lean beef, chicken, and fish.

Replacing foods high in saturated fats with those high in essential fatty acids was hard for Nadine to get used to, but she was determined to improve her diet for herself and her kids. She started eating a handful of nuts and seeds each day and used olive oil on her salads and when cooking vegetables. I introduced her to smoked tofu, which she loved and continues to eat almost every day in a sandwich or on a salad. I also introduced her to edamame (boiled soy beans), and she realized that it was a delicious and wholesome snack both she and her kids could happily and healthfully devour.

Within 2 weeks, Nadine felt much less bloated, her energy level increased, and her excess water weight came off. She continued to go grocery shopping at least once a week, armed with a shopping list loaded with wholesome foods for quick and balanced meals and snacks. Soon, she began making and packing lunch for herself and her kids (when necessary). Making lunch helped her stay on track with her food life, plus it saved her quite a bit of money.

By week 5, Nadine recognized that she needed to find time for exercise, so she started doing workout videos a few times a week while the kids napped. Exercise made her feel great, got rid of her blahs, and gave her even more energy. She also lost 16 pounds and felt much happier and more satisfied with her life than she had in years.

spread—with or without a little low-fat canola mayonnaise. It's a much healthier fat than butter.) High in protein and good fat, nuts and seeds should definitely be in your Real Food Life, but keep them in the refrigerator so they won't turn rancid. Peanut butters with hydrogenated oils and added sugar should go, but they should be quickly replaced by all-natural peanut butter (stir it when the oil separates). Keep cashew butter, almond butter, or soy nut butter in the refrigerator, too.

Random stuff. Everybody's fridge is full of random stuff, but what's the best for your Real Food Life? Here are a few tips.

❱ Sugar-added jellies and jams are truly pointless when there are so many delicious all-fruit spreads out there. Buy the best-quality items you can find and use them sparingly—the flavor will really come through.

❱ Hummus, a delicious, nutrient-rich chickpea and garlic spread, is a great sandwich food or dip (with crackers or vegetables). Consider making this a new food staple—try the recipe on page 284.

❱ Throw out low-fat dressings that are loaded with additives and sugar; they also often contain the wrong types of fats. (I suggest alternatives in the shopping list on page 186.) Check out the recipe chapter for homemade dressing ideas.

❱ Throw out full-fat mayonnaise; keep low-fat mayonnaise, low-fat canola mayon-

naise, low-sodium chutneys, mustards, ketchup, and relishes.

Freezer

The freezer is a marvelous tool for your Real Food Life. You can stock it with homemade meals that keep you on track and healthy convenience products for satisfying, quick meals-at-the-ready. As with the cupboards and refrigerator, ask yourself, "Will this help me toward my goals or keep me from achieving them?" Then, decide what to keep and what to toss.

Frozen dinners. Do you see many frozen dinners and side dishes? Are they extremely high in bad fats, sodium, and preservatives that you can't even pronounce?

Unless you're an expert label reader, it's sometimes hard to determine how healthful a prepared dinner is. One good rule of thumb: If a product contains hydrogenated oils, artificial colors, artificial flavors, and more than 10 grams of fat, you should toss it. Refer to the shopping list for frozen meals and sides that are lower in fat and sodium and taste great.

Frozen veggies and fruit. How many different kinds of frozen vegetables or fruit are in your freezer?

Frozen fruit and vegetables are great to keep on hand. They're loaded with vitamins and minerals and they're super-convenient. Toss frozen berries into a smoothie or a cup of yogurt; nuke a package of spinach with a sprinkle of garlic salt.

Frozen meat. Do you have any frozen meats? Breakfast meat?

With the exception of ham, all so-called breakfast meats—sausage links and patties, bacon, scrapple—are extremely high in saturated fat. Toss them. Keep the frozen chicken, frozen fish, and lean meats for handy meals, soups, or stews. Frozen veggie burgers and veggie hot dogs are also great for fast and easy meals.

Frozen desserts. How many different ice creams, ice cream products, and frozen desserts do you have? Are they full of fat?

We all need a special treat, but do we really need it in every flavor? If you can limit yourself to serving sizes, keep a maximum of one full-fat, extra-rich ice cream on hand as a super-special treat. Otherwise, toss all the extra-rich iced desserts and replace them with sorbet, sorbet bars, frozen low-fat yogurt, and soy milk desserts.

2. Go Grocery Shopping

When I work with clients, part of my consultation includes a fun, educational trip to the grocery store. Typically, we'll go to their local supermarket or health food market and spend some time browsing through the aisles, reading labels, and choosing tasty foods that will pave the way to their Real Food Life.

Don't think that just because you don't cook at home, you won't benefit from the shopping trip. Part of being responsible to your Real Food Life goals is to give yourself the tools to achieve them. I'm not mandating that you cook, but you should take at least one trip to the grocery store to stock your larder with healthy, quick meals and snacks.

From your work on the kitchen makeover, you should now have a list of items you need to replace (for example, a bottle of olive oil to replace unhealthful corn oil). If you're already in the habit of cooking at home, you probably have a decent number of staples—particularly items like onions, pastas, seasonings, and canned goods—even after doing the kitchen makeover.

Or perhaps you're like many of my clients, left with a can of seltzer and a jar of pickles. In that case, this first food shop may be very big. Staples last, so if you buy a bunch now, you won't need to buy them again for quite some time.

Sadly, I won't be there to accompany you on your shopping trip, but below I've detailed a strategy that will help you navigate through the different areas of your store. Actually, a good maxim of food selection is Shop the Walls—that's where the fresh produce, dairy, and meat sections are. Everything in the middle of the store has been processed in some way.

Take along a copy of my shopping list,

(continued on page 188)

The Get a Real Food Life Shopping List

Use this handy list as a reminder of your shopping strategies while you're in the store. If your market doesn't stock the items recommended, speak to a clerk—often they'll be happy to add different foods if they think customers are interested.

Fruits and Vegetables

Prewashed salad greens
Baby carrots
Cherry or grape tomatoes
Garlic, onions, ginger
Dark green vegetables (kale, collards, spinach, broccoli)
Cauliflower, asparagus, string beans
Bananas, apples (make sure they're hard), oranges, other seasonal fruits
Lemons, limes
Fresh herbs

Bread, Crackers, and Bread Products

English muffins (Thomas's Honey Whole Wheat or Oat Bran)
Crackers (Finn Crisp, Wasa, Ryvita, Woven Wheats)
Whole Grain Bread (Matthews, The Vermont Bread Company, The Baker, or Branola)
Muffins (choose small, low-fat, high-fiber ones)
Health Valley Breakfast Bakes (fruit-filled breakfast pastries)

Dressings and Sauces

Salad dressing (Consorzio, Paula's, Blanchard and Blanchard, Walden Farms, Cardini's, or other all-natural, low-fat, low-sugar, low-sodium brands)
Barbecue sauce (Peter Luger's, Newman's Own, or other all-natural brand)
Canned tomatoes (Pomi, Muir Glen, Tutorosso, or other all-natural, low-sodium brand)
Bottled tomato sauce (Muir Glen or other organic or all-natural brand)
Salsa (Guiltless Gourmet or other all-natural brand)

Cereals

Honey Puffed Kashi, Kashi Good Friends, Kashi Go Lean
Health Valley Oat Bran Flakes
Uncle Sam's Cereal
Wheatabix

Health Valley Puffed Corn (tastes like waffles with syrup)
Toasted Wheat Germ

Staples, Condiments, and Grocery Items

Low-fat mayonnaise (Hellmann's or Best Foods)
Ketchup (low-salt)
Bragg's Liquid Aminos (to flavor just about anything)
Mustard (Gulden's brand and Dijon)
Worcestershire sauce
Vinegar (red wine, balsamic, apple cider, rice wine)
Hot sauce (Pickapepper, Tabasco, or another all-natural hot sauce)
Canned tuna in spring water or olive oil
Canned salmon
Canned sardines (with bones)
Fat-free chili (Health Valley or another organic or all-natural brand)
Canned or bottled low-sodium soup (Health Valley, Walnut Acres, or another organic or all-natural brand)
Bagged beans (Bean Cuisine)
Canned beans (Eden Farms or other low-sodium or sodium-free brand)
Spices, herbs, and seasonings, including black pepper, cayenne pepper, cinnamon, cumin, garlic powder, kosher or sea salt, oregano, paprika, pure vanilla extract, and rosemary
All-natural nut butter
Jam or all-fruit spread (St. Dalfour, Wilkens and Sons, Dickenson's, or other all-fruit or mostly fruit brands)
Seltzer (plain and flavored)
Green tea, chamomile tea
Caffix (chicory beverage)

Snack Foods

Dried veggies (Just Veggies or Eat Your Vegetables brands)
Dried fruit (apricots and raisins)
Pasta chips
Pretzels (Harry's Fat-Free or another fat-free, all-natural variety)

(continued)

The Get a Real Food Life Shopping List (cont.)

Snack Foods *(cont.)*

Small bags of Power Puffs or Pirate Booty (or other Robert's American Gourmet item)

Small bags of Terra Chips

Nuts or seeds (walnuts, Brazil nuts, sunflower seeds, pumpkin seeds)

Dairy and Refrigerated Foods

Fat-free or 1% milk

Fat-free plain yogurt (organic tastes best)

Stonyfield Farm or Horizon low-fat yogurt

Friendship 1% fat whipped cottage cheese (or other 1% cottage cheese)

Parmesan Reggiano (a small chunk of real Parmesan is worth the money)

Fromage blanc or Quark cheese

Low-fat cream cheese

SmartBeat cheeses (nondairy cheese singles)

Veggie Singles (soy cheese slices)

Low-fat Swiss, Jarlsberg, or Alpine Lace cheese

Eggs (enriched with omega-3, if you can find them)

Hummus (or try recipe on page 284)

Low-fat whole wheat tortillas

and feel free to adjust it to your tastes. It includes a number of different brands that may be available in your store.

Start your grocery carts!

Produce Aisle

Most supermarkets open onto the produce section—what a lucky break! Whichever eating plan you're embarking on, fruits and vegetables are a mainstay.

Fruit. Buy enough to get three servings a day for the week. While you'll have the best selection in spring and summer, there are fresh, tasty fruits available throughout the year. Also consider frozen fruit and fruit canned in its own juices.

❿ Apples, bananas, and oranges are especially transportable, making them great for snacks on the run.

Soy Foods

Veggie/soy hot dogs (Tofu Pups, Lightlife Smart Dogs, Wonderdogs, New Menu)

Yves Veggie Cuisine product line (www.yvesveggie.com)

Tree of Life Tofu (flavored tofu blocks)

Light Life product line (I like their soy hot dogs.)

Smoke and Fire naturally smoked, flavored tofu (www.smokeandfire.com)

Soy milk (fat-free or regular, any flavor)

Frozen Foods

Soy/veggie burgers (Boca Burgers or Gardenburgers)

Vegetable-based organic frozen dinners (choose Cascadian Farm or another similar brand)

Frozen shrimp or lobster (plain)

Frozen soy beans (also called edamame)

Whole grain waffles (Van's)

Frozen dessert (Häagen-Dazs sorbet, Tofutti bars, Sharon's Sorbet)

Frozen fish sticks (Natural Sea brand breaded with whole grain crumbs)

Frozen chicken nuggets or soy "chicken" nuggets (Health Is Wealth or other organic brand)

Frozen fruits and vegetables (organic is best; otherwise plain, no sauce)

Frozen organic French fries (Cascadian Farms or another organic brand)

◗ Consider precut melon and pineapple—what could be easier?

◗ Tropical fruits, like mango and papaya, are available year-round. Let them ripen until they're soft to the touch, peel, remove the seed, and serve.

◗ Fragile berries should be eaten within a day or two of purchasing. Wash them just before using, or they'll rot.

◗ A squeeze of fresh lemon or lime brightens the flavor of drinks, salads, and other foods.

Vegetables. With the large number of prewashed and precut vegetables on the market, getting your five servings a day should be a snap. If the vegetables don't look fresh, remember that frozen ones and plain canned ones can be just as nutritious.

❯ Choose sturdy vegetables that cook quickly and make tasty leftovers, such as broccoli, cauliflower, green beans, or a hardy green such as kale, bok choy, or Swiss chard. Steam, microwave, or sauté it with a little olive oil and a clove or two of crushed garlic.

❯ Choose prepackaged salad greens and spinach.

❯ Celery, cucumbers, and baby carrots are proven kid-pleasers.

❯ Buy veggies that lend themselves to snacking, like baby carrots, precut celery stalks, and cherry tomatoes.

❯ Stock up on staples such as yellow onions and fresh ginger. They last for weeks in your refrigerator.

❯ Fresh herbs add flavor and freshness to sandwiches, soups, omelettes, and even prepared dishes. If you're not sure which you like, start with basil and add it to spaghetti sauce, then branch out into parsley or cilantro next week.

Bread Aisle

If none of the whole grain breads included on the shopping list are sold at your store, choose a product that lists whole wheat or another whole grain flour as one of the first two ingredients.

❯ Try breads that have sunflower seeds, pumpkin seeds, sesame seeds, or flaxseeds in them for added fiber and vitamin E.

❯ If you prefer eating a carbohydrate-based meal plan, you might consider more than one variety of bread.

Grains, Beans, and Canned Goods Aisle

Don't be afraid to stock up here. Rices, grains, and pasta last for years on the shelf—and unopened cans line the shelves of markets for months.

❯ Try some whole wheat pasta. While the taste is different than semolina-flour pasta, each serving yields a potent fiber dose.

❯ Any brown rice variety, including the quick-cooking type, is better than white rice.

❯ Stock up on several cans of beans—chickpeas, kidney, black, white—choosing lower-sodium or salt-free varieties (such as Eden's Organic) whenever possible.

❯ Stock up also on low-fat soups (check the label if you're not sure of the fat content) and canned tomatoes.

Condiments Aisle

Most condiments—except mayo—have a very long shelf life, even after opening. Condiments are flavor boosters that enhance cooked foods, homemade dressings, and salads and sandwiches. Buy products with all-natural ingredients whenever possible.

❯ If you're replacing your oil, or stocking your kitchen for the first time, consider buying a bottle each of extra-virgin olive oil, canola oil, and toasted (or Asian) sesame oil.

▶ Instead of the big cylinder of salt, look for sea salt, kosher salt, or reduced-sodium salt.

▶ Vinegar adds a sharp, tart flavor to salads and cooked foods with no fat and very few calories. Buy many different kinds—they last forever.

▶ All-fruit spreads last for a year or two in the fridge after opening.

Dairy Aisle

Fresh dairy foods like milk and yogurt are perishable, so don't feel compelled to buy a lot of them. Always look at the expiration date and choose the latest one. (As an alternative, consider shelf-stable cow's milk or calcium-added soy milk.) If you store cheese well-wrapped in the fridge, it'll last for weeks.

▶ You should always have some milk on hand to drink straight-up or use on cereal—choose fat-free, low-fat, or soy (with calcium added).

▶ Opt for plain, low-fat or fat-free yogurt, and avoid those with artificial sweeteners. Organic yogurt tastes especially good.

▶ Buy a whole chunk of Parmesan cheese—the flavor is so superior to the pre-grated kind, it will blow you away. To make it last *a year*, wrap it first in a slightly damp paper towel and then tightly in foil.

▶ Be sure to get a carton of eggs, enriched with omega-3 if available. Hardboiled eggs make a great snack on the go.

▶ Fromage blanc (French for "white cheese") and Quark are both low-fat or fat-free soft spreadable cheeses; buy them as an exotic replacement for cream cheese. They're particularly tasty on toast with a little jam.

▶ The dairy aisle also features most of the fresh soy items. Packaged tofu and soy products have expiration dates, so read and heed them.

Meat and Fish Aisle

Meat freezes well, especially in big freezers. Avoid gray or "dead"-looking meat, and if it's prewrapped, make sure it's not sitting in a pool of its own liquid. If you're buying fish, plan on cooking it that same night—otherwise, freeze it or buy prefrozen.

▶ Skinless chicken breasts, parts, or whole birds are extremely versatile and lower in fat than most other meat.

▶ For beef, opt for flank steak (I love it marinated in barbecue sauce and then grilled or broiled), filet mignon, or ground sirloin—all are lower in fat. Better yet, have the butcher grind the sirloin to order. It'll taste fresher, and you'll know it's the cut you want.

▶ Try ground turkey or chicken breast as a beef substitute.

▶ If you buy whole fish, like trout or bass, look for clear, sparkling eyes—gray, cloudy eyes mean the fish is old.

Frozen Food Aisle

If you're lucky enough to be blessed with a large freezer, go crazy! Frozen foods are designed for convenience and last up to a year.

▶ Frozen soy foods like veggie burgers and hot dogs cook in under 10 minutes—some varieties of veggie burger are even toaster-ready!

▶ Frozen veggies and fruits can pinch-hit for fresh when the produce aisle is looking less than up-to-snuff.

▶ Frozen shrimp is as good as fresh; in fact, most of the "fresh" shrimp you bought in your life was actually defrosted before it was sold to you.

▶ Avoid frozen dinners as much as possible. They're processed to death and usually filled with fat and salt. If you need a quick meal, look for organic or vegetarian meals. Always scan the label to avoid hydrogenated and saturated fats and excess sodium.

As you're putting away your groceries, take a moment to see how your shelves and fridge look now—do you see more color? More shapes and varieties of food? You should feel good—you've accomplished another giant step on the road to getting a Real Food Life.

Get Real Check-In

Assess your progress by checking off each of the following items you achieved during week 3.

❏ Instant Makeover #3: I replaced a half-hour of TV-watching with extra sleep time.

❏ I added an extra glass of water—I'm up to 7.

❏ I achieved my week 3 mini-goals.

❏ I set my week 4 mini-goals.

❏ I gave my kitchen the Real Food Life Makeover (the long or short version).

❏ I went grocery shopping.

❏ I kept my food journal each day.

❏ I rewarded myself for my intentions and my efforts.

Weekly Words: Write a couple of paragraphs in your journal about how you felt throwing away food—was it difficult, liberating, a little of both? Discuss how your new kitchen will help you achieve your ultimate goal.

Week Four:

10 COOKING FOR YOUR REAL FOOD LIFE

During this week, you will:

▶ Accomplish Instant Makeover #4: Replace corn oil with olive or canola oil

▶ Add one extra glass of water (reach 8 glasses a day)

▶ Follow your week 4 mini-goals

▶ Keep week 4 of your food journal

▶ Refine your eating plan

▶ Cook your first Real Food Life meal

▶ Learn how to plan for future Real Food Life meals

▶ Complete week 4 of your Get Real Check-In

For some people, cooking is a passion they can't live without.

And then there are most of my clients.

Many of them are intimidated by cooking—they weren't taught how to do it, don't own cookbooks, and don't feel comfortable making food for themselves. As a result, they eat out often, relying on other people to prepare their meals and ultimately feeling disconnected from their food.

Cooking is a great way to learn exactly what you're putting into your mouth. When you cook, you learn a key Real Food Life skill without even thinking about it: portion control.

Instant Makeover #4:

Replace corn oil with olive or canola oil

Forget all those years of brainwashing—fat can be healthy! The trick is, you have to favor the good kinds of fats (and it won't hurt to avoid the bad ones altogether).

Replacing corn oil with olive or canola oil stacks the good fat odds in your favor. Monounsaturated fats, like those found in olive and canola oils, lower the "bad" cholesterol in your blood. The polyunsaturated fats in corn oil do, too, but they also lower your "good" cholesterol. (Saturated fats— those found in animal products and fried foods—raise your total cholesterol and increase your risk of heart disease.) When eaten in excess, polyunsaturated fats may promote cancer; monounsaturated fats protect against it.

Eating a lot of food with corn oil also increases the proportion of certain fatty acids in your body. If you eat too much corn oil, you can cancel out all the good you're doing by eating foods rich in omega-3 fatty acids, such as salmon, sardines, and flaxseed.

If you're not a fan of olive oil's distinctive flavor, try canola oil, which offers a very versatile flavor that many can't distinguish from corn. Buy it and try it today!

Because you measure so often when you're cooking, you learn to develop an "eye" for portions. You'll no longer be mystified by a cup of vegetables or a teaspoon of butter— you'll have a mental picture of what they look like from your travels as a cook.

Cooking comes down to control. *You* decide whether to use corn or olive oil. You decide to lightly sprinkle salt as opposed to pouring it on. You decide to select the leanest cuts of chicken, and you probably won't dip it in butter (the way they do in restaurants). Your food is literally in your own hands, putting you in the driver's seat of your Real Food Life.

Before we get to cooking, take a moment at this halfway point to assess where you are with your Real Food Life. Reflect on the changes you've made by asking yourself the questions that follow—the answers will guide you through the second half of your Real Food Life Plan.

1. Refine Your Eating Plan

By now, keeping your journal has become a fully entrenched habit. You've probably grown to be an eager student of your own eating habits. Isn't it empowering to draw the direct connection between what you put in your mouth and how it makes you feel?

Let's take some time here in week 4 to revisit your food journal in more depth. Reflecting on where you are now, the compelling changes you've made, and how different your Food Life feels now can bolster your dedication to reaching your ultimate goals.

Turn to a fresh page in your journal, ask yourself the following questions, and note the answer that sounds most like how you feel.

Am I hungry throughout the day? If the answer is yes, try one of these suggestions:

▶ *You may have cut out too many complex carbohydrates from your diet.* Try increasing your complex carbohydrate intake by 1 or 2 servings for a few days (noting how you feel in your journal). If you feel "fuller" by eating more carbohydrates, continue with that amount of carbs in your diet.

▶ *You may not have enough fiber in your meals.* Pick up a box of Kashi or Health Valley cereal (or another low-sugar/high-fiber brand). Have a bowl for breakfast or eat it as a snack with some low-fat yogurt.

▶ *You may have lowered your fat intake too much.* Since fat slows the emptying of the stomach, a fat-free or low-fat meal will cause you to feel hungry quicker. Two servings of fat a day might not be enough, so add another and see how you feel after a few days.

▶ *You may not be drinking enough water.* Dehydration can cause false hunger and make you feel tired and lethargic. You might be reaching for food instead of the needed glass of water.

Am I feeling tired much of the time? If the answer is yes, try one of these suggestions:

▶ *You may not be taking in enough calories.* Carefully examine your food journal to see if you're falling short in any category or several. Add a snack to boost your caloric intake. If that doesn't help, try increasing your food plan by one serving in each food group to boost your caloric level.

▶ *You may be on the three-squares plan.* If you're not already doing the grazing plan, try eating six mini-meals each day. Many of my clients love this way of eating because it makes them feel like they're eating all day long and they feel they have more energy.

▶ *You may not be eating enough protein.* Protein helps slow down the emptying of the stomach, yielding sustained energy that lasts all afternoon. If you don't eat at least a little bit of protein with your carbohydrates, you'll feel hungry and tired quickly thereafter.

▶ *You may not be eating enough complex carbohydrates.* Complex carbs are the main source of energy for all bodily functions. A lack of complex carbs will make you lethargic and probably constipated (because of lack of fiber), which can also slow you down.

▶ *You may not be eating balanced meals.* Salads with lean meats and grains are great for getting a balance of complex carbs and proteins. Or skip the meats and try adding a soy alternative. Edamame beans (frozen fresh soybeans) are a great

LIVING A
REAL FOOD LIFE

This High School Senior Bade Farewell to Her Binges

Name: Carly
Real Food Life Issues: bingeing, always hungry

When I met Carly, she was a college-bound high school senior. She had no concentration at school, which had nothing to do with senioritis. She told me that she felt she had too little energy. Plus, she was chronically constipated. Carly always felt hungry—as many teens do—but she could never enjoy the food she ate because eating to the point of fullness made her feel guilty. The pressure to be thin, to fit in, and to wear the latest belly-revealing outfits caused her to shun food—at least in public. She admitted to me that, in private, she regularly binged on cookies, candy bars, potato chips, and fast foods. She would alternate these binges with starving herself. Here's where I found her:

September 18

I did it again. I always think I'm going to be able to stop myself, but then I get in the middle of a box of cookies and I just think, "Why bother stopping? I'm already a fat pig." And then I just eat and eat and eat until I've worked through my whole stash and I feel like I'm going to explode. Then all I want to do is lie around with my pants unbuttoned and moan. It's like that Thanksgiving feeling, but at least then, everyone's doing it!

It's always so much more fun when we all eat together, especially at Heather's house. Her mom doesn't think twice about all the food that disappears, she just buys more! My mom's always hanging around, bugging us, embarrassing me—I can tell she's afraid I'll gain weight. I just don't get how Heather and Lisa

way to get protein and carbs all in one!

Am I emotionally unsatisfied with what I'm eating? If the answer is yes, try one of these suggestions:

▶ *You may be stuck in the "diet" mentality.* If you're constantly pining for your old food life or "foraging" for food during the day, not satisfied with your meals, you need to change your *can eat everything I do—sometimes so much MORE—and still look like little twigs? Lisa told me her mom uses laxatives when she needs to fit into a cocktail dress for a party—I wonder if she's doing the same thing...? That would be a very gross way to lose weight...but who knows? Maybe I'll try it...*

After Carly told me about her starving and bingeing, I explained the health risks associated with those behaviors. I explained that bingeing and starving interfered with her body chemicals and contributed to the symptoms she wanted to relieve. We worked together to set up a nourishing eating plan with enough calories so she didn't feel constantly hungry. This kept her from bingeing, which would have started the whole bingeing/starving cycle all over again. Her eating plan consisted of a variety of complex carbohydrates (she especially loved oatmeal for breakfast), lean proteins (turkey sandwiches for lunch and seafood dinners), fruits, vegetables, and essential fatty acids (she was crazy for sunflower seeds and loved avocados).

Right off the bat, I had her drink 8 cups of water each day. We also made sure she ate plenty of fruits and vegetables every day, and much to her relief, by week 2 she no longer suffered from constipation. By week 3, Carly realized she no longer felt constantly hungry and she had much more energy. She started to recognize that the punishing cycle of starving and then bingeing on unhealthy foods really did play a part in her symptoms.

I also gave Carly some cooking ideas she could use at college. I taught her how to make simple and fast foods like poached salmon, Veggie Trio (see page 269), and Middle Eastern Tabbouleh Salad (see page 291), all of which can be done with a microwave or hot plate. I also shared strategies for ordering sensible foods at restaurants and at the cafeteria.

In the first 8 weeks that we worked together, Carly noticed dramatic improvements. For the first time since her adolescence began, she was able to recognize what "full" felt like, and she knew that it was normal to feel that way. Her attention span improved dramatically and resulted in better grades (even for a college-bound senior). But most important, Carly realized that she hadn't binged once since she began working with me, and that felt really great to her.

eating plan. Getting a Real Food Life should empower you and help you get rid of the soul-draining diet mentality that is hazardous to your emotional relationship with food.

▶ *You may be more of an emotional eater than you thought.* Your Real Food Life should not make you feel deprived. You can eat and should eat plenty of the foods that make you feel good. But you also need to remind yourself that if you listen to your body more and recognize that you have many food choices, your food life can become much more emotionally satisfying.

▶ *You may not be experimenting enough.* Experiment with the different food options I've recommended in the various eating plans. If you're eating a meal and feel something is missing, if something isn't tasty enough or it's not satisfying to you, engage your food awareness, review your food journal, analyze what's going on, and remedy it.

▶ *You may not be getting enough essential fatty acids.* Fat feeds your brain, so if your diet is too low in fat, it can make you feel emotionally unsatisfied. Try eating more deep-sea, cold-water fish, like salmon, herring, and mackerel.

▶ *You may not be satisfying your cravings.* First, identify the craving. Remember, you can have any food you want in your Real Food Life, but limit less wholesome choices to small quantities. Or try a "healthier" version of your craving—a turkey burger instead of a hamburger, chocolate sorbet instead of chocolate ice cream. You'll satisfy your craving and support your Real Food Life at the same time!

Am I bloated? If the answer is yes, try one of these suggestions:

▶ *You may have eaten pasta.* Pasta is a common culprit in bloating. Next time you eat it, take note of how you feel a few hours afterward and the next day. If it's causing discomfort and bloating, eat it as a treat instead of a staple.

▶ *You may have eaten a lot of high-fiber foods.* High-fiber foods, such as beans, whole grains, and lots of vegetables, can take a while for your body to get used to, and until then, they can cause discomfort. If you find you're experiencing a lot of gas after high-fiber meals, cut back and add them in more slowly. Until your body gets used to them, try just a small portion of beans on top of your salad or as a side dish. Also, rinse beans well, which eliminates some of the enzymes that cause gas and bloating, or use Beano (a bottled enzyme) on cooked vegetable and bean dishes.

Am I finding the plan inconvenient? If the answer is yes, try one of these suggestions:

▶ *Your plan is too time consuming or hard to follow.* If so, you need to start adapting it until you find what works for you and your lifestyle. A successful Real Food Life can change and vary depending on your situation, the season, your inclination, and your mood.

▶ *You don't like doing one shop a week.* Try doing a big shop every other week, with smaller trips to the market for fresh items as needed.

▶ *You dine out often and find it hard to stick to your plan.* Almost every restaurant has healthful options, if you know what you're looking for. Take time to consider the dining-out information on page 228.

Drawing from the suggestions that seemed to resonate with you, use this information to inform the decisions you make in the next step: cooking!

2. Cook Your First Real Food Life Meal

At its essence, your Real Food Life is all about eating nourishing foods that you love. Once you embrace your Real Food Life fully, cooking to support that love won't feel like a labor. Even if you're a die-hard dining-out junkie, trust me—there will come a time when you'll want to prepare your favorite foods for yourself, just the way *you* like them, rather than relying on restaurants or take-out menus.

Whether you're a beginner or an experienced cook, being comfortable in the kitchen will help you support your healthy eating habits for years to come. I have helped clients who literally didn't know how to boil water have success in the kitchen, so I know you can have success, too. The best way to settle in is to roll up your sleeves and experiment with some of the recipes in this book (starting on page 259).

To counter your kitchen fear, I've noted some steps to lessen your anxiety. Follow the Top Ten Tips I've included below, which will make sure every experience in the kitchen is a successful one.

1. As with all worthwhile pursuits, preparation is key. Read the recipe all the way through to see if you have all the ingredients on hand; if not, write the missing ingredients on your shopping list. A read-through also gets you familiar with the recipe, gives you an idea of how long it will take to make, and lets you know if you need special tools.

2. Go shopping for ingredients you need to make the recipe.

3. Read the recipe all the way through once again, so you'll understand the methods and steps involved.

4. Place all the ingredients on the counter. This visual is a great double check to make sure you have enough of the ingredients you'll need, including the ones you may have assumed you had on hand.

5. Collect all necessary kitchen tools—cutting board, sharp knives, pots, pans, and so on.

6. Wash, dry, chop, cut, dice, preheat—set the stage for the main event. Just as your favorite TV chefs measure and place their ingredients in various bowls before beginning, you will be able to cook quickly, smartly, and efficiently if you follow this method. This way, you can motor through your recipe without having to stop and prepare another ingredient.

7. Commence cooking. As you go, follow the recipe step-by-step. Nothing should come as a surprise to you now since you've already read it twice.

8. Mini-sermon: Be safe and cook smart. Never leave a cooking pot unattended.

You don't have to watch it like a hawk, but don't leave the house when something is cooking in the oven or on the stove.

9. Adjust the recipe, if necessary. If you prefer your vegetables crisp-tender, feel free to cook them for less time than called for in the recipe. Likewise, if you want something cooked more, increase the cooking time by a minute or two.

10. Try to embrace cooking as fun and therapeutic. I find that cooking helps me calm down, and it gives me enormous pleasure to see my family enjoying something I made for them. As a bonus, cooking helps me take care of my Real Food Life because I prepare the foods that fit into the program I've made for myself.

Are you a beginner? If so, start with soup. It's easy to make, hard to burn, and requires minimal technique, yet you still get to practice your cooking skills. And since soup is a dish that pretty much cooks itself, you don't have to worry about "messing it up."

Soup is also a great way to get in more of the vegetables you may be short-changing in your Real Food Life. For example, if you want to eat more yellow and orange vegetables, preparing Roasted Acorn Squash Soup (see page 280) is a great way to accomplish that. Squash is very high in beta-carotene and cooks up very creamy and smooth, but it's still very low in calories. A big pot is a winning appetizer or great side dish.

Are you lacking in confidence? If you aren't that comfortable in the kitchen, there's nothing like some practice to build up your confidence. Try making at least one or two meals during week 4, and build from there. Take a trip to a local kitchen store and purchase a few new gadgets to reinforce your commitment to cook. Consider getting a garlic press, a steamer basket, and maybe a new knife. You will be amazed at how easy cooking can be if you have the right tools.

Are you an experienced cook? Shoot for making at least three meals for yourself during week 4. This is a great way to incorporate new foods into your Real Food Life (such as soy products, fresh fish, and more vegetables). The more you cook for yourself, the more you reinforce your new good food habits.

Regardless of your skill level, you're sure to reap health benefits from taking the time to cook. Please try many of the tasty recipes I've included, starting on page 259. These recipes, the same ones I make for my family, have been tested by a panel of professionals to ensure that they'll work in every home kitchen. Pick out some to try, and don't be afraid to experiment with some new flavors. Each recipe will be wholesome and tasty and will help you get the most out of your Real Food Life.

3. Planning Your Future Real Food Life Meals

For all cooks, time is often the biggest obstacle to making home-cooked meals. Cooking's

Kitchen CURES

Cheat a Cold or Flu

Stuffed up? Feeling achy? Show your cold or flu who's boss with these powerful strategies that will have you feeling better faster than you can say "achoo."

- Cayenne and other hot peppers (dried and fresh) keep mucus flowing and help with congestion and headaches. So kick up the heat in your next meal.
- Garlic helps stimulate the immune system and inhibits the growth of bacteria. If you don't mind garlic breath, eat several raw cloves a day until your symptoms subside. (They're very tasty added to soups and salads.) If bad breath is a concern, take enteric-coated garlic capsules in 300-milligram dosages three times a day for as long as your cold symptoms last.
- Ginger combats inflammation, so drink ginger tea, add fresh ginger to your food, or eat a few pieces of crystallized ginger.
- Drink lots of fluids: water, tea, soup. They will keep you hydrated, help mucus to flow, and flush out your body.
- Eat plenty of fruits and vegetables, including those rich in beta-carotene, such as apricots, sweet potatoes, carrots, and broccoli. Beta-carotene helps maintain mucous linings in the nose and lungs.
- Vitamin C in its many forms will help. It lowers levels of histamine, a chemical that's responsible for the stuffiness associated with colds and flu. It also appears to strengthen white blood cells, which are essential for fighting infection. Load up your plate with citrus fruits, berries, and tomatoes. Also take a supplement of 500 to 1,000 milligrams.
- Getting plenty of rest, including at least 8 hours of sleep, can help your body fight off infection.
- Chicken soup really helps! It clears mucous membranes and contains loads of nutrients that boost the immune system. Check out my recipe on page 275.

biggest trick is to find shortcuts and time-savers. For me, two of the best all-around timesaving tools are two things you already own: a refrigerator and freezer. With those, and a little planning, you can really save time and energy when you're short on both but still want to enjoy wholesome home-cooked foods. When you plan your meals ahead of time, you enable yourself to fix a meal in a minute, just by defrosting it and reheating it.

Here are some great ways I've found to use your refrigerator and freezer to their fullest, most timesaving capacity.

Cook ahead. Double your recipes and freeze the extra for another day. If you have some extra time, make a batch of spaghetti sauce or dishes that freeze well, like stews, soups, or casseroles such as lasagna or Eggplant Parmesan (see page 303).

Pre-portion. Immediately after cooking, place the food in individual serving containers—sealable freezer bags work great. If you plan on eating them within a few days, stick them in the fridge; otherwise, they'll keep in the freezer for up to 6 weeks (longer for soup). Defrost and reheat for a quick, easy meal.

Prepare extra basics. Whenever I cook my own burgers from ground turkey breast, I always make and freeze a few extra. With a vegetable or two and a grain or starch, this is a yummy, fast meal.

Freeze soup. I always double the quantity of a soup recipe and freeze individual- or double-size portions to have as a meal or part of a meal later on. Be aware, though, that not all soups freeze well. Don't freeze soups with potatoes in them—they get mealy and don't reheat well.

Pre-bake muffins. Muffins freeze well, so split a batch—keep some out for the next few days and freeze the rest. These muffins can be part of a breakfast on the run, a snack in the afternoon, or a dessert in the evening. (See the recipe on page 319.)

Get Real Check-In

Assess your progress by checking off each of the following items you achieved during week 4.

❏ Instant Makeover #4: I replaced the corn oil I had been using with olive or canola oil.

❏ I added one extra glass of water—I'm at my goal of 8!

❏ I achieved my week 4 mini-goals.

❏ I set my week 5 mini-goals.

❏ I reanalyzed my Food Plan and made appropriate adjustments.

❏ I cooked my first Real Food Life meal.

❏ I learned how to plan for future meals.

❏ I kept my food journal each day.

❏ I rewarded myself for my intentions and my efforts.

Weekly Words: Write a couple of paragraphs in your journal about what it felt like to cook your first Real Food Life meal. Did you like it more than you thought you would? Discuss how making this a habit will help you reach your ultimate goal.

Week Five:

FINE-TUNING YOUR REAL FOOD LIFE

During this week, you will:

- ▶ Accomplish Instant Makeover #5: Replace white or "wheat" bread with 100 percent whole wheat bread
- ▶ Follow your week 5 mini-goals
- ▶ Keep week 5 of your food journal
- ▶ Pack your own lunch
- ▶ Diversify your diet
- ▶ Add exercise to your Real Food Life
- ▶ Complete week 5 of your Get Real Check-In

"Let's do lunch!"

Who doesn't love to hear that sentence? Lunch offers a wonderful opportunity to catch up with your friends. Breaking bread bonds us to each other in a way few other activities can.

Just like other meals, lunch offers you a great opportunity to practice the principles of your Real Food Life. Packing your lunch helps you stay in control. In week 5 of your Real Food Life plan, I'll offer you numerous tips on how to lunch intelligently.

By this point, you should be eating better and finding that your new habits are feeling more familiar and comfort-

Instant Makeover #5:

Replace White or "Wheat" Bread with 100 Percent Whole Wheat Bread

Many of my new clients share the same uncomfortable malady: constipation. But within a few weeks, they're feeling regular and less bloated. Why? They've simply started eating more fiber-rich whole grains.

If you didn't already do so in your Kitchen Makeover, toss out that squishy, lifeless white bread or so-called wheat bread that's merely white bread colored to look healthier. To your body, the refined carbohydrates in these products act like pure sugar. Replace them with 100 percent whole wheat bread, which is packed with constipation-relieving fiber. Whole wheat bread also does a better job of filling you up and satisfying your hunger. Plus, it's higher in the vitamins and minerals that keep your body young and healthy.

Since you have been gradually increasing your intake of high-fiber foods for the past several weeks, your body should be used to the fiber by now. If not, try Beano to prevent intestinal distress. It really helps.

---

able. You're shopping smarter and making more sensible eating choices with your newfound knowledge and strategies. Your body should also be adapting to the better food you're giving it. You should be feeling more energetic and healthy. Celebrate the fact that you're well on your way to getting a Real Food Life!

I hope that you've also grown more adventurous in your food selections and are feeling more confident about your choices. With some well-placed inspiration and a little bit of creativity, there's no reason why your Real Food Life should ever be boring. In week 5, I'll talk about a number of ways you can diversify your diet. The world of wholesome food is a never-ending garden of riches—there is no end point,

no "perfect" diet. Continue to experiment with new foods and keep your tastebuds guessing!

Finally, we'll talk about exercise. While this book focuses primarily on foods, exercise is a huge part of your Real Food Life. Food is fuel, simple as that. Ideally, the amount of energy you take in is equal to the amount of energy you expend. On the flip side, the more energy you expend, the more choices you'll have for your Real Food Life.

In addition to burning calories, exercise has a million other immediate benefits—it drains stress from your body, makes your clothes fit better, gives you an inner buzz that's better than any drug or drink. Exercise in some form should be part of your daily life, and I'll give you lots of suggestions on how to incorporate more movement into your daily routine. Challenge yourself to find some way to move your body every second you're not sleeping, even if it's just fidgeting in your chair!

1. Pack Your Own Lunch

If there's a common element that most of us share regarding lunch, it's that we usually eat it every day. What's different is *where* we eat it. We might eat it in cafeterias, restaurants, fast-food joints, take-out stands, or simply wherever we can grab a bite.

Lunch can be a challenge if you're always relying on someone else, whether it be a restaurant or cafeteria, to keep your food needs in mind. Remember that portions at restaurants are usually much larger than what you actually need to eat—often they could take the place of two or three meals. Restaurants also ladle on sauces, dressings, and unhealthy fats that you wouldn't dream of using in your own cooking. Fast food and takeout may fit into any lunchtime break, but you can easily eat much more than you need to or will feel good about later.

Hitting the lunch circuit with friends and coworkers can also cause overeating because in our minds, socializing often equals indulgence. Friends or coworkers may unwittingly sabotage your efforts to eat healthfully. You might feel peer pressure to order or share a "bad" meal or dessert with your friends.

Packing your lunch helps you avoid these scenarios. If it has been years since you've packed a lunch for yourself, it's time to give it a try. Ideally, you should try to bring your own lunch 4 days a week.

This doesn't mean that you have to eat solo, like Cinderella stuck inside eating gruel while her sisters are out having a ball. Plan lunch dates with your friends and encourage them to order their lunch to go, and you can all eat outside in a park. Or, in a cafeteria, you can certainly share the table with buddies who have bought their lunches. When your friends see how tasty and fulfilling bringing a lunch can be, more than likely they'll start "brown bagging" it along with you.

Need more convincing? Think how full and contented your pocketbook will be. Bringing lunch can save you in the neighborhood of $1,000 a year. Save money, gain energy—seems like a good deal to me!

Keep these tips in mind to make your lunches fun and healthy.

Sandwiches. Sandwiches are generally the best and most portable lunch item you can make.

❥ During your weekly shop, buy a loaf of whole wheat bread, a pound of deli-sliced turkey breast or roast beef, a head of romaine lettuce, and a few ripe tomatoes. There are your sandwich fixings for the week. (Pack the sliced tomatoes separately to

(continued on page 208)

Lunch Lists

Agreasy cheeseburger and fries from the fast-food joint down the street. Questionable beef stew from the cafeteria. Take heart! You don't need to be tied down to unhealthy lunch choices like these anymore. Read on for a plethora of nutritious lunch options—whether you're brown-bagging your lunch, dining in a cafeteria, grabbing something at a fast-food place, or ordering takeout. There are even choices for afternoons when you want extra energy.

What to Bring

If you bring lunch every day instead of going out or ordering in, you'll save at least 100 calories a day (which translates to 10 pounds a year) and at least $1,000. Try packing some of the following healthful brown-bag options.

- Turkey or roast beef sandwich on whole grain bread, with lettuce, slices of tomato, and 1 tablespoon low-fat mayonnaise and/or mustard
- Egg salad sandwich (1 whole hard-boiled egg with 3 hard-boiled egg whites, with chopped apple and low-fat mayonnaise on a whole grain roll)
- Salad greens with 1 scoop of either egg salad, curried tuna salad, or chicken salad made with low-fat mayonnaise
- Leftovers, such as roasted chicken and a vegetable
- Peanut butter and jam on whole wheat bread
- 4 tablespoons hummus inside 1 whole grain pita bread with baby carrots and lettuce
- 1 low-fat yogurt and one blueberry Lifeline muffin (or see muffin recipe on page 319)
- 1 pint vegetable soup (Health Valley brand, or see recipe on page 281) with a whole grain roll or a salad or both
- Frozen entrées that contain fewer than 300 calories

To accompany your brown-bag lunch, try one of these tasty options: 1 cup of Pirate Booty or Veggie Booty, 1 small bag of baked Lay's potato chips or 1 small bag Terra chips, 1 small box of raisins, 15 animal crackers, or 1 piece of fruit

What to Eat at a Cafeteria

Most cafeterias offer at least some healthful lunch options—you may just need to seek them out. Here are some ideas to get you started.

- Salad bar salad (heavy on the raw and steamed veggies) with a drizzle of olive oil and vinegar or 1 tablespoon Russian dressing; with half a grilled chicken breast (about 4 to 5 ounces), or a medium-size piece of roasted chicken (4 to 5 ounces), or 3 to 4 ounces tuna, or a large spoonful of beans (not drenched in oil)

- 1 medium baked potato with a sprinkle of cheese, and a green salad drizzled with olive oil and vinegar
- 1 cup vegetarian chili with whole grain crackers
- Small portion of hot roast beef (3 ounces) with two vegetables
- Roast beef or turkey sandwich on whole wheat bread with lettuce, tomato, and mustard
- 1 veggie burger on a small whole grain roll, with lettuce, tomato, and a small pack of ketchup; a salad with a drizzle of olive oil and vinegar or 1 tablespoon Russian dressing
- 1 piece grilled or roasted chicken with ½ cup cooked brown rice (or 1 slice whole wheat bread); a salad with a drizzle of olive oil and vinegar or 1 tablespoon Russian dressing

Fast-Food Picks

Fast-food restaurants are starting to get the message that many of their customers want healthier options. Check out the following list, which includes items offered at many fast-food establishments.

- Grilled chicken sandwich (no mayonnaise)
- Roast beef sandwich (no mayonnaise or low-fat mayonnaise only) with lettuce, tomato, and mustard
- Baked potato with 2 tablespoons of cheese
- Green salad with low-fat dressing
- Veggie burger
- 2 slices thin-crust pizza (take off half the cheese and add veggies if they're available) and a salad with a drizzle of low-fat dressing
- Salad with grilled chicken
- Yogurt parfait
- For your drink choice, choose water or low-fat or fat-free milk

Safe Bets to Order In

Just because food is being delivered to your doorstep doesn't mean that it has to be un-healthful. When you call to place your order, explore what healthful alternatives might be available that aren't listed on the menu. Most restaurants will be happy to prepare something special—you just need to request it.

(continued)

Lunch Lists (cont.)

Safe Bets to Order In (cont.)

- Steamed mixed veggies with tofu, chicken, or shrimp and a sprinkle of black bean sauce or garlic sauce; small portion (½ to 1 cup) brown rice
- 2 sushi rolls (12 pieces) (maki) with green salad and a cup of miso soup or 1 cup of edamame
- Grilled chicken breast paillard with chopped green salad and 1 tablespoon olive oil and lemon juice with a small whole grain roll
- Pasta e fagioli (pasta and bean soup) with a green salad dressed with a little olive oil and lemon or vinegar and a small low-fat bran muffin
- Grilled chicken fajita made with 2 small tortillas (just a dab of sour cream or omit it altogether) with 1 tablespoon guacamole, lettuce, and tomatoes
- 2 slices thin-crust pizza (with half the cheese removed) and a mixed salad

Lunches to Energize

These lunches are low in complex carbs and high in protein, so they won't make you feel sleepy after eating them.

- 8 ounces (the size of 2 decks of cards) grilled fish (salmon and tuna are especially good choices); sautéed vegetables
- 1 Unfried Chicken Breast (see page 311) with steamed veggies and tzatziki (garlic and herb yogurt) dressing
- 1 Turkey Burger (see page 297) in a small whole wheat pita with a green salad
- 1 cup chicken and walnut salad (with 1 tablespoon low-fat mayonnaise) on lettuce with whole grain crackers
- 1 serving Roasted Vegetables (see page 267) with leftover barbecued flank steak (about 3 ounces) with one slice of whole grain toast
- 1 can Health Valley vegetarian chili and a green salad

keep your sandwiches dry during the day.)

❱ Keep a jar of all-natural peanut butter and low-sugar jam or fruit spread on hand. A bonus: PB&J sandwiches don't need to be refrigerated.

Salads. Salads offer a great way to get a bunch of your vegetable servings at one time.

❱ Pre-bagged lettuce is simple for instant-gratification salads.

▶ Toss in some baby carrots, slices of cucumber, and some cherry tomatoes. Then add tofu, leftover chicken, or canned tuna.

▶ Rinsed canned beans, like kidney beans or chickpeas, give salads staying power.

▶ Be sure to add a whole wheat roll for a perfect balance of carbohydrates that will keep you going strong all afternoon.

Leftovers. Often what was just okay the night before will be a treat for lunch the next day.

▶ Keep that leftover pasta. Any addition of vegetables and high-quality protein, such as chicken, meat sauce, or baked tofu, will make it filling and delicious. You can even eat it cold!

▶ Make a large pot of soup on the weekend and bring it with you to warm up in the microwave for lunch through the following week.

▶ When you make dinner, make extra for yourself for the next day's lunch. That goes for vegetable dishes as well as main courses.

Convenience foods. Instead of relying on the vending machines or take-out stands, make your own fridge a convenience shop.

▶ Add easy-to-pack lunchtime foods to your shopping list: freshly sliced turkey, cooked chicken, precut carrots, hummus, single-serving packs of applesauce, nuts, and fruits and vegetables are always great to bring along.

▶ Reusable microwave- and freezer-safe plastic containers are the lunch-packer's best friend. Use these to carry your food with no fear of spilling, and reheat it in the same container.

▶ Buy yogurt and cottage cheese in individual serving sizes to take with you.

▶ Fruit is the perfect fat-free lunch dessert. It's wrapped in its own natural packaging, generally comes in a single-serving size, and is sweet enough to use as a dessert.

Packing tips. A little preparation is the key to making your packed lunch appealing at any hour.

▶ Pack your lunch the night before and stick it in the fridge. You'll spare yourself one extra task during your morning rush.

▶ Wash and cut up a mound of different raw vegetables and store them in the refrigerator. When you're packing lunch, place a few handfuls in a sealable plastic bag (with low-fat salad dressing, hummus, or fat-free black bean dip in a small sealable container), and you have an easy, healthful snack or lunch side dish.

▶ If you have access to a microwave, check out healthful varieties of frozen organic or vegetarian dinners. All you have to do is heat and eat, giving you extra time for a walk or to run errands over lunch.

▶ The night before, cook one or two soy or vegetable burgers or hot dogs and bring them in the next day with crackers. Or if you have access to a freezer and microwave at work, just pack the frozen burgers or dogs and cook them right before eating.

2. Diversify Your Diet

Eating a rich assortment of healthy foods is the fun and pleasurable cornerstone of any Real Food Life.

Because you're adjusting your eating habits, a natural instinct is to start limiting yourself to a few reliable foods that fit your program and are easy to make. But if you don't explore your possibilities, you put yourself at risk of getting into an eating rut. And if you get into a rut, you're more likely to be tempted by a high-calorie food because you feel you owe yourself some pleasure for all the drudgery you've endured.

In addition, every food has its own set of nutrients, so eating many different types of foods will ensure you're getting the widest possible variety of vitamins and minerals. So if you find yourself looking at the same meals day after day, mix it up. Here's how:

Experiment! Take a food that you enjoy and try a new recipe for preparing it. Start with some of the recipes beginning on page 259. If you always gravitate toward grilled chicken, for example, try your chicken roasted, baked, or slivered into a salad.

Include fish in at least two meals a week. If you have a hard time preparing fish for yourself, order it each time you eat out and see which varieties you enjoy the most. Then, try variations on these themes at home. Fish tastes great when it's prepared simply, and it cooks quickly, so it's the perfect food for your Real Food Life.

Add zing with different spices and flavorings. For a whole new taste sensation, add different spices, herbs, or flavorings to your usual dishes. Curry powder, five-spice powder, paprika, cumin, hot sauce, and low-sodium soy sauce are some of my favorite flavor boosters. Adding curry powder to canned tuna along with low-fat mayonnaise, apples, and raisins creates an entirely new, zesty type of tuna salad. Tiptoe through your cookbooks to find new recipes using new flavors that still fit into your Food Life.

Add new greens. If you've never had dandelion greens or kale, give them a try. Wash the leaves and cut off tough stems, chop the leaves, and then steam until wilted. Place in a bowl and season with lemon juice, a drizzle of olive oil, and a dusting of black pepper. Then toss well. Greens are delicious and brimming with nutrients.

Satisfy your sweet tooth with kiwifruit. Not only is kiwifruit sweet and tangy, but this fuzzy green fruit has more vitamin C than an orange. Or how about a mango, a candy-sweet and filling tropical fruit? You can even try new fruit combinations blended into smoothies. Strawberry-banana or blueberry-peach are two great combinations.

Go international! Have you ever eaten hummus? I love this Middle Eastern bean dip. (You may have noticed I can't stop talking about it!) It's usually available in the refrigerator section of most supermarkets, near the cheese and other dairy foods. Or try my recipe on page 284. Sample some with sliced tomato and whole wheat crackers for a tasty, satisfying snack or light lunch.

Spruce up your salads. Add chopped walnuts, raisins, pears, or apples. They'll add a new dimension in taste and texture to your usual bowl of lettuce. Also, try a different dressing than usual (see the recipes on pages 262 and 263 for some ideas).

3. Add Exercise to Your Real Food Life

Your body was meant to operate. Your legs are there so you can walk or run. Your arms aren't just attachments dangling from your body—they're to help you swim and lift weights. If you want your arms, legs, heart, and lungs to last for a long lifetime, you have to give them work to do.

Regular exercise also relieves stress, helps you sleep better and longer, and makes you feel better about yourself. After any workout, even a 20-minute walk, I always feel better and feel like I have accomplished something important on my own that no one can take away from me.

You'll find that exercise also goes a long way toward keeping you on track with sensible eating. Once you've made the connection between what you put into your mouth and how much energy it takes to burn it up, you'll realize that a 300-calorie soda would require you to run several miles to shed those calories.

When you exercise, you also increase your lean muscle mass. This, in turn, increases your metabolism and makes you burn more calories even when you're at rest. So this week, I want you to start moving your body any way possible, as often as possible. Simply try to incorporate as much movement into your everyday routine as you can. If you have never exercised before, call your doctor back to make sure she agrees you're ready to start doing some physical activity (she'll probably sing out a hearty, "You bet!").

Any movement, even a 5-minute walk, is better than sitting still. Exercise helps you live longer, feel healthier, and have more energy than any other single activity you could do, including several of the huge changes you've made in your eating plan. Do it today.

Here are some creative ways to slip some exercise into your routine.

▶ Walk everywhere that's less than a mile away, provided it's a safe, well-lit route.

▶ If walking all the way isn't possible, park your car before you get to your destination and walk at least 10 minutes from your car and 10 minutes back.

▶ Get up into the attic, down into the basement, or out to the garage and give it the cleaning you keep meaning to do. It's not work now—it's exercise!

▶ Similarly, get out in the yard and pull weeds, prune, or do any other gardening activity.

Kitchen CURES

Ease Sore Muscles with These Simple Strategies

Whether you overdid it at the gym, spent the day rearranging furniture, or got involved in any other activity that made your muscles ache, check out the pointers below. They'll ease the ache and help you to prevent soreness in the future.

- Sore muscles mean that your muscle fibers have torn. This is a natural and desirable state that prompts muscles to repair themselves and become stronger. Overly sore muscles aren't good, however. Working out to the point where your muscles are achingly sore actually slows down the healing process and, of course, prevents you from continuing your exercise regimen.
- Work out different muscle groups on different days, so that each group gets a day of rest between workouts.
- Protein helps repair muscles and aids in the healing process, so eat a little extra protein when your muscles feel sore.
- Treat yourself to some fresh pineapple. Bromelain, an enzyme found in pineapple, can help the healing process.
- Calcium and magnesium help repair connective tissue and the skeletal system. Be sure to eat foods that contain both of these nutrients. Try low-fat or fat-free dairy foods, seafood, soy foods, and nuts and seeds.
- Antioxidant-rich foods can help speed up the muscle-healing process, so have some dark green, leafy vegetables; legumes; oatmeal; asparagus; avocados; mangoes; or tomatoes.
- On days you work out, drink an additional 4 to 5 cups of water (yes, that means 12 to 13 total cups); it may help relieve soreness later.
- Don't forget to stretch your muscles. Stretching helps to maintain flexibility and relieve soreness.

▶ Always use the stairs instead of the elevator. If you're really adventurous, try doing the steps two at a time—it will help build muscle.

▶ Carry your baby instead of using the stroller.

▶ Go dancing. Hit a disco and step out to your favorite tunes from the 1970s and 1980s.

Or go the opposite direction and try a ballroom dancing class.

❿ Go roller-skating or swimming. If it has been years since you've tried either of these, you might have forgotten how much fun they are. Be sure to wear protective gear when you pull on those skates, though.

❿ Hop on your bike instead of getting into the car if you're going relatively short distances. Again, put on that helmet.

❿ Try yoga. This ancient exercise method combines meditation, breathing, and stretching in ways you never tried before, unless perhaps you carpool in a Volkswagen Beetle.

❿ Join a gym and hire a trainer to develop a personalized program for you. This way, you'll get personalized instruction on how to use the equipment, and the trainer can teach you fun routines you might never have discovered otherwise.

❿ If you already have a gym membership, simply experiment with a new machine or piece of equipment on your own each week. Be sure to read the directions first or get help from a staff member.

❿ Follow an exercise video. This is an easy way to sweat off some pounds in the comfort of your own home. You can choose step aerobics, martial-arts routines, abdominal exercises, or countless other styles. Use it at least three times a week.

❿ Find an exercise partner. Draft a friend, coworker, or family member to join you in your quest for fitness. Having someone expecting your company can motivate you when you're feeling sluggish, and having a friend along will make the time pass more quickly.

Get Real Check-In

Assess your progress by checking off each of the following items you achieved during week 5.

❑ Instant Makeover #5: I replaced white or "wheat" bread with 100 percent whole wheat bread.

❑ I achieved my week 5 mini-goals.

❑ I set my week 6 mini-goals.

❑ I packed my own lunch.

❑ I diversified my diet.

❑ I added exercise to my Real Food Life.

❑ I kept my food journal each day.

❑ I rewarded myself for my intentions and my efforts.

Weekly Words: Write a couple of paragraphs in your journal about how your reassessment of your goals last week affected your behavior this week. Do you feel reinvigorated? Discuss how checking in regularly with your mini-goals will help you reach your ultimate goal.

Week Six:
REFINING YOUR REAL FOOD LIFE

If eating were a sport, you'd be going pro right about now.

That doesn't mean you're eating a lot or even that quickly. Just like an athlete, you've developed highly sensitive techniques to make the most of the natural power of your body. By the time you enter week 6 of your Real Food Life, you've mastered most of the skills we nutritionists (or coaches!) hope our clients will embrace. If certain hurdles have stood in your way in the past— cravings, binges, unhealthy choices— you've since sailed over them with ease, once and for all.

You have more energy, your skin and hair feel and look better, you're

Instant Makeover #6:

Replace one cup of coffee with one cup of green tea

Even if you're the biggest java junkie and green tea isn't one of the brews you would normally choose, you owe it to yourself to give it a try. If you're currently drinking a lot of coffee—or soda—each day, replace just one of those servings with a cup of green tea.

This drink, made from the unfermented leaves of the tea plant, is milder and less bitter than black tea. It has half the caffeine of coffee, and drinking a cup or two per day may reduce your risk of cancer. In fact, a cup of green tea offers you as many health-enhancing antioxidants as one or two servings of vegetables.

Keep a stash of green tea bags handy, and walk right on past the steaming coffee pot or quarter-gobbling soda machine. At the end of the day, you'll have taken in less nerve-jangling caffeine and reinforced your protection against disease.

---

more alert, and you have a better overall sense of well-being. You know that accepting responsibility for your food choices increases your ability to make other changes you desire. You may not realize this about yourself, though.

That's the purpose of week 6—to review your plan thus far, remind yourself of how far you've come, and regroup for the future. First, let's look at the history of your food journal.

1. Compare Your Food Journal from Weeks 1, 3, and 5

For a humble little notebook, your food journal is really a powerhouse of information. As your constant companion for the past 5 weeks, your journal has helped you learn about your cravings and energy dips, understand the importance of portion control, even out the imbalances in your diet, and gain more control and energy in your Real Food Life. Not bad for less than $5!

Let's review three key weeks in your journal, so you can see how far you've come, realize how much you've learned, and readjust your program for the next 3 weeks. (You can either just think about these questions or write your answers to them in your journal.)

Week 1: Remember that during week 1, you were just observing your former food life, your personal eating style, and any shortfalls in nutrition. Normally my clients are blown away by the difference a mere 5 weeks makes. Prepare yourself—it could be a bit surprising.

❯ What kinds of breakfasts were you eating? Were they loaded with sugar? Were you eating breakfast at all?

❯ What kinds of lunches were you eating? Did you *ever* bring your own lunch? Did you frequent the drive-thru or the deli?

❯ What happened during the afternoons? Were you snacking on chocolate or quaffing loads of coffee?

❯ What did dinners look like? Huge wads of calories, drenched in heavy fat sauce? Nary a trace of fresh vegetables or quality protein?

Week 3: By week 3, you'd started implementing changes into your plan. You did your Kitchen Makeover and went grocery shopping. Perhaps your journal already reflected some changes, large and small.

❯ How often did you eat out in week 3?

❯ Were your meals after the Kitchen Makeover different from the ones before it?

❯ Had you already begun eating more balanced meals (for example, more lean proteins if you were a carbohydrate-based eater, or more high-quality carbohydrates if you were a protein-based eater)?

❯ Had you settled into a loose schedule that felt good for your type (three-squares style or grazing style)?

❯ Had you begun setting (and keeping) mini-goals?

Week 5: Now look at your journal from this past week—do you notice a big difference?

❯ What foods had you eaten before that are now entirely absent? Why?

❯ What foods have been showing up a lot more often? Why?

❯ How many meals did you prepare for yourself in week 5 versus week 3? Versus week 1? What do you notice about the nutritional quality of those meals versus the takeout or restaurant food that used to take its place?

❯ Have you noticed a difference in your energy level? Your bathroom habits? Your cravings?

❯ Have your mini-goals affected your eating habits since week 2?

❯ Are you making progress toward your ultimate goal?

The biggest change my clients typically notice at this point is how many of the foods they used to eat regularly have been replaced with more wholesome, nutritious, and balanced foods. Congratulate yourself on this accomplishment because it's a big step toward achieving your Real Food Life. Changing your Food Life takes energy and thought, and you should know that you are well on the way to feeling even better and more alive and making choices with positive health benefits.

2. Review Your Ultimate Goal

Sometimes my clients are real overachievers—they find halfway through their

Food Life Plans that they've already achieved their ultimate goals.

I'm kidding, of course. There's nothing "over" about this—in fact, there's nothing stopping you from making and achieving hundreds of ultimate goals. In fact, continual goal-setting is a good principle to take with you beyond the Real Food Life plan. Goal-setting, in eating and in the rest of life, keeps us in touch with what we really want. It's a great way to help us measure current choices, feel accomplished, and remain enthusiastic about healthy habits. Instead of "giving up" decadences that may taste or feel good in the moment, you're gaining all the personal power—and energy and vitality— that comes from controlling your own Real Food Life.

When my clients achieve their first goal, I counsel them to immediately create a new goal, one that will keep them motivated until the end of the program and beyond. Look back to week 1's quiz and see if there are other issues you'd like to tackle. Perhaps you started out wanting more energy, but now you want to get serious about weight loss. Perhaps you've already lost a few pounds, and now you want to tackle your sugar addiction.

Don't worry—you still get "credit" for your first goal! Turn to the first page of your journal. Next to the ultimate goal, write "ACHIEVED." Draw a star or smiley face next to it—something to denote that you set a goal

and achieved it. And most important, *give yourself your reward*. Whatever you planned at the beginning, make sure you do it now. (This is a critical, often-skipped step in the program, but I urge you to do it. Nothing reinforces good habits like promises kept to yourself.)

Underneath your first goal, write down your next ultimate goal, and pick a new, completely different but equally enjoyable reward for this one. You can continue doing this kind of goal-setting motivation with yourself for the rest of your Real Food Life. Think of this as your body's extra credit—with no limits!

3. Eat More—Strategically

This one sounds easy, huh?

As I recommend with all my clients at this point in the food program, I want you to start adding a little more food to your eating plan. If you have experienced some weight loss in the first few weeks, at this point you may reach a weight plateau. However, even if you haven't been trying to lose weight, now is the time to increase the number of calories you consume.

Many of us were raised with a diet mentality that told us if fewer calories were good for weight loss, almost none would be better. Nothing could be farther from the truth. Remember, when you eat too few calories, your body wants to conserve energy and so slows everything down—especially your metabolism. You don't want your body to conserve energy. You want your body to know there is a constant supply of energy coming in so it will always burn calories efficiently.

Note: If you're comfortable with your food amounts and don't want to add extra food, this isn't a required component of getting a Real Food Life. My experience, however, is that people enjoy additional food—go figure!—especially when it leads to additional energy and no weight gain.

Start with favorites. Choose a food group you love and can't get enough of, like complex carbohydrates. Take this opportunity to try something you've been neglecting because you didn't want to use your precious allotment of servings—perhaps a new whole grain like bulgur wheat.

Branch out. If you started out as a primarily carbohydrate- or protein-based eater, try branching out into the other side. Many people who start off in one camp find their tastes changing as their bodies do.

Enjoy your weekends. If you eat a mostly balanced and wholesome diet during the week, your body has learned to efficiently process the food. Eating just slightly more—no more than 200 extra calories—on the weekends will tell your body to work extra hard to burn those extra calories.

On page 158, we discussed what a serving of carbohydrates or protein is, so remember: Adding one more serving daily to your food intake isn't a license to overeat.

4. Look at Daily Food Issues

As you continue on with your Real Food Life, you might come up against some challenging eating situations. Brimming with nachos, cookies, or fountains of cocktails, social gatherings are often food-centric, chock-full of staples of your old food life that no longer fit in your plan.

For those key moments when you find yourself dealing with more of these challenges than you'd like, I've collected some surefire strategies to keep your plan on track. Two tricks that work no matter what the occasion: Before you go, review your goals, envision the situation you're about to walk into, and mentally practice what to eat to stay within your plan. Second, by all means, don't "save your appetite" for the party—in fact, do the opposite. Have a snack. Arriving full and satisfied will make those cheese puffs a lot less appealing.

Remember, your Food Life is your own. By week 6, you have a very clear picture of how good you feel when you eat wholesome foods. Use that feeling to motor your body past those cheese puffs.

Meals at a Friend's or Family Member's House

Good times, good friends, good food—they all seem to go together. When the gang's all here, there can be enormous pressure to fit in and eat what everyone else is eating. Here are some strategies to help you stay in control.

(continued on page 222)

LIVING A
REAL FOOD LIFE

This Corporate Executive Exercised—And Ate—
His Way Back to Health

Name: John
Real Food Life Issues: weight gain, exhaustion, indigestion

John is a workaholic financial executive in his mid-thirties. His competitive industry dictated his 14-hour workdays. Like many workaholics, he regularly used food as a stress-reliever and coffee as a stimulant. He ate when he felt tense, he ate at meetings, he ate when the stock market went up or down, and he ate and drank when he went out with his friends or business associates, which was at least three times a week. Here's where I found him:

August 25

I am so glad to be home in the air conditioning. Just the walk from the office building to my car is so disgusting in this heat—I sweat, my legs rub together. I feel like I'm going to pass out. To make matters more humiliating, my pants barely fit me anymore. I had to slip out of a meeting sideways a few days ago because I was afraid the seam in the seat was about to give.

I don't know what my problem is. It's not like I'm doing anything differently. I might not have been addicted to peanut M&M's back in college, but I sure drank a lot more beer! I'm dreading my high school reunion. I know people are going to come up to me and say stuff like, "Hey, looks like you're not starving in finance!" Well, screw 'em. I work hard, I play hard. That's the way the system works. You don't get to where I am spending your whole day at the gym.

When I met him, John was used to eating whatever was around, or whatever was fast—and a lot of it, at that. Since his life revolved around work, he no longer found the time to go running, to go to the gym, or to play tennis with his friends. Between the volatile financial market, no time to eat properly, and long hours sitting in an office, John gained 20 pounds in the few months before he came to see me. His weight gain caused his blood pressure to go up, decreased his energy level, and exacerbated his chronic indigestion.

After he turned over his food journal to me, I noticed that John was a serious coffee junkie and he drank hardly any water—both of which contributed to his indigestion and promoted dehydration. The dehydration, in turn, resulted in a lack of energy. John's first Real Food Life change was to cut back on coffee to no more than 2 cups a day and to increase his water consumption to at least 8 cups a day, with a cup or two of green or ginger tea to help with his indigestion. Two weeks later, his chronic indigestion was practically eliminated.

Then John focused on cutting out the hot dogs, pizza, and other fast foods that tempted him around his office and on his way home from work late at night. He replaced his usual snacks with a few pieces of fresh fruit and a handful of nuts, which satisfied his hunger but also gave his body vital nutrients without loading up on bad fats.

Since snacking was a major part of John's life that he wasn't willing to give up, we devised a bunch of healthy, energy-producing snacks that he could reach for in times of hunger (and, occasionally, when particularly stressed). His snack list included hummus with whole wheat crackers and baby carrots, canned low-fat soup, and leftover chicken and vegetables (which he really loved). All of these filled his belly, gave him energy to keep going, and kept him satisfied.

To also help with his energy level, especially in the morning, I suggested that John eat breakfast. So for the first time in years, he ate a morning meal, usually in the form of a low-fat yogurt, fresh fruit, and a piece of whole wheat toast with jam and a little low-fat cream cheese. He quickly recognized that breakfast did give him energy all morning long.

He also came to realize that stress at work and lack of sleep were major factors in his overeating and tiredness. First he left 15 minutes earlier, then half an hour earlier, and then an hour or so. He also started sleeping 6 to 7 hours a night instead of his usual 4 to 5. Plus, he began exercising. He had a weekly tennis match with a friend and also started running once a week. He then added a weekly workout at the gym. The exercise not only helped him sleep better but also relieved much of his anxiety.

Within 4 weeks of starting his new food life, John had more stamina, experienced less stress, and wasn't constantly eating. By the end of 8 weeks, he had lost 17 pounds, his blood pressure was almost back to normal, his indigestion was gone, and he had energy to spare.

▶ Whatever the menu is, be prepared and plan your food intentions. For example, tell yourself, "I'm going to have only cut-up veggies with a little dip and a glass of wine before dinner. At dinner, I will eat very small portions of the healthiest items being served. I'll stop eating when I'm comfortably full."

▶ Don't let anyone bully you into eating something you don't want. If someone puts food on your plate that you didn't want, leave it. If they get annoyed, tell them you're trying to stick to an eating plan and that you'd love it if they could support and respect that.

▶ Compliments go a long way—begin them early and continue often. Talk about how great the food smells, rave about the first few bites, and slow down when you've had enough. If someone comments on what's left on your plate, simply say, "I wish I could eat more!" Let them assume you mean you're absolutely stuffed.

Holidays

The holiday season need not result in an all-or-nothing feeding frenzy. A little mental preparation will keep you on course.

▶ Remember that no food is taboo. You can eat any holiday food you want as long as you keep yourself accountable in your food journal and the portion sizes remain in keeping with your Real Food Life eating plan.

▶ Create a plan of action before you go to holiday gatherings. If holiday meals whip you into a food frenzy, before you get there write down your food intentions and the strategies you will use to combat the eating situations.

▶ Overhaul your favorite recipes to make them fit into your food life. Many times old favorite recipes can easily be "retooled" to fit into your new style of eating. If you can't redo it yourself, check the December issue of the women's or cooking magazines—the story of cutting fat from holiday favorites shows up every year.

▶ The best defense is a good offense—prepare your counterstrike by bringing food with you to homes or parties you know will not offer any options that fit in with your plan. You can sample the other dishes, but eat your own food in abundance and without compromise.

Traveling for Business

You don't have to remain a prisoner of the mini-bar or dinner cart. Prepare for your Real Food Life the way you'd prepare for your trip—plan ahead and pack well.

▶ Before you go, buy some wholesome foods you can take with you on the plane, train, car, or bus. Portable snacks such as crackers, nuts and seeds, a sandwich, and dried or fresh fruits can fit into everyone's food life.

▶ Pack a meal as if you're bringing lunch to work. Any food you take along will be much better than the food available on the train or plane. Or call ahead to ask for a vegetarian or heart-healthy meal.

Kitchen CURES

Natural Fixes for Diarrhea

Diarrhea has been the topic of more than its share of jokes, but when you have a bad case of it, it's no laughing matter. Check out the following strategies for all-natural relief.

- Brown rice is binding, so it reforms stools and can calm the stomach. It can also help replenish your stores of B vitamins, which can get lost through diarrhea. Eat small portions throughout the day.
- Take an acidophilus supplement to help rebuild good bacteria in your intestines.
- Diarrhea is dehydrating, so be sure to drink at least 10 glasses of water and a few cups of green tea throughout the day.
- Chicken soup will rehydrate your body and calm your stomach.
- Ginger tea is excellent for relieving cramps and abdominal pains. Drink this soothing beverage all day long.
- Bananas and applesauce will help as well.
- Avoid dairy foods for a few days because they can aggravate loose stools.

▶ Avoid the mini-bar in your hotel room because it's there to tempt you (and make you spend too much on small indulgences). If you can't resist, give the key back to the main desk. Or call ahead or ask the check-in clerk to have the mini-bar emptied out for you. Then fill up the empty space with healthful snacks such as yogurt, low-fat cheese, seltzer water, and fruit.

▶ If the buffet is too tempting, stick to room service—especially at breakfast.

▶ Make fish your automatic selection when you eat out. Not only is it filling and nutritious, but if you're eating out a lot, you'll get to try a number of different types and preparation methods. Order vegetables along with your meal, which will also keep you satisfied.

Vacations

Sure, vacations are all about fun. But how much fun will it be to arrive back with a souvenir 5 pounds or rebound sugar cravings? Your Real Food Life should be flexible enough to let you enjoy just about any location. Enjoy yourself, but always be on the lookout for healthful choices.

▶ Foods you have successfully eliminated in your Real Food Life may be front and center on vacation. Eating a small amount of these foods is fine, but be warned: Your body may not be used to them, and they may actually make you feel sick. People who have cut back on rich foods or red meats can get stomachaches or diarrhea when they eat a lot of them again.

▶ Don't go crazy with alcohol—it dehydrates you, fills you with empty calories, and weakens your resolve. If you've cut back on drinking lately, the effects will be swift and overwhelming. At the very least, make sure you drink 8 ounces of water for every alcoholic drink you have—and exercise the following day to sweat it out.

▶ Shun ideas such as "Come on, you're on vacation, eat what you want!" Remember, you will eat all your Real Food Life choices—you just don't have to eat unhealthful foods.

A Word on Unexpected Friend or Family Hostility

As you progress with your new food life and start to feel and look great, some people—even people who love you—may become jealous or threatened. They'll show it in unexpected ways, like encouraging you to eat foods you don't include in your Real Food Life. Perhaps they will become critical of your appearance and try to sabotage your efforts at getting a Real Food Life.

Over the years, I've regularly heard variations on "My wife thinks I look too thin," "My mother doesn't understand why I need to eat before dinner," or "My boyfriend always asks me if I should be eating from my food plan."

Remember, first and foremost, this is not your issue—it's theirs. Maybe they also want to eat better and are jealous that you have been successful; maybe they think once you become healthier, you won't need them anymore. These are not rational feelings, but they are honest feelings. Lost in the confusion of these feelings, they may not even be aware that their actions are undermining your efforts.

Keeping these thoughts in mind, try not to lash out at them. Realize they are just dealing with their own "stuff," and it's not your job to help them feel better—they have to do it for themselves.

Share with them your food intentions and explain to them that their behavior isn't helping you achieve your goals. It's your responsibility to yourself to speak up and tell them what your needs are. After counseling many clients, I've discovered most friends and family members aren't conscious of their sabotage. After talking it out, sabotage turns into support.

Friends and family members may get upset or frustrated with you, but this is a time when you need to assert what you want. You are taking care of yourself, your health, and your food life—those who love you will eventually come around. They may even join you.

Get Real Check-In

Assess your progress by checking off each of the following items you achieved during week 6.

❏ Instant Makeover #6: Each day, I replaced a cup of coffee or soda with a cup of green tea.

❏ I achieved my week 6 mini-goals.

❏ I set my week 7 mini-goals.

❏ I compared my food journal from weeks 1, 3, and 5.

❏ I reviewed my original goals and realized what I've accomplished. I retooled my goals as necessary.

❏ I devised a plan for eating more.

❏ I examined some food issues.

❏ I kept my food journal each day.

❏ I exercised for at least 10 minutes on 3 separate days.

❏ I rewarded myself for my intentions and my efforts.

Weekly Words: Write a couple of paragraphs in your journal about what it felt like to look at some key friend and family food issues. Were there any situations that really popped up? Discuss how being honest and assertive with your close friends and family will help you achieve your ultimate goal.

13

Week Seven:

DINING OUT IN YOUR REAL FOOD LIFE

During this week, you will:

▶ Accomplish Instant Makeover #7: Replace your afternoon coffee or sweet with a 10-minute walk and a healthful snack

▶ Follow your week 7 mini-goals

▶ Keep week 7 of your food journal

▶ Devise a Real Food Life dining-out strategy

▶ Read guidelines for ordering at restaurants

▶ Devise your own junk food strategy

▶ Add a food you've been fearing to your eating plan

▶ Exercise for at least 15 minutes on 3 separate days

▶ Complete week 7 of your Get Real Check-In

When we first see each other, many of my clients confess an overdependence, even an addiction, to restaurant food. And, really, who doesn't love to eat out? You sit down and people literally *serve* you. No wonder everyone who's stressed on a regular basis—from stay-at-home moms to CEOs—loves the indulgence of dining out.

Yet, once you've spent a couple of weeks on the Real Food Life plan, you may be justifiably wary about straying back into restaurants again. "They're full of fat!" I hear you saying. "Think of the portions!"

Sure, sure, think of all that. But

Instant Makeover #7:

Replace Your Afternoon Coffee or Sweet with a 10-Minute Walk and a Healthful Snack

Why exactly are you eating that midafternoon chunk of cake or piece of chocolate? Sure, it gives you a nice treat to sweeten a dragging afternoon, and maybe it gives you a bit of energy to see you through until dinnertime. But it's sure not contributing to a Real Food Life.

Instead, take yourself in a different direction by heading out the door for a 10-minute walk. The exercise will firm your legs and backside and strengthen your heart and lungs.

Breathing some fresh air and getting blood pumping through your body during your jaunt down the street or around the block is almost guaranteed to perk you up more than that sugary snack would have.

When you return from your walk, have a healthful snack such as half a cantaloupe, half a small honeydew melon, or a low-fat bran muffin with a bit of almond butter. The combination of a 10-minute walk and a nutritious snack will help you sail through the rest of the afternoon.

---

your Real Food Life is just that—a *life*. You still have to get out there and live it.

That's why we're focusing this week on how to handle the curves and steep cliffs of even the trickiest menus and the most tempting junk food. It's all a question of balance and choices. Every menu has at least *one* thing that fits in with your plan. Below you'll discover the treasure map to finding it.

1. Dine Out Using Real Food Life Strategies

By week 7, I'm sure you've already gone into restaurants. Maybe you scoured the menu, trying to find something that would fit in your plan. Maybe you thought you'd nailed it, and then your skinless breast of chicken showed up in a bath of butter.

Never fear—you have many weapons in your arsenal. Your power as a restaurant patron lies in your order. Take time to do it well. Try a few of these tricks for getting *exactly* the foods you want in restaurants.

Prepare Your Plan of Attack

It's amazing how much trouble you can get in even before your ordered meal hits the table. Take a proactive stance against the unhealthful food assault catapulting in from all sides.

Spoil your appetite. Before you leave for

dinner, eat something substantial like a bowl of soup, a piece of leftover chicken, a piece of toast with low-fat cheese and leftover vegetables, or a yogurt with fruit and nuts. If you're following your Real Food Life at home, no matter what you eat, it will never be equivalent in calories and fat to an indulgent restaurant appetizer.

Know where you're going. Become familiar with the dining guidelines for different kinds of restaurants (see page 230) and try to know what you're going to eat before you even walk in the door. Don't let the menu sway you. If you've been to the restaurant before and you can resist the temptation, don't even open the menu. Order what you'd like and let the waiter sort it out. It's your meal—have it *your* way.

Avoid the bread basket. The bread basket is one of the leading culprits of overeating at restaurants. I almost always send it back, because out of sight is out of mind. If that sounds horrible to you, take one slice of bread and enjoy it with your meal. Just keep in mind that bread can tack on an additional 500 calories, not even including the butter or olive oil that usually accompanies it.

Limit yourself to one alcoholic drink. Alcohol, whether in the form of cocktails, wine, or beer, can weaken your resolve for exercising thoughtful moderation with your food. Plus, it dehydrates you and doesn't give you any nutritional benefit. So, when you go out, try to limit yourself to just one drink— or order a bottle of fancy water instead.

Drink water. Bet you've never heard this from me before. (Ha!) I know I'm sounding like a broken record, but drink water before, during, and after every meal, regardless if it's at a restaurant, at home, or anywhere else.

Place Your Order with Confidence

Many of my clients start out being intimidated by waiters. They worry that they're holding the waiter up with their questions and requests. Don't be shy about questioning the waiter. And don't worry about wasting his time—it's his job.

Be constantly aware of portion sizes. Trust me: You won't need an appetizer and an entrée in many restaurants today. Some restaurants have been known to serve up to *seven* times the normal serving size for a meal.

Plan to leave food on your plate—or have the waiter wrap up half of the portion before your serving even comes to the table. Appetizers are generally more realistic portion sizes. Look for your favorite and order it as a meal with a side salad, or order two appetizers—one that is more vegetable-based.

Ask, ask, ask. And continue asking. Is it fried? What kind of sauce comes with it? What sides are served with each dish? Can I get brown rice instead of white?

Always request sauces and dressings on the side. When you do this, you'll realize how little sauce and dressing you really need.

Don't order something new when you're very hungry. If you do, you'll likely order too much food, you'll probably overeat, and you'll regret it later. If you're starving, order a standby that you know is good for you (see the list below).

Order plenty of vegetables. Get a large mixed salad, or order vegetables sautéed in a little bit of olive oil or steamed with sauce on the side (so you can lightly dip them in the sauce).

Sip some soup. Soup is a good high-volume food that will fill you up. Look for vegetable, broth-based, and bean soups. Avoid cream-based soups and chowders.

Finish with a Flourish

Don't put down your guard after the waiter scurries off to the kitchen with your order. You'll still need to exercise some caution when your perfectly ordered meal arrives in front of you.

Stay alert. It's easy to get caught up in an engaging conversation and eat everything on your plate without even thinking about it. So stay alert. After you've eaten your allotted amount, have the waiter wrap up your leftovers. The bonus is that you have lunch (or dinner) for the next day already prepared.

Finish up meals with refreshing green or herbal teas. Ginger tea can help with digestion, and green tea is good for your overall health. Many restaurants are now serving a variety of exotic teas, so help yourself to some! Some teas are so fruity that they're a perfect replacement for dessert.

2. Know What You're Up Against: The Restaurant Guidelines

Here are some tried-and-true tips for ordering at specific types of restaurants. These suggestions will help you keep your food life right on track.

American

Appetizer Recommendations

▶ Steamed asparagus or artichoke
▶ Mixed salad (with vinegar or lemon juice and olive oil dressing on the side)
▶ Shrimp cocktail
▶ Vegetable-based soups
▶ Grilled vegetables (light on oil or without it)
▶ Steamed mussels in a light broth
▶ Melon
▶ Fruit salad

Main Course Recommendations

▶ Grilled fish or chicken with a small sweet potato or rice
▶ Grilled chicken breast with a large salad (sauce and dressing on the side)
▶ Grilled or roasted chicken or turkey breast sandwich
▶ Grilled shrimp with rice
▶ Pasta and tomato sauce (appetizer portion)
▶ Roast chicken
▶ Roast beef
▶ Barbecued chicken breast with a baked potato (try eating half the portion)

BEST BITES

Top Foods to Keep in Your Desk or Locker

When you get an attack of the midday munchies, feast on one of the foods listed below. It will keep you humming along through the afternoon.

- Nuts and seeds—particularly soy nuts
- Dried fruit
- Any fresh fruit
- Whole wheat crackers or rice cakes and all-natural peanut butter
- Pop-top canned tuna packed in water
- Ginger tea and green tea
- Robert's American Gourmet Pirate Booty or Terra chips (small bags)
- Carrots

- Steamed vegetables and rice dressed with lemon juice or vinegar and olive oil
- Grilled tuna or swordfish steak with a small portion of rice and lightly steamed vegetables
- Grilled whole fish with herbs (no oil or butter)
- Grilled filet mignon with grilled vegetables
- Vegetarian chili with a small bowl of brown rice
- Large salad (with beans, sprinkle of cheese, and 1 hard-boiled egg, and dressed with lemon or vinegar and olive oil)

Chinese

- Try to get your own small bowl of steamed brown rice.

- Eat small amounts of food along with the rice.
- Ask for no MSG in your food.
- Use only low-sodium soy sauce.
- Drink water before, during, and after the meal.

Appetizer Recommendations

- Steamed shrimp, chicken, or vegetable dumplings
- Steamed vegetable bun
- Steamed spring roll with rice paper
- Grilled vegetable sticks (satay or skewers)
- Grilled chicken sticks (chicken satay or chicken skewers)
- Small bowl of hot and sour or wonton soup (if you're sensitive to salt, you might want to avoid this)

Main Course Recommendations

- Grilled shrimp
- Steamed fish in ginger sauce (try to have very little sauce)
- Peking-style chicken (remove excess fat and skin)
- Steamed shrimp or chicken with vegetables (sauce on the side)
- Dry-sautéed string beans (take from the beans at the top of the pile when served to avoid all the sauce)
- Steamed Chinese broccoli with oyster sauce on the side
- Steamed scallops with sauce on the side
- Steamed mixed vegetables and tofu with sauce on the side
- Stir-fried bok choy, spinach, broccoli, or other green with garlic

Indian

- Avoid curries at all costs—they're made with coconut milk and butter (ghee) and are loaded with saturated fat.
- Do not order samosas, poori, or paratha. These are loaded with oil.

Appetizer and Main Course Recommendations

- Small portion of raita (yogurt and cucumber)
- Mixed salad
- Chicken and vegetable kabob
- Rice pilaf (small portion)

- Dal (lentils)
- Tandoori chicken, fish, or vegetables
- Chicken or fish tikka
- Naan bread (a small portion)

Italian

- When you sit down, don't eat bread; in fact, have the waiter remove it from the table.
- Drink water before, during, and after the meal.
- Order an appetizer-portion for your main course.

Appetizer Recommendations

- Mussels in a light tomato broth
- Mixed salad (with balsamic vinegar or lemon juice and olive oil on the side)
- Grilled mixed vegetables (light on oil)
- Seafood salad (light on oil)
- A small portion of pasta with tomato sauce (eat only half an entrée portion)
- Caponata (have only a small amount if it is very oily)
- Grilled portobello mushrooms
- Steamed artichoke or asparagus with dressing on the side
- Minestrone soup
- Pasta e fagioli (pasta and bean soup)

Main Course Recommendations

- Pasta with shrimp or chicken in tomato sauce
- Pasta with clams in tomato sauce

- Pasta with mushrooms, peas, and beans in tomato sauce
- Grilled salmon or red snapper (no oil)
- Grilled chicken breast with salad or cooked vegetables (no oil)
- Gnocchi in a light tomato sauce
- Half a vegetable pizza with a very small amount of cheese
- Shrimp marinara

Japanese

- Ask for low-sodium soy sauce.
- If the restaurant offers brown rice, order that instead of the white rice.
- Fresh lemon juice or rice wine vinegar are tasty, low-sodium alternatives to soy sauce for dressing sushi, sashimi, or salad.
- The avocado in sushi rolls is a great way to get some good fat.

Appetizer Recommendations

- Steamed vegetable, chicken, or shrimp dumplings
- Japanese salad with seaweed (dressing on the side)
- Yakitori (grilled chicken skewers)
- Edamame (cooked fresh soybeans)
- Oshitashi (cold boiled spinach salad)
- Tofu with soy dressing

Main Course Recommendations

- Soba noodles (made from buckwheat) with sauce on the side

- Sushi and sashimi (all kinds)
- Grilled fish or chicken (no soy sauce)
- Steamed vegetables with chicken or seafood
- Beef negimaki (grilled beef slices stuffed with green onion)

Mexican

- Avoid sour cream and cheese.
- Pass up nachos, chimichangas, and taco salads since all of these are loaded with saturated fats.
- Eating some guacamole is fine—but limit your chips to about 10.
- Avoid dishes made with ground beef or ground pork.
- Avoid refried beans unless they're low-fat (they are often made with beef or pork fat).
- Many Mexican restaurants use beef or pork fat even in vegetarian dishes, so be sure to ask, and order accordingly.

Appetizer and Main Course Recommendations

- Vegetarian chili (lard-free)
- Soft taco stuffed with grilled chicken, with salsa, lettuce, and tomato (with a sprinkle of cheese but no sour cream)
- Soft taco with bean or vegetable filling (make sure the filling is low-fat)
- Vegetable or chicken burrito with rice and beans (with a sprinkle of cheese but no sour cream)

Kitchen CURES

Banish a Bad Mood

When you're in a foul mood, do yourself—and those around you—a favor by following the tips below.

- Start exercising! Working out releases endorphins, brain chemicals that naturally help lift moods.
- Carbohydrates release serotonin, a mood-enhancing brain chemical. So try some brown rice, quinoa, fruit, or vegetables.
- If you're on a high-protein diet, get off it now. The lack of carbs—as well as the general lack of variety in food choices these diets entail—will throw off your energy level and put you in a bad mood.
- Make sure you're getting enough calories. Eating fewer than 1,500 calories a day will decrease your energy level and put you in a bad mood.
- Essential fatty acids—especially omega-3's—protect the nervous system and may lift your mood. To take advantage of these beneficial fats, top your next salad with a handful of nuts or seeds and some extra-virgin olive oil.
- Caffeine can make you irritable and moody if you drink too much, so cut back on caffeinated beverages or cut them out of your diet completely. Reduce your intake gradually, though, to avoid headaches and fatigue, two common withdrawal symptoms.
- Cut back on sugary foods. They can jumble up blood sugar levels and create huge mood swings.
- The B vitamins play a role in your moods. Take a B-complex vitamin or eat foods containing the Bs, such as bananas; avocados; fish; beans; eggs; and dark green, leafy vegetables.

▶ Chicken or beef fajita (with only a little fried onions and peppers)

▶ Chicken or vegetable quesadilla (with a sprinkle of cheese)

▶ Grilled chicken with lemon and rice

▶ Grilled chicken salad with dressing on the side

▶ Grilled shrimp with rice

▶ Sliced roast pork (a small portion with sauce on the side and the fat cut off) with rice and beans

Middle Eastern

▶ Avoid falafel, or limit yourself to only one fritter (they're delicious, but they're deep-fried).

▶ Order whole wheat pita bread (if available).

▶ Limit pita bread to one.

Appetizer and Main Course Recommendations

▶ Bean salads

▶ Stuffed grape leaves (avoid if they're extremely oily)

▶ Stuffed tomatoes

▶ Tabbouleh (bulgur wheat and herb salad)

▶ Hummus (chickpea dip)

▶ Baba ghanoush (eggplant dip)

▶ Mixed vegetable salad (with lemon and a sprinkle of olive oil)

▶ Grilled chicken or fish and rice

▶ Fish, chicken, lamb, or vegetable kabobs

▶ Couscous (small portion)

3. Devise a "Junk Food" Strategy

It lurks. In vending machines, at gas stations, in supermarket checkouts, at almost every coffeehouse, and even on your coworker's desk—everywhere, surrounding us at all hours of the day, is junk food.

Of course, junk food may be in the eye of the beholder. What I consider to be junk food may not be what you consider to be junk food. Since I'm the nutritionist, I'll define it my way—by reading the label. Simply put, if you feel you'd need a chemistry degree to identify more than five of the ingredients that are listed on the label, the item is probably junk food.

Choosing "Good Junk"

We can't ignore processed foods—we do live in the real world, after all. In fact, I actually like some of them. They're convenient and often taste really good. Throughout this book, I recommend certain processed foods. But the ones I approve of are generally less harmful to your health than others.

In general, stay as close to nature as possible. Many packaged foods are very processed, so be careful and read the labels; see what's in them and then decide if you want to eat them. Can they boast of any fiber or soy?

People often turn to junk foods because they crave a flavor or a texture and they think nothing else will satisfy. Instead of the usual junk, try one of these more healthful options.

▶ If you crave sweet and creamy, try a low-fat yogurt, a cup of sorbet, or a Tofutti pop.

▶ If you crave sweet and chewy, try some dried fruit—it's nature's candy.

▶ If you crave crunchy, try baby carrots or edamame.

▶ If you crave salty and crunchy, try all-natural pretzels, dried vegetables, or lightly salted roasted pumpkin seeds (called pepitas in many markets).

▶ If you crave burgers or hot dogs, try vegetarian soy alternatives. Many people don't notice a big difference in taste.

Where you can, try to find healthful alternatives to what you crave. If you miss the chips on the side, try thinly slicing pears or apples for that crispy crunch that goes well with a sandwich. All foods do fit into a Real Food Life, so if you have a craving, just be smart. If it's a food you wouldn't typically regard as healthful, go easy on it—you'll feel better later.

4. Add a Food You've Been Fearing

I see it all the time with my clients—people are very "afraid" of certain food groups and go out of their way to avoid eating from that group. A huge part of having a Real Food Life is feeling confident to eat from any food group (unless, of course, you are a vegetarian and don't eat meat, or if you're allergic to a food group).

Carbohydrates for Protein Lovers

Attention, protein lovers: Carbs aren't evil. Carbohydrates are the body's major source of energy and the only source of fuel for the brain and muscles. Foods with carbs can also be great sources of fiber, which is necessary for optimal functioning of the digestive system.

To get more carbohydrates in your diet, start adding 1 slice of whole wheat bread, 2 whole wheat crackers, or a cup of whole grain cereal to your meal plan each day for a week. Gradually add an additional serving of complex carbohydrates each day for a week until you feel comfortable both physically and emotionally. When you find the amount that feels good to you, stick with it. Everyone, even the protein lover, needs a bare minimum of 2 servings of complex carbohydrates every day.

Proteins for Carbohydrate Lovers

Carb crunchers often forget that protein is the basic building material for the brain, heart, muscles, blood, skin, hair, and nails and is essential for growth and development.

Start with a few small servings of protein each day. For example, have a cup of beans or cooked fresh soybeans (edamame) plus a small piece of chicken or lean beef each day for a week. Or have an egg and a slice or two of low-fat cheese every day for several days (try to limit the eggs to no more than seven each week, or four if you have diabetes or high cholesterol or are overweight).

Even carb lovers should have a minimum of 4 ounces of protein each day. Eating this amount of protein will mean that you'll be less sore after exercise and you'll feel satisfied longer after a meal. Adding a small handful of nuts and/or seeds each day will also help you get some protein with the added bonus of essential fatty acids.

Big Meals for Grazers

Grazers are often pleasantly surprised to find that when their bodies are well-nourished, they can process and digest larger meals without any problems. Don't be afraid to try eating a large meal once in a while. You may even discover that a larger meal actually suits you when you are so busy you don't have the time or access for your regular mini-meals.

Quality Protein from Plant Sources

I often see that vegetarians get a majority of their daily calories from fruits, vegetables, and grains, unconsciously avoiding protein. Because grains are quick, easily available, and contain some protein, vegetarians often rely on them, not realizing that they might not be getting as much high-quality protein as they need.

Try to have a daily 4-ounce serving of tofu—flavored, plain, cooked or not. This satisfying, quality vegetable protein source is nutritionally equivalent to meat—without the saturated fat. Another way to get quality plant-based protein is to have a meal of whole grains and legumes, such as low-fat beans with brown rice (see recipe on page 286). You should also try a protein- and calcium-filled low-fat regular or soy yogurt as part of a meal or a snack a few times a week.

Don't Fear Fat

Fat has gotten a bad rap. Fat helps stave off hunger, makes food more appetizing, and— oh, yeah—allows the body to function.

While saturated animal fats such as those found in full-fat dairy products and fatty cuts of meat, trans fats, and hydrogenated fats can all promote chronic health problems, most vegetable fats actually promote good health. Get a little daily fat, even if you're watching your weight. Just make sure it's the right fat.

You'll find that it's easy to incorporate health-boosting omega-3's into your diet each day with the following tips.

▶ Try some all-natural nut butters such as walnut, almond, or peanut butter.

▶ Eat fish three or four times a week.

▶ If you prefer, get your omega-3's from canned fish such as sardines, salmon, or tuna.

▶ Try one of the easy fish recipes from this book each week.

▶ Soybeans (edamame) or roasted soy nuts, wheat germ, walnuts, flaxseeds (freshly ground) or flaxseed oil, and pumpkin and sesame seeds all have omega-3's.

▶ Choose eggs enriched with omega-3's, if they're available in your market.

To incorporate monounsaturated fats into your diet, try the following foods.

▶ Olives and olive oil, almonds, and peanuts (and almond and peanut butter) are rich in monounsaturated fat.

▶ The avocado is a fruit that's treated like a vegetable, and it can supply a part of your

(continued on page 240)

LIVING A
REAL FOOD LIFE

She Overcame Her Fear of Protein— And Gained Energy in the Process

Name: Melissa
Real Food Life Issue: fear of protein

Melissa is in her midtwenties and works long hours at her job in the fashion design industry. In her field, there is a high priority on being thin and good-looking, and she is determined to maintain this standard for herself. Her diet was very poor, however, and as a result, her hair was thinning and falling out, her skin was very dry, and she lacked muscle tone even though she worked out several times a week. She felt tired and hungry all the time. Here's where I found her:

> *April 18*
>
> *This afternoon, I was in a stall in the ladies room when I heard my boss come in with the shoot manager to check their hair before going into a big meeting. My boss started shredding the new receptionist, calling her "bubble butt" and cackling about how she'd probably applied her makeup with a putty knife. Please God, don't let her be saying the same things about me! I have been so good, following this vegetarian diet I found on the Internet, but I'm getting so frustrated! All I want to do is lose a measly 5 pounds, and then I have to look at that plastic-y Carlotta—who you just KNOW had lipo—while everyone tells her how good she looks! I can barely get through the day as it is—how can I eat even less food? But then I think about my boss and "bubble butt" and I'm scared to put a single thing in my mouth . . .*

Melissa confessed that she didn't have time to cook for herself. She was also afraid to eat many different types of food because she thought everything, especially fish, chicken, and meat, would make her gain weight. I immediately identified two things Melissa would need to do to get a Real Food Life: She had to start eating better foods for her overall health, and she needed to realize that high-quality protein wouldn't make her gain weight.

After Melissa kept a food journal for a week, it was easy to see that she ate very little protein and virtually no fat or oil, which is a key source of essential fatty acids. Most of her calories came from carbohydrates such as fruits and vegetables, which she thought would keep her thin since they contained hardly any fat. She was scared that protein and fats would cause her to gain weight and make her "out of control" with food.

After reviewing her journal, I helped Melissa understand the importance of eating from all food groups. Usually my clients need a push in the fruits and vegetables department, but Melissa was just the opposite. She needed to incorporate a variety of foods into her diet, and while vegetables and fruits were certainly a part of that, they wouldn't be able to supply her body with all the essential nutrients it needs. Because many of her meals were eaten outside of her apartment, we focused on foods she could enjoy that were easy to find. Since she loved vegetables, we explored salad bars, and I pointed out easy, complete meals that were also nutritious and that would help her maintain her energy level and make her feel better. She also stocked up on wholesome snacks to keep at her desk so she could eat throughout the day without having to focus on three main meals.

We gradually added a little protein to her diet in the form of beans, soy foods, and low-fat cheese, which she ate in small amounts throughout the day to keep her hunger in check. This also got her used to eating a greater variety of foods. We then added some nuts, seeds, and a little olive oil to her daily food plan. Nuts and seeds took some time for her to get used to, so we started with just two walnuts a day and increased the amount until she felt comfortable eating a handful daily. By week 3, we added 3 to 4 ounces of canned tuna or poached shrimp to her daily eating plan. She had forgotten how much she loved both of these.

Within 4 weeks, Melissa noticed that she had much more energy, which helped her get more out of her workouts. She had more vigor during and after her long workday. Melissa also noticed that she had started craving more balanced meals. Soon she was adding tuna and grilled chicken to her salads. She also soon realized that her balanced diet didn't make her gain weight at all. In fact, by week 8, she became aware that she woke up with more energy than she had had in years, and she saw her body finally becoming more toned. She loved that meals now satisfied her for hours after eating. She also noticed that her hair was shinier and her skin was more supple and moist. Most important, she felt more confident about her food life—and better about herself.

daily fat. Add some avocado to your salad, or mash some on a slice of whole wheat toast with or without low-fat mayonnaise (regular or canola) and sliced tomato.

Finally, experiment with different oils.

▶ Try using a few drops of toasted (dark) sesame oil in your cooking or salad dressing. It adds a sweet, typically Asian taste (this oil is intense, so you don't need a lot).

▶ I put a teaspoon of walnut oil on my salad; it has a mild nutty flavor.

▶ Use canola or extra-virgin olive oil to lightly sauté vegetables such as baby carrots, broccoli, zucchini, and cauliflower.

▶ Dress steamed vegetables with a little high-quality extra-virgin olive oil.

▶ Oils do become rancid after 6 months to a year, so unless you're feeding a lot of people, buy small bottles.

▶ To preserve their flavor, oils should be kept out of the light and away from heat. Store them in a cool cupboard or in the refrigerator to extend their shelf life.

Get Real Check-In

Assess your progress by checking off each of the following items you achieved during week 7.

❑ Instant Makeover #7: I replaced my afternoon coffee or sweet treat with an invigorating 10-minute walk and a healthful snack.

❑ I achieved my week 7 mini-goals.

❑ I set my week 8 mini-goals.

❑ I read the guidelines for ordering at restaurants.

❑ I ate out using the Real Food Life strategies.

❑ I learned how to eat junk food.

❑ I added a food I was afraid of—and survived!

❑ I kept my food journal each day.

❑ I exercised for at least 15 minutes on 3 separate days.

❑ I rewarded myself for my intentions and my efforts.

Weekly Words: Write a couple of paragraphs in your journal about what it's like to feel educated in restaurants. Does it limit your options? Does it make the whole experience less of a mystery? Discuss how learning these strategies will help you achieve your ultimate goal.

Week Eight:
EMBRACING YOUR REAL FOOD LIFE

14

You like fish, right? I've certainly talked about its benefits enough. Perhaps you know the maxim: "Give a man a fish, and he'll eat for a day. Teach a man to fish, and he'll eat forever."

Week 8 is all about making sure you have the fish on the line.

For the first 7 weeks, we've laid the foundation for your Real Food Life: You've learned your carb/protein quotient, your meal style, your favorite eating times, the foods you crave and why. You've examined your Real Food Life from every angle—except the ones that haven't popped up yet.

That's where week 8 comes in.

Instant Makeover #8:

Replace Two Meat-Based Meals with Bean-Based Meals

If you barged into many homes around the world at meal time, you might be surprised to see that the food dishes in many cultures don't revolve around a pile of burgers or fried chicken or pork loin. Instead, you'll see lots of beans, vegetables, grains, and the like—with maybe just a bit of meat as a treat or a condiment, not the main course.

Bring good health—and some international flair—to your own table by replacing two meat-based meals with meals that use beans as their main dish. Think south of the border: a zesty, spicy chili, full of kidney beans and chunks of tomato. Or Mediterranean: a bowl of hummus, topped with a bit of olive oil and dotted with ripe olives, which you can dip out with pieces of pita bread. Your options are endless.

By doing this, you'll be cutting out sizable amounts of saturated fat, which is the bad, artery-clogging fat found in meats. You'll also be offering your body plenty of great bean-based fiber, which helps fill you up with fewer calories and keeps your digestive system working well.

Together, we'll look at some of the traps that ensnare new Food Lifers, and I'll give you strategies to escape from them. We'll develop a Real Food Life ritual that will help to reconnect you to your goals and remind you why you set them in the first place. And finally, we'll create an action plan, so you can go forth and conquer what's left of your food demons, confidently and permanently.

But first, take a moment to really savor this accomplishment. You've devoted 2 months of your life to taking responsibility for everything you put into your body. You are probably enjoying the fruits of your labor with more energy, greater mental focus, and better control over your emotions. Congratulations!

1. Discover Your Personal Traps and Outsmart Them

As you move ahead in your Real Food Life, you may be faced with new challenges. Since we're getting close to the end of your 8 weeks of coaching, I want to make sure you are well-fortified to deal with some challenges you might face now or in the future.

Even though you're nearing the end of your first 8 weeks, your life in the coming months will certainly present some food challenges you haven't thought of yet. I see this with clients all the time—after several months of working with me, they may have difficulty with one or a couple of aspects of their food lives. That's perfectly normal. A Real Food Life isn't rigid; it's adjustable and constantly evolving.

In your journal, right now, write down this sentence: "All challenges are manageable." When you come up against a challenge in the future, revisit this rule. Make the challenge concrete by writing about it in your journal. Then focus on just one challenge every week or two.

Keep reminding yourself that it may take time to overcome challenges—you may not even conquer them for good, but you can contain them and find strategies to live with them. Try out some of these strategies for dealing with common food challenges.

Trap #1: You Don't Have Time for a Real Food Life

First of all, you *do* have time. I don't care if you are the President, you always have time to take care of your food life. What you need is to figure out what's standing in your way, and then deal with each issue one by one. Ask yourself these questions:

▶ Do you eat out too often and find you make bad food choices? Reread chapter 13 and think about if your problem occurs before, during, or after ordering.

▶ Are there too many temptations in your daily life? Use your food journal to help you decipher those temptations. Reread pages 35 to 41 for tips to combat emotional eating.

▶ Is it hard to find foods that fit your food life and that your family likes, too? If you feel like you're cooking twice, once for yourself and again for your family, you are probably overwhelmed by the time you're spending in the kitchen. Explain why you have made the changes you have and ask for your family's support, whether it be helping you with the cooking or simply being willing to try new things.

If you have time for a bad food life, you have time for a Real Food Life. It just takes time to form your new habits. Train yourself to acknowledge that every food decision is about taking care of your body and your emotions. Once you do, finding time for your food life will come automatically. Don't give up.

Trap #2: Eating Enough Fish Is Difficult

Yes, there was a lot of bad fish served in the 1970s and early 1980s. Get over it. It's time to discover how good fish has gotten.

In the past decade or so, fish has really taken off. A booming "fish farming" industry has made fresh fish available to local markets, and the quality has vastly improved. Here are some great strategies for fitting more fish into your diet.

(continued on page 246)

Living a
Real Food Life

The Pounds Came Off—And His High Cholesterol Plummeted—When He Changed His Way of Eating

Name: David
Real Food Life Issues: carbohydrate addict, overweight, high cholesterol

David is in his midforties and has his own consulting business. He can make his own hours, so he can work out daily. Nevertheless, when we met, he was carrying an extra 30 pounds and had suffered from back problems caused by the extra weight. David came to see me very reluctantly. The only reason we met was on the orders of his doctor, who told David that unless he lowered his cholesterol and triglyceride levels, he would need to go on medication. Here's where I found him:

March 19

Beat Nate at handball again today. He really needs to work on his serve. I tried to show him how to get a better spin on it, but he just brushed me off. I guess that made him think he could lecture me about water. The way he slugs down liter after liter, you'd think we were stuck out in the desert somewhere. He said I was going to get sick if I didn't rehydrate. Poor sap–I didn't have the heart to tell him water was going to make him blow up like a balloon.

When we met, David said this would be the only time he would see me. I convinced him to keep a food journal for a week and come back to me at least once more. When he sent over his journal, I saw that most of his meals were big portions of fat-free refined carbohydrates, such as cereals, baked goods, and spaghetti. He wrote in his journal that he always felt hungry. He told me he ordered in most of his meals—even his breakfast of a bagel with jelly and a banana and his dinner of pasta and tomato sauce. His afternoon snacks were often half a box of cereal. Other than his daily banana, he ate no fruit, and he ate hardly any vegetables or high-quality protein. He also consumed virtually no fats or oils. Most alarmingly, *David drank no water at all* because he believed water would bloat him and cause him to gain more weight. The only things he did drink were a cup of coffee in the morning and a diet soda in the evening.

When he came back to see me, I shared the analysis of his food journal. When I told him that by making changes in his diet, he could really improve his health, he shrugged. With a little more goading, I finally convinced him to change his food life for just 8 weeks. I told him he had nothing to lose, except some of the extra weight and the bad cholesterol levels. So, with that, he complied hesitantly.

First, I asked him to take a daily multivitamin and a B-complex supplement to help protect against high homocysteine levels. My next suggestion was to increase his water intake dramatically. Since he wasn't used to drinking water, we had to do this gradually. During the first week, he had just 1 cup a day; for the second week, he drank 2 cups a day and so on. It wasn't until week 6 that he finally came to understand why water was important to his overall health and energy. At first he called twice a week to make sure the water wouldn't cause him to gain weight; he now drinks at least 10 cups a day and recognizes that drinking a lot of water makes his workouts more productive.

Next, I had him pull out all his delivery menus. We went through each of them, and I showed him how to order sensible dishes and how to eat realistic portions. I had him cut way back on refined carbohydrates and replace them where he could with whole grains. We also added protein to each meal. For example, instead of the bagel, jelly, and banana breakfast, I now had him order a hard-boiled egg, whole wheat toast, and a fruit salad. Instead of dinners of pasta and tomato sauce, I had him order the flattened grilled chicken breast topped with arugula, tomatoes, and lemon juice.

Instead of half a box of cereal for a snack, David began to eat whole grain crackers with hummus or even a single bowl of cereal with fresh fruit cut into it. He also started eating a salad every day dressed with olive oil and lemon, and he ordered grilled fish dinners. And always, David would try to leave about half of what was delivered to him on his plate.

By week 8, David had lost 15 pounds and his back pains had subsided almost completely. Further, when his cholesterol and triglyceride levels were checked a month later, they had come down enough for his doctor to hold off on the medication. David realized that his new food life made him much less hungry and his fears of protein and water were almost gone. He also realized that the changes in his diet he had been so loath to try really improved his health and sense of well-being. Now, 20 months later, David has happily stuck with his new way with food.

▶ Even if you don't cook fish at home, order it whenever you go out for dinner.

▶ Canned tuna is just about the easiest fish there is. Open a can, drain it, chop up some green onions or celery, add a tablespoon of low-fat mayo, and voilà! A fish lunch or dinner.

▶ If you really cannot abide any seafood at all, be sure to eat other sources of omega-3 fatty acids and monounsaturated fats. Enriched eggs, soybeans, and nuts and seeds and their oils all have some form of these necessary and "good" fats.

Trap #3: Vegetables Are Too Much Work

Is breathing too much work? Vegetables are as essential for a Real Food Life as oxygen. They are chock-full of nutrients that you need for good living. You should strive for at least 5 servings daily. Here are some tips to help you work more vegetables into your Real Food Life.

▶ Use frozen vegetables! They're already cleaned, cut, and ready to use. All you have to do is steam, microwave, or lightly sauté them in olive oil with a little garlic.

▶ Chop up a ripe tomato and cucumber, dress with 2 teaspoons of olive oil and balsamic vinegar, and there you have it: a vegetable salad (which counts as at least one or two servings).

▶ Buy bags of prewashed, cut romaine lettuce. Open up the bag, pour in a tablespoon of olive oil, a healthy dash of lemon juice or vinegar, and as many herbs and spices as you want. Shake. You have an instant, perfectly coated salad. Toss in some sliced peppers, and you'll have a few servings of vegetables!

▶ Buy prewashed and peeled baby carrots, grape tomatoes, and chopped cauliflower and broccoli from the salad bar. If time or expense are your stumbling blocks, figure out a way to get over that—veggies are worth every second and every cent you spend on them.

Trap #4: There's No Time for Breakfast

You know you need to give your metabolism a kick start in the morning with breakfast. If you feel too taxed by your morning routine to eat, try these quick and easy ways to fit breakfast into your Real Food Life.

▶ Take a piece of fruit, a yogurt, or a muffin (see the recipe on page 319) with you to eat in your car or on the train or bus.

▶ Toast a piece of whole wheat bread and top it with a slice of low-fat cheese. Toasting bread takes 3 minutes.

▶ Pour a cup of dry cereal into a bowl. Add fat-free milk. This is the definition of fast food.

BEST BITES

Top Foods to Eat before a Big Exam

Bone up on the following superfoods, which may help you to think more clearly and focus more intently for that big exam.

- Fish: grilled, sautéed, poached, or canned
- Brown rice
- Nuts and seeds
- Sweet potatoes
- A variety of mixed vegetables, either in a soup or salad
- Avocados

▶ If you really can't stomach food in the morning, try drinking breakfast. Smoothies or soy shakes are the perfect way to get wholesome nutritious food without ingesting anything too heavy.

▶ Reheat and eat leftovers from last night's dinner. Sure, it's odd, but it's a quick and tasty way to get a morning meal.

Trap #5: You Still Feel Hungry All Day

If you still feel hungry by week 8, you need to find foods that will satisfy you. Consult your journal and see what types of foods you're eating and how long they sustain you before you're hungry again. Focus on the foods that keep hunger at bay for the longest amount of time, and experiment with eating those types of foods. Also, try these tips.

▶ Make sure it's not dehydration that you're feeling. Always drink at least eight 8-ounce glasses of water each day.

▶ Your diet may be too low in fat, so check your intake. If you're hovering at the lower level, this may be making you hungrier faster. (Nut butter on an apple or whole wheat bread is a quick, healthy way to get some good fat.)

▶ You may not be getting enough protein. Protein lingers in your stomach longer than carbohydrates alone, so be sure to eat a little protein with your carbohydrates to keep yourself feeling fuller, longer.

▶ Add more high-water and high-fiber snacks to your eating plan. Try a cup of soup, melon, berries, yogurt, tomatoes, cucumbers, asparagus, broccoli, carrots, or high-fiber cereal with milk.

Trap #6: Regular Exercise Is Hard

Many people find exercise to be their Real Food Life Achilles' heel. If they work long hours or have many commitments, exercise will often take a backseat in their lives.

▶ If you feel overscheduled, make an appointment in your calendar to exercise and don't break it. Then you'll stop trying to "fit it in," because it will be right there, in your schedule.

▶ Set exercise as one of your mini-goals every week. Start by setting a goal of exercising just once a week. Then—here's the critical part—just do it. Put one foot in front of the other until you walk around the block. Next week do it twice. And so on.

▶ Take classes at the gym that will keep you interested in exercise. You might discover you really enjoy yoga, Pilates, spinning, or weight-lifting classes. Make friends—just knowing people at the gym will help keep you exercising.

▶ Walking, running, and many other solitary exercises are great for clearing your head. If your exercise time doubles as your private mind-clearing alone time, that's okay. We're all time-pressured, and free time must often serve double duty.

▶ Hobbies can be exercise, too. Gardening, biking, running around the yard with your children, walking in the park, even walking around the mall is exercise. Just keep your body moving.

▶ An exercise partner—a spouse, pet, or friend—can make time pass more quickly while you are exercising and will keep you motivated to stick with it.

2. Give Yourself Your Ultimate Reward

You have worked hard and have probably achieved your ultimate goal—maybe even several of them—by now. No matter how often you reach and surpass your goals, take the moment to give yourself the reward you promised yourself when the goal was set.

It's easy to brush it away and pretend it doesn't matter, but what you've done is nothing short of revolutionary. Seize this revolutionary spirit and forever burn it in your brain with the reinforcement of the reward you promised yourself at the outset.

Many of my clients are tempted to forgo this part—don't! Get out there and buy yourself that new dress or CD player. You earned it, you deserve it.

3. Establish a Real (Food) Life Ritual

Many of my clients really become attached to their weekly check-ins. They like the idea of a quiet oasis of time in their otherwise hectic

Kitchen CURES

Solve Your Energy Crisis

When you're so tired you feel like you need someone to pick you off the couch, try one of these natural pick-me-ups instead. You'll be surprised by the extra energy you gain.

- If you're feeling lethargic, drink lots of water. It hydrates your cells, prevents dehydration, and provides instant energy.
- Avoid sugary foods, including most so-called energy bars. After giving you an initial burst, sugar will stop energy dead in its tracks.
- Carbohydrates provide almost all of the energy for your muscles and brain—so eat a variety of fruit, vegetables, and whole grains daily. When you need a pick-me-up, try eating a complex carbohydrate along with protein. Good choices include a sliced apple with a tablespoon of all-natural nut butter or a handful of nuts with a handful of raisins.
- Add foods that are rich in B vitamins to your diet. Good choices include oranges, yogurt, chicken, bananas, soybeans, and cheese.
- Graze. Eating smaller meals more often will provide a constant stream of energy. Your body will be able to use the food more efficiently, so you won't experience extreme highs and lows in your energy levels.
- Exercise. Physical activity helps blood to flow through your muscles and your brain, and it releases endorphins (which make you feel good) and hormones that provide sustained energy.
- Eat enough. Eating too few calories will make you feel tired. At the very least, you need 1,500 calories each day.
- Get at least 8 hours of sleep a night. If you're feeling particularly tired during the day, take a 20-minute nap, if possible. (Napping longer than that can leave you feeling groggy and cranky.)
- Turn the television off and read before you go to bed. Watching TV can promote active sleep, which can leave you feeling more tired in the morning.

week, time to think just about themselves, their growth, and their goals.

I'll encourage you as I encourage them—please continue. Pick a place in your house where you will try to sit every week at the same time to revisit your goals and set new ones for the coming week. If you feel that you've gotten a handle on your Real Food Life, use the time for yourself in another way.

At a time not so long ago, a Real Food Life was just one of your hopes and dreams—now it's your reality. Take these same skills and apply them to the rest of your life. By doing your check-in in the same place every week, you'll be physically reconnecting with the person who sat in that chair those many months ago. Use that person's strength to buoy you through the rest of life.

4. Create a Food Action Plan for the Future

All the pieces of your newly acquired food knowledge are really the tools of your Real Food Life. By learning what foods are necessary for the human body, figuring out which work best for you, and identifying and avoiding food "gimmicks," you have all the tools you'll need to continue your Real Food Life into the future.

Just as you learned to set mini-goals, deal assertively with food pushers, and manage temptation, you've also come to realize that a

Real Food Life is about experimenting with food, knowing your body, and using practical strategies to solve food challenges.

You've begun to recultivate your natural instinct with food, eating when you're hungry, feeding your body nourishing foods, and avoiding foods that make you feel sluggish, tired, and bloated. You are now empowered to be your own nutritionist, armed with the knowledge you need to make good food choices that need only to suit you—nobody else.

You now know that every individual has his or her own food needs and that a one-size-fits-all eating plan doesn't suit anyone. You now know how to take responsibility for your own food life because you have begun to discover what works for you and what doesn't.

To create a plan of action for your future food life, you must recognize that eating plans are dynamic and ongoing. Just as change is part of life, it is also part of your food life. Your own way of dealing with food will change and grow as you continue to listen to your body and learn about its needs. Permanent change takes time and is the result of many small changes.

Any of the tools here—the mini-goals, the ultimate goals, the Instant Makeovers, the checklists, the check-ins—any of these can help you formulate your own action program. Start at the beginning—where are you now? Where do you want to go?

I'm going to leave you with just a few

remaining strategies. You already have everything you need to succeed in the future—consider these the icing on the cake.

Continue with the principle of starting small. Try new foods by sampling. Go to a wholesome salad bar and take small amounts of new foods, including new vegetables and fruits. Take note of what you like. Many supermarkets also have healthful prepared foods. Ask the clerk for samples of new foods that catch your eye.

Don't be afraid of food. There are so many wonderful foods out there that can be part of your food life.

Try a new recipe every week. Review the recipes in this book for dishes that will fit anyone's Real Food Life. Or treat yourself to a new cookbook that is chock-full of healthful recipes that fit in with your new style of eating. Remember, this eating plan is for the long haul. You need to enjoy every bite you take.

Visit the local farmers' market. I love going to the farmers' market. Walking around admiring the bounty of fresh produce makes me happy and gives me inspiration for eating and cooking well.

Pick up this book often. Often a well-timed paragraph can answer just the challenge you've been encountering. Come back to any week if you need additional reinforcements or fresh ideas for your Real Food Life. And don't forget all the yummy recipes that are sure to keep your food life interesting.

Get Real Check-In

Assess your progress by checking off each of the following items you achieved during week 8.

❑ Instant Makeover #8: I replaced two meat-based meals with bean-based meals.

❑ I achieved my week 8 mini-goals.

❑ I kept my food journal each day.

❑ I exercised for at least 20 minutes on 3 separate days.

❑ I learned about the traps I've been setting for myself—and this time, I didn't bite!

❑ I gave myself my ultimate reward for my intentions, my efforts, and my success!

❑ I established my Real Food Life ritual.

❑ I devised an action plan for the future of my Real Food Life.

Weekly Words: Write a couple of paragraphs about what it feels like to finish. Are you proud of yourself? (You should be!) Tentative about the future? Discuss the three most important changes you've made, how they make you feel, and how they will keep you focused on what really defines your Real Food Life.

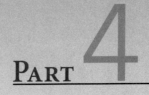

The Real Food Life
Life
RECIPES

15 THE REAL FOOD LIFE STARTER KIT

One of the most empowering steps you can take toward achieving a new food life is to begin cooking for yourself rather than relying on restaurants, take-out places, and packaged foods. Consider the recipes that follow, then, to be your starter kit for achieving and maintaining your Real Food Life: They're nutritious, they're fast, and they use *delicious*, healthful ingredients that will delight and satisfy you.

Cooking is one of the most empowering things you can do for yourself. It lets you connect with your food directly because it allows you to choose and prepare the foods you know will make your body happy. When you cook wholesome meals, you are nourishing yourself, both in body and soul. And when you cook for friends and family, you're giving them a gift of nourishment and love. Most of all, cooking should be fun! It's an activity you can share with your friends, family, and children.

If you're a novice when it comes to cooking, take a deep breath and relax. Generally speaking, cooking is not an exact science. If you do mess up a dish, it's not the end of the world—it's an education. If you make a mistake and the outcome isn't what you expected, think of it this way: It's only one dish (or one meal) out of thousands you will eat in your life, and you shouldn't accept it as a defeat. Just try again (or try another recipe). The likelihood, though, is that you won't make a mistake in the first place.

Like many home cooks, I learned to cook not by taking a class, but by reading cookbooks, watching my mom cook, and watching cooking shows. I've had my share of mistakes along the way. But I truly believe that the more you cook, the more intuitive you become with cooking. Once you gain a little confidence in the kitchen, cooking will come more naturally and you'll be able to look at a recipe and adapt it to your tastes.

I personally use all the recipes that follow, so you know that they're going to taste good! Further, these recipes have been "tested" in the homes of my clients and friends. As if that weren't enough, they were also tested by a panel of professionals to ensure that they'll work in every kitchen. I'd say that makes them pretty much guaranteed successes!

Before you begin, please read through the following pointers. They will make your time in the kitchen more pleasant and help you to work quickly and efficiently through any recipe.

◗ Before you start, read the recipe all the way through. I learned this lesson the hard way, but you don't have to. If you read the entire recipe, you know what steps you have to follow and approximately how long the recipe will take.

◗ Before you cook, have everything ready. In professional kitchens, this is called *mise en place*, which is just a French phrase meaning to be prepared. Have all the washing, rinsing, drying, chopping, and measuring done before you start, so you can cook efficiently. The pros do it, I do it, and so should you.

◗ When you're shopping, always choose the healthiest, most abundant-looking fruits, vegetables, and herbs. If a produce item doesn't look fresh, it's not. The freshest and best ingredients make the best final dishes.

◗ If the selections in the produce aisle look tired and old, use frozen produce (making sure there are no added sugars, salts, syrups, or artificial ingredients in the products you choose), substitute with related produce that looks better, go to another store, or do without. If you cook with old ingredients, your dishes won't taste their best.

◗ I love herbs and use them in practically everything. I particularly like fresh herbs—if you're used to only dry herbs, try some fresh varieties. They add a lively flavor and, well, *freshness* to everything they touch.

◗ When a recipe calls for herbs but you don't like the ones listed, feel free to substitute with herbs you do like.

◗ Whenever a recipe calls for fruits or vegetables, it is very important to wash them well under running water for at least a minute. Bacteria and dirt can cling to produce, but a thorough washing gets rid of them. There are a number of produce sprays on the market that really help clean fruits and vegetables well. They're definitely not a requirement and cost about $5 for a bottle, but they do save time and get your fruits and vegetables very clean. Look for them in the produce section of your supermarket.

◗ Before using raw chicken, red meat, or fish, rinse them very well. This will help to get rid of bacteria, which could otherwise promote food poisoning. Dry the chicken, meat, or fish with paper towels, which you then should throw away immediately.

◗ After handling raw fish or chicken, be sure to wash your work surfaces, knives, and hands thoroughly. Raw chicken in particular has a lot of bacteria, and you can cross-contaminate other foods if you use the same knife or cutting board without washing it in hot, soapy water first.

◗ I think it's fine to use canned beans in recipes. However, try to buy low-sodium or sodium-free varieties. They may not be labeled as such, but if you read the label, you can determine the brand lowest in sodium. Regardless of sodium content, beans should always be rinsed well—under running water for 3 to 5 minutes or soaked in a bowl of cold water for 5 minutes—and drained before using.

◗ Many of the following recipes call for liquid aminos. This is a chemical-free seasoning liquid protein concentrate made from soybeans. It is similar to soy sauce, but is lower in sodium, isn't fermented, and doesn't taste nearly as salty. I use it because it really does give a nice flavor to food, adding a depth of flavor to dishes without extra salt. It's sold simply as "Bragg Liquid Aminos," and it's available in health food stores and from the company's Web site (www.bragg.com).

◗ If you can't find liquid aminos, or don't want to use them, you have the option of using salt instead. When I use salt, which is rare, I use kosher salt or sea salt.

◗ Many recipes call for extra-virgin olive oil. I love the flavor, but if you find it too assertive, choose the lightest olive oil available. Many cooks use regular olive oil to cook with and extra-virgin in dressings. I use extra-virgin for everything.

◗ Many recipes call for canned tomato puree. I use this ingredient a lot because it's convenient and adds lots of body, flavor, and moisture to dishes. The brands I prefer are Muir Glen, Tutorosso, and Pomodoro. If you can't find these, try to get one without added sugars, salt, or additives.

◗ Some recipes call for vegetable or chicken broth. For canned broth, I'll use almost any type that's labeled low-sodium. For dried bouillon, I prefer Vogue brand (available at health food stores) because it's lower in sodium than most other brands. If you can't find it, try to get the lowest-sodium variety available.

▶ Many recipes call for a food processor or blender. These are great time-saving devices. If a food processor isn't in your budget, alternatives are a mini–food processor (which costs about $35) or an immersion or hand-held blender (which costs between $15 and $35). I love my hand-held blender—it makes extremely quick work of soups, shakes, smoothies, sauces, and dressings.

▶ Recipes are meant to be adjusted to suit the cook and the eaters. Tweak each recipe to suit your tastes: You love onions? Add more. You don't like bell peppers? Don't use them, or replace them with more of an ingredient you do like.

▶ Most of the recipes make 2, 4, or 8 servings. You can double the small recipes to serve more people, or cut the bigger ones in half to serve fewer. But remember, leftovers make quick meals for the next day!

Lemony Carrot Salad

6	large, thick carrots
	Juice of 1 lemon
2	teaspoons white vinegar
1	tablespoon olive oil
2	teaspoons sugar
¼	teaspoon salt
	Ground black pepper

Makes 4 servings

Per serving: 58 calories, 1 g protein, 14 g carbohydrates, 4 g total fat, 1 g saturated fat, 0 mg cholesterol, 3 g dietary fiber, 171 mg sodium

1. Grate the carrots on the wide-holes side of a box grater.

2. In a medium bowl, combine the carrots, lemon juice, vinegar, oil, sugar, salt, and pepper to taste. Toss well and serve.

Asian Sesame Slaw

1	medium head green or red cabbage (about 2 pounds)
3	large carrots (or 4 medium)
2	tablespoons sesame seeds
½	cup rice wine vinegar
2	teaspoons toasted (dark) sesame oil
2	tablespoons honey
2	tablespoons reduced-sodium soy sauce

Makes 8 servings

Per serving: 72 calories, 2 g protein, 12 g carbohydrates, 2 g total fat, 0.5 g saturated fat, 0 mg cholesterol, 4 g dietary fiber, 99 mg sodium

1. Shred the cabbage and carrots using a box grater or the shredder attachment in a food processor.

2. Toast the sesame seeds in a small nonstick skillet over medium heat, stirring often, about 3 minutes, or until the seeds start to turn brown and become fragrant.

3. In a large bowl, combine the cabbage, carrots, sesame seeds, vinegar, sesame oil, 1 tablespoon of the honey, and 1 tablespoon of the soy sauce. Toss well.

4. Add the remaining 1 tablespoon each of honey and soy sauce to taste, if desired. Refrigerate for at least 1 hour or up to 1 day before serving to allow flavors to develop.

Herbed Tomato Salad

Salad

6	ripe plum tomatoes
1	scallion (green onion)
1	small bunch fresh basil (about 1 cup of leaves)
1	small bunch fresh dill (about 15 sprigs)

Dressing

1	clove garlic
¼	teaspoon salt
	Juice of ½ lemon
1½	tablespoons extra-virgin olive oil
1	tablespoon water
1	teaspoon Dijon mustard
2	teaspoons fresh basil or ½ teaspoon dried
2	teaspoons fresh oregano or ½ teaspoon dried
	Ground black pepper

Makes 2 servings

Per serving: 99 calories, 3 g protein, 11 g carbohydrates, 6 g total fat, 1 g saturated fat, 0 mg cholesterol, 2 g dietary fiber, 55 mg sodium

1. *To make the salad:* Chop the tomatoes. Slice the scallion into ¼" pieces. Cut the stems off the basil and dill and discard. Roughly chop the herb leaves. In a large bowl, combine the tomatoes, scallion, basil, and dill.

2. *To make the dressing:* Peel the garlic and chop finely. In a small bowl, stir the salt and lemon juice until the salt dissolves. Add the garlic, oil, water, mustard, basil, oregano, and pepper to taste. Mix well. Pour 2 to 3 tablespoons of the prepared dressing onto the salad. Toss well and serve. Store leftover dressing in a covered glass jar in the refrigerator for up to 5 days.

Chunky Potato and Scallion Salad

3 medium red potatoes (1 pound)
2 scallions (green onions)
¼ cup low-fat mayonnaise
1 tablespoon fat-free plain yogurt
¼ teaspoon salt
Ground black pepper

This salad is a snap to prepare, and it boasts delicious homestyle flavor. Best of all, the fat content is reduced by using low-fat mayonnaise and fat-free yogurt instead of the traditional full-fat mayo.

Makes 4 servings

Per serving: 126 calories, 3 g protein, 20 g carbohydrates, 4 g total fat, 0.5 g saturated fat, 5 mg cholesterol, 2 g dietary fiber, 144 mg sodium

1. Cut the potatoes into 1" to 2" pieces. Place in a 2- to 4-quart pot and cover with water. Boil for 15 to 20 minutes, or until the potatoes can be easily pierced with a knife point or fork. Drain and set aside to cool.

2. Slice the scallions into ⅛" pieces.

3. In a small bowl, combine the mayonnaise, yogurt, salt, and pepper to taste. Whisk well.

4. In a large bowl, combine the cooled potatoes, scallions, and mayonnaise mixture. Toss well. Refrigerate until ready to serve, or serve immediately.

Caesar Salad

Dressing

2	tablespoons extra-virgin olive oil
1/3	cup white wine vinegar
3	tablespoons balsamic vinegar
2	tablespoons fat-free plain yogurt
1–2	small cloves garlic
2	teaspoons Dijon mustard
2	anchovy fillets (optional)
2	teaspoons Worcestershire sauce
1/2	teaspoon salt or liquid aminos
	Ground black pepper
2	tablespoons grated Parmesan cheese

Salad

1	head romaine lettuce
1/2	pint cherry or grape tomatoes

Makes 4 servings

Per serving: 112 calories, 3 g protein, 8 g carbohydrates, 8 g total fat, 2 g saturated fat, 3 mg cholesterol, 1 g dietary fiber, 402 mg sodium

1. *To make the dressing:* In a blender or food processor fitted with the chopping blade, combine the oil, white wine vinegar, balsamic vinegar, yogurt, garlic, mustard, anchovies (if using), Worcestershire sauce, salt or aminos, and pepper to taste. Blend or process until smooth. Stir in the cheese.

2. *To make the salad:* Remove and discard the outer leaves of the lettuce. Wash and thoroughly dry the lettuce. Tear or cut the lettuce into bite-size pieces. In a large bowl, combine the lettuce and tomatoes. Top with the dressing. Toss well and serve.

Fresh Vegetables and Blue Cheese Dressing

Dressing

8	ounces fat-free sour cream
1/2	cup low-fat mayonnaise
1/4	cup white wine vinegar
2	cloves garlic
1/2	teaspoon ground white or black pepper
3/4	cup (3 ounces) crumbled blue cheese

Salad

6	large carrots or 50 baby carrots
6	ribs celery
1/2–1	pound green beans
2	red or yellow bell peppers
2	cups broccoli florets
1	pint cherry or grape tomatoes

You can use any fresh or gently cooked vegetable you like. Asparagus spears, sugar snap peas, and endive are great, too.

Makes 8 servings

Per serving: 178 calories, 7 g protein, 21 g carbohydrates, 8 g total fat, 2 g saturated fat, 15 mg cholesterol, 4 g dietary fiber, 258 mg sodium

1. *To make the dressing:* In a blender or food processor fitted with the chopping blade, combine the sour cream, mayonnaise, vinegar, garlic, pepper, and 1/2 cup of the blue cheese. Blend or process for about 1 minute, or until smooth. Pour into a medium bowl. Stir in the remaining 1/4 cup blue cheese. Cover with plastic wrap and refrigerate.

2. *To make the vegetables:* If using large carrots, peel and cut into 1/2" x 3" pieces. Discard celery leaves and cut ribs into 1/2" x 3" pieces. Cut off ends of green beans. Remove seeds from the pepper and cut into 1/4"-thick strips.

3. Arrange the vegetables on a serving platter and serve with the dressing as a dip.

Greek-Indian Cucumber Salad

2 medium cucumbers
2 cloves garlic
8 ounces low-fat plain yogurt
2 ounces fat-free sour cream
1 teaspoon lemon juice
½ teaspoon salt
Pinch of dried red-pepper flakes
Ground black pepper

1. Peel the cucumbers. Halve them lengthwise and scoop out the seeds with a spoon. Cut the cucumber halves into thin slices and place in a medium bowl. Peel the garlic and chop finely.

2. In a medium bowl, combine the garlic, yogurt, sour cream, lemon juice, salt, red-pepper flakes, and black pepper to taste. Mix well. Add the cucumbers and mix well.

3. Let sit for 15 minutes and serve, or refrigerate for up to 8 hours and serve.

This salad is sort of a hybrid between the Indian raita *(made with cucumbers and yogurt) and the Greek* tzatziki *(also made with cucumbers and yogurt). It's a great dish for a hot summer night. The low-fat yogurt and fat-free sour cream provide a rich, creamy taste for just 1 gram of fat per serving.*

Makes 4 servings

Per serving: 76 calories, 5 g protein, 12 g carbohydrates, 1 g total fat, 1 g saturated fat, 4 mg cholesterol, 2 g dietary fiber, 323 mg sodium

Incredibly Tasty Mediterranean Roasted Peppers

2	tablespoons olive oil
4	red bell peppers
2	cloves garlic
16	cherry tomatoes
	Ground black pepper
1	cup fresh basil leaves

Makes 4 servings

Per serving: 90 calories, 1 g protein, 7 g carbohydrates, 7 g total fat, 1 g saturated fat, 0 mg cholesterol, 2 g dietary fiber, 6 mg sodium

1. Preheat the oven to 350°F. Coat a 13" x 9" roasting pan with 1 to 2 teaspoons of the oil. Set aside.

2. Carefully halve the red peppers, keeping the stems intact. Cut out the seeds and ribs without piercing the pepper. Peel the garlic and chop finely.

3. Arrange the pepper halves, skin side down, in the pan.

4. Place two tomatoes in each pepper half, along with a little garlic, a sprinkle of the remaining oil, and black pepper to taste.

5. Roast for 30 minutes. Remove from the oven. Add 3 or 4 torn basil leaves to each pepper half. Return to the oven and continue to roast for 15 to 30 minutes longer, or until the edges are charred and the peppers are soft but remain intact. Remove from the oven and let cool. Serve at room temperature or cold.

Roasted Baba Ghannouj

1	large eggplant
1	clove garlic
2	tablespoons low-fat mayonnaise
1	tablespoon fat-free plain yogurt
½	teaspoon ground cumin
3	tablespoons lemon juice
½	teaspoon salt or 1 teaspoon liquid aminos
	Ground black pepper
3	tablespoons chopped parsley

This recipe calls for roasting the eggplant in a 500° oven. Do not be alarmed. Yes, the oven is hot, and you might smell a little burning, but you need this hot an oven to get the rich, smoky flavor from the eggplant.

You can serve this dish as a side dish or a sandwich spread, or use it as a dip with crackers or pitas.

1. Preheat the oven to 500°F. Pierce the eggplant in several places with a fork or sharp knife. Place the eggplant on a baking sheet lined with foil. Roast for about 35 to 40 minutes, or until the skin starts to blacken and the flesh softens. Remove from the oven and let cool. When the eggplant is cool enough to handle, either scoop the flesh from the skin (it's fine if some skin is left in) or chop roughly and place in a medium bowl.

2. Peel the garlic and chop finely. Stir into the eggplant. Add the mayonnaise, yogurt, cumin, lemon juice, salt or aminos, and pepper to taste. Stir to combine, making the mixture as smooth or chunky as you like. Sprinkle with the parsley.

Makes 4 servings

Per serving: 81 calories, 3 g protein, 16 g carbohydrates, 2 g total fat, 0.5 g saturated fat, 0.5 mg cholesterol, 1 g dietary fiber, 371 mg sodium

Roasted Vegetables

3 medium yellow squash
3 medium zucchini
2 large beets, peeled
4 large carrots
1 medium eggplant
4 tablespoons fresh herbs (such as thyme, rosemary, basil, parsley, tarragon, or any combination of these) or 1½ tablespoons dried
½ teaspoon salt or dash of liquid aminos
2 tablespoons olive oil
1 pint cherry or grape tomatoes

You can include any seasonal vegetable you'd like. Mushrooms, broccoli, cauliflower, yellow and red bell peppers, and fennel are all nice options.

Makes 8 servings

Per serving: 94 calories, 3 g protein, 14 g carbohydrates, 4 g total fat, 0.5 g saturated fat, 0.5 mg cholesterol, 5 g dietary fiber, 156 mg sodium

1. Preheat the oven to 450°F. Coat a large baking sheet or baking dish with cooking spray.

2. Cut the squash, zucchini, beets, carrots, and eggplant into 1" to 2" pieces and spread over the prepared baking sheet or dish. If using fresh herbs, cut off the stems and roughly chop the leaves. Sprinkle the vegetables with the herbs and salt or aminos. Drizzle with the oil.

3. Roast for 30 minutes. Then stir the vegetables and add the tomatoes. Cook for 40 minutes longer, or until the vegetables are browned.

4. Serve immediately or let cool for about 30 minutes. Transfer cooled leftovers into covered containers and refrigerate for up to 4 days.

Layered Potato and Zucchini Pie

4	medium Idaho potatoes
4	medium-large zucchini
2	large Spanish (yellow) onions
3	tablespoons fresh basil or 4 teaspoons dried
½	cup (2 ounces) grated Parmesan cheese
¼	cup all-purpose flour
2	cans (14 ounces each) evaporated fat-free milk
½	teaspoon salt
	Ground black pepper

Makes 8 servings

Per serving: 217 calories, 15 g protein, 35 g carbohydrates, 2 g total fat, 1 g saturated fat, 9 mg cholesterol, 3 g dietary fiber, 387 mg sodium

1. Preheat the oven to 350°F. Coat a 13" x 9" baking dish or roasting pan with cooking spray. Set aside.

2. Slice the potatoes into ⅛" to ¼" pieces. Slice the zucchini into ¼" to ½" pieces. Peel the onions and cut into ⅛" to ¼" pieces. Set the vegetables aside. If using fresh basil, cut off the stems and roughly chop the leaves. Set aside.

3. Layer a third of the potatoes in an overlapping manner in the bottom of the pan. Layer a third of the zucchini on top of the potatoes. Then layer a third of the onions on top of the zucchini. Sprinkle with 2 to 3 tablespoons of the cheese, 2 tablespoons of flour, and 1½ tablespoons of fresh basil or 2 teaspoons dried. Then make a second layer of each vegetable, using half of the remaining amount, and sprinkle with 2 to 3 tablespoons of the cheese, 2 tablespoons of flour, and 1½ table-spoons of fresh basil or 2 teaspoons dried. Finally, make a third layer with each of the remaining vegetables. Top the pie with the remaining cheese and pour the evaporated milk over all. Sprinkle the salt and pepper to taste over the top.

4. Cover with aluminum foil and bake for 1 hour, or until the vegetables are tender. Remove the foil and cook for 20 minutes longer, or until browned.

5. Cool for at least 20 minutes, then cut into portions and serve. (If you don't let the pie cool first, it is difficult to serve in slices.) Transfer cooled leftovers into covered containers and refrigerate immediately.

Veggie Trio

2 medium carrots, peeled
½ red bell pepper
2 pounds fresh asparagus
1 tablespoon mustard
3 tablespoons balsamic vinegar
1 teaspoon lemon juice
1 teaspoon dried basil
1 tablespoon extra-virgin olive oil
¼ teaspoon salt

Makes 4 servings

Per serving: 115 calories, 22 g protein, 16 g carbohydrates, 4 g total fat, 1 g saturated fat, 0 mg cholesterol, 3 g dietary fiber, 201 mg sodium

1. Finely grate the carrots using a box grater or food processor. Remove seeds from the pepper and cut into ¼"-thick strips.

2. Cut off and discard the woody ends of the asparagus. Wrap the asparagus loosely in waxed paper, or place on a microwaveable dish covered with plastic wrap. Microwave on high power for about 2 minutes, or until the asparagus turns bright green and softens slightly. Remove, let cool, and cut into 1" pieces.

3. In a small bowl, combine the mustard, vinegar, lemon juice, basil, oil, and salt. Whisk well.

4. In a large bowl, combine the carrots, pepper, and asparagus. Add the dressing. Toss and serve.

Eggplant Caponata

1 clove garlic
1 medium onion
1 tablespoon olive oil
1 large eggplant
1 rib celery
3 ounces tomato paste
2 cups canned tomato puree
2 tablespoons red wine vinegar
1 tablespoon capers
1 teaspoon dried oregano
1 teaspoon dried basil
½ teaspoon salt or 2 teaspoons liquid aminos
¼ cup oil-cured olives, pitted and chopped (optional)
Ground black pepper

Makes 8 servings

Per serving: 85 calories, 3 g protein, 17 g carbohydrates, 2 g total fat, 0.5 g saturated fat, 0 mg cholesterol, 2 g dietary fiber, 504 mg sodium

1. Peel the garlic and chop finely. Peel the onion and cut into ¼" to ½" pieces. Coat a 2- to 4-quart pot with the oil. Add the garlic and onion, and cook over medium heat, stirring often, until the onion starts to brown. Add water, 1 tablespoon at a time, as necessary to prevent burning.

2. Peel the eggplant and cut into 1" chunks. Add the eggplant to the garlic-onion mixture. Cook together for about 15 minutes, or until the eggplant starts to soften.

3. Cut the celery into ¼" to ½" pieces. Add the celery, tomato paste, tomato puree, vinegar, capers, oregano, basil, and salt or aminos to the pot. Reduce the heat to low. Add the olives (if using). Cover and cook for 35 minutes, or until tender. Add the pepper to taste. Serve warm or at room temperature. Refrigerate cooled leftovers.

Pureed Sweet Potatoes

4	medium sweet potatoes
2	teaspoons cinnamon + additional to taste
2	tablespoons honey
2–4	tablespoons fat-free milk

Makes 4 servings

Per serving: 174 calories, 2 g protein, 41 g carbohydrates, 0.5 g total fat, 0.5 g saturated fat, 1 mg cholesterol, 4 g dietary fiber, 23 mg sodium

1. Peel the sweet potatoes and cut into 1" to 2" chunks. Place in a 2- to 4-quart pot and cover with water. Boil for about 20 minutes, or until soft.

2. Drain well. In a food processor fitted with the chopping blade, add the sweet potatoes, 2 teaspoons cinnamon, and honey. Process until smooth. If the mixture seems too thick, add 2 tablespoons of milk and process for a few seconds longer. Keep adding milk, by the tablespoonful, until the desired texture is achieved. Sprinkle with additional cinnamon, if desired, and serve immediately.

"Unfried" French Fries

4	medium Idaho potatoes (about 2 pounds)
1	teaspoon dried oregano
1	teaspoon dried basil
½	teaspoon dried rosemary
1–2	tablespoons olive oil
	Ground black pepper

Makes 4 servings

Per serving: 201 calories, 5 g protein, 38 g carbohydrates, 4 g total fat, 0.5 g saturated fat, 0 mg cholesterol, 4 g dietary fiber, 17 mg sodium

1. Preheat the oven to 450°F. Coat a nonstick baking sheet with cooking spray. Set aside. Fill a 4-quart pot with water and bring to a boil.

2. Scrub the potatoes well (do not peel). Cut the potatoes into ½"-thick wedges. Boil in the water for 7 minutes. Drain the potatoes and rinse under very cold water to stop the cooking process.

3. Arrange the potatoes in a single layer on the baking sheet. Sprinkle with the oregano, basil, rosemary, and oil. Coat them with the cooking spray.

4. Bake for 45 to 55 minutes, turning the potato wedges every 15 minutes, or until evenly browned on all sides. Add the pepper to taste. Serve immediately or let cool.

Roasted Rosemary Potatoes

4	medium red potatoes (about 1 pound)
2	tablespoons olive oil
5	cloves garlic, finely chopped
1	tablespoon dried rosemary
¼	teaspoon salt or 1 teaspoon liquid aminos
	Ground black pepper

Makes 4 servings

Per serving: 151 calories, 3 g protein, 21 g carbohydrates, 7 g total fat, 1 g saturated fat, 0 mg cholesterol, 2 g dietary fiber, 143 mg sodium

1. Preheat the oven to 400°F. Scrub the potatoes well. Cut the potatoes into ½" to 1" squares (irregular chunks are fine, too, as long as they're more or less the same size).

2. Coat a 9" pie plate or 8" x 8" baking pan with the oil. Add the potatoes and garlic. Sprinkle with the rosemary and salt or aminos. Toss well.

3. Bake for 20 minutes. Stir well and bake for 30 minutes longer, or until browned.

4. Add the pepper to taste. Serve hot.

Sautéed Broccoli and Garlic

1	clove garlic
1	large head broccoli or 3 cups broccoli florets
2	tablespoons olive oil
¼	teaspoon salt or 1 teaspoon liquid aminos
1	tablespoon white wine or squeeze of fresh lemon juice

Makes 4 servings

Per serving: 81 calories, 2 g protein, 4 g carbohydrates, 7 g total fat, 1 g saturated fat, 0 mg cholesterol, 2 g dietary fiber, 152 mg sodium

1. Peel the garlic and chop finely. Cut off and discard the thick broccoli stalks, leaving about 1" of stalk attached to the florets.

2. Coat a large nonstick skillet with the oil and place over medium heat. Add the garlic and cook for about 1 minute, or until the garlic becomes fragrant. Add the broccoli and cook for 3 to 4 minutes, stirring occasionally, or until the broccoli turns bright green and the stems soften slightly. Add the salt or aminos and the wine or lemon juice.

3. Serve immediately or when cooled. Transfer cooled leftovers into covered containers and refrigerate immediately.

Asian Red Lentil Soup

2	large Spanish (yellow) onions
1	clove garlic
2	tablespoons olive oil
1	1" piece fresh ginger
2	teaspoons coriander seeds or 1 medium bunch fresh cilantro
1	teaspoon ground cumin
1½	cups red lentils
1	cup canned tomato sauce
½	teaspoon salt or 2 tablespoons liquid aminos
1	teaspoon dried basil
1	teaspoon dried oregano
6	cups water

Makes 8 servings

Per serving: 112 calories, 6 g protein, 21 g carbohydrates, 4 g total fat, 0.5 g saturated fat, 0 mg cholesterol, 8 g dietary fiber, 219 mg sodium

1. Peel the onions and garlic. Chop the onions into rough ½" to 1" pieces. Chop the garlic finely. Warm the oil in a 6- to 8-quart pot over medium heat. Add the onions and garlic, and cook, stirring often, for about 10 minutes, or until the onions just start to brown. Add water, 1 tablespoon at a time, as necessary to prevent burning. Meanwhile, peel the ginger and chop finely.

2. Add the ginger, coriander seeds (if using), and cumin. Cook on medium heat for about 1 minute, or until the spices get very fragrant.

3. If using fresh cilantro, cut off the stems and chop the leaves roughly to make about 1½ cups and set aside.

4. Add the lentils, tomato sauce, salt or aminos, basil, oregano, fresh cilantro (if using), and water to the pot. Bring to a boil, then reduce the heat to a simmer for 30 minutes.

5. Puree in a blender or food processor fitted with the chopping blade, or use an immersion blender directly in the pot. Serve immediately. Transfer cooled leftovers into covered containers and store in the refrigerator or freezer.

French Onion Soup

2	large Spanish (yellow) onions
2	medium red onions
2	cloves garlic
2	tablespoons olive oil
1	cup white wine
3½	cups low-sodium beef, chicken, or vegetable broth
3½	cups water
2	teaspoons dried basil
2	teaspoons dried oregano
	Parmesan cheese

*T*his recipe depends on the browning of the onions for good flavor and color, so don't rush cooking the onions. Allow them to brown and not burn.

Makes 8 servings

Per serving: 92 calories, 3 g protein, 8 g carbohydrates, 4 g total fat, 0.5 g saturated fat, 0 mg cholesterol, 1 g dietary fiber, 279 mg sodium

1. Peel the Spanish and red onions and the garlic. Cut the onions into ¼" slices. Chop the garlic roughly. Warm the oil in a 6- to 8-quart pot over medium heat. Add the onions and garlic and cover the pot. Cook over medium-low heat, stirring occasionally, for about 30 minutes, or until the onions start to brown. Add water, 1 tablespoon at a time, as necessary to prevent burning.

2. Stir in the wine, scraping up any browned bits from the bottom of the pot. Add the broth, water, basil, and oregano. Simmer on low heat for 30 minutes. Serve immediately sprinkled with Parmesan cheese to taste. Transfer cooled leftovers into covered containers and store in the refrigerator or freezer.

Chicken Soup

4	large carrots
2	medium zucchini
2	ribs celery
1	small bunch fresh dill
1	small bunch fresh parsley
12	ounces boneless, skinless chicken breasts
1	large Spanish (yellow) onion
2	cloves garlic
2	tablespoons olive oil
2	bay leaves
1	teaspoon dried basil
1	teaspoon dried oregano
2	tablespoons low-sodium chicken bouillon granules
4	cups low-sodium chicken broth or defatted fresh chicken stock
4	cups water
	Ground black pepper

Makes 8 servings

Per serving: 126 calories, 13 g protein, 9 g carbohydrates, 4 g total fat, 1 g saturated fat, 25 mg cholesterol, 3 g dietary fiber, 298 mg sodium

1. Peel the carrots and cut them into ½" pieces. Cut the zucchini and celery into ½" pieces. Cut off the dill and parsley stems and roughly chop the dill fronds and parsley leaves (about ¾ cup each). Set aside.

2. Rinse the chicken and blot dry with paper towels. Cut the chicken into 1" pieces and set aside.

3. Peel the onion and garlic. Chop the onion into rough ½" to 1" pieces. Chop the garlic finely. Warm the oil in a 6- to 8-quart pot over medium heat. Add the onions and garlic and cook, stirring often, for about 10 minutes, or until the onions just start to brown. Add water, 1 tablespoon at a time, as necessary to prevent burning.

4. Add the carrots, celery, dill, parsley, chicken, bay leaves, basil, oregano, bouillon, chicken broth or stock, and water. Cook over medium-low heat for 45 minutes. Then add the zucchini and pepper to taste and cook for 15 minutes longer, or until the chicken is cooked through. Remove and discard the bay leaves. Serve immediately, or transfer cooled leftovers into covered containers and store in the refrigerator or freezer.

Smokin' Fish Chowder

1	large Spanish (yellow) onion
1	clove garlic
2	tablespoons olive oil
1	pound carrots
1	medium zucchini
1	yellow squash
2	ribs celery
½	cup chopped fresh dill
½	cup canned creamed corn
½	cup fresh or frozen corn kernels
1	bay leaf
	Ground black pepper
¼	cup dry white wine
¼	teaspoon salt or 1 tablespoon liquid aminos
6	cups water
¼	pound smoked trout or mackerel
½	pound cod, sole, flounder, halibut, or salmon fillet, small bones removed

Makes 8 servings

Per serving: 145 calories, 11 g protein, 15 g carbohydrates, 5 g total fat, 1 g saturated fat, 23 mg cholesterol, 3 g dietary fiber, 220 mg sodium

1. Peel the onion and cut into ⅛" slices. Peel the garlic and chop finely. Warm the oil in a 6- to 8-quart pot over medium heat. Add the onion and garlic and cook, stirring often, for about 10 minutes, or until the onion just starts to brown. Add water, 1 tablespoon at a time, as necessary to prevent burning.

2. Meanwhile, peel the carrots and chop into ¼" to ½" pieces. Chop the zucchini, squash, and celery into ¼" to ½" pieces.

3. Add the carrots, zucchini, squash, celery, dill, creamed corn, fresh or frozen corn, bay leaf, pepper to taste, wine, salt or aminos, and water. Simmer over low heat for 30 minutes. Meanwhile, cut the smoked and fresh fish into 1" pieces.

4. Add the fish. Cook for 5 to10 minutes longer over low heat, or until the fresh fish is cooked through. Remove and discard the bay leaf. Serve immediately. Transfer cooled leftovers into covered containers and store in the refrigerator or freezer.

Creamy Carrot Soup

6 large carrots
1 2" piece fresh ginger
1 large bunch fresh parsley
1 small bunch fresh cilantro
3 large Spanish (yellow) onions
2 cloves garlic
2 tablespoons olive oil
8 cups water
3 tablespoons low-sodium soy sauce or liquid aminos
¼ cup low-sodium chicken or vegetable bouillon granules
Peel of 1 orange, with no white pith
Ground black pepper

Makes 8 servings

Per serving: 98 calories, 2 g protein, 14 g carbohydrates, 4 g total fat, 1 g saturated fat, 0 mg cholesterol, 4 g dietary fiber, 253 mg sodium

1. Peel the carrots and chop into 2" to 3" pieces. Set aside. Peel the ginger and chop finely. Cut off the parsley and cilantro stems to make about ¾ cup each of loosely packed leaves. Cut the leaves roughly. Set aside.

2. Peel the onions and garlic. Chop the onions into ½" to 1" pieces. Chop the garlic roughly. Warm the oil in a 6- to 8-quart pot over medium heat. Add the onions and garlic and cook, stirring often, for about 10 minutes, or until the onions just start to brown. Add water, 1 tablespoon at a time, as necessary to prevent burning.

3. Add the carrots, ginger, water, soy sauce or aminos, and bouillon. Cook over low heat for 25 minutes. Add the parsley and cilantro, orange peel, and pepper to taste. Continue cooking for 15 minutes longer. Remove the orange peel.

4. Puree in a blender or food processor fitted with the chopping blade, or use an immersion blender directly in the pot. Blend until creamy and medium-thick. If the soup is too thick, add more water. Serve hot, warm, or cool.

Roasted Tomato and Basil Soup

3   pounds whole ripe plum tomatoes, halved, or 2 cans (28 ounces each) Muir Glen Fire-Roasted Whole Tomatoes

2   cloves garlic

1   large Spanish (yellow) onion

1   tablespoon olive oil

½   cup loosely packed chopped fresh basil leaves

2   cups canned low-sodium tomato puree

½   teaspoon salt or 2 tablespoons liquid aminos

1   teaspoon dried oregano

6   cups low-sodium chicken or vegetable broth or water

If you want a creamy version of this soup, add a 14-ounce can of evaporated fat-free milk at the end.

Makes 8 servings

Per serving: 99 calories, 5 g protein, 17 g carbohydrates, 2 g total fat, 0.5 g saturated fat, 0 mg cholesterol, 4 g dietary fiber, 381 mg sodium

1. If using fresh tomatoes, preheat the oven to 450°F. Coat a 13" x 9" baking pan with cooking spray. Place the tomatoes, cut side down, in the baking pan. Peel the garlic and chop finely. Sprinkle the tomatoes with half of the garlic.

2. Coat the tops of the tomatoes with cooking spray and roast in the oven for about 1 hour, or until the edges of the tomatoes are well-roasted and start to blacken. If the tomatoes start drying out while cooking, add a little bit of water to the bottom of the pan. Remove from the oven and set aside. When the tomatoes are cool enough to handle, slip off the skins. Coarsely chop the tomatoes. (If using canned tomatoes, just coarsely chop them and save their liquid.)

3. Meanwhile, peel the onion and cut into rough ½" to 1" pieces. Warm the oil in a 6- to 8-quart pot over medium heat. Add the onions and remaining half of the garlic (or 2 chopped cloves of garlic if using canned tomatoes). Cook, stirring often, for about 15 minutes, or until the onion turns light brown. Add water, 1 tablespoon at a time, as necessary to prevent burning.

4. Add the roasted or canned tomatoes with their liquid, basil, tomato puree, salt or aminos, oregano, and broth or water. Cook over medium heat for 30 minutes, stirring often to break up the tomatoes. Serve hot or warm. Transfer cooled leftovers into covered containers and store in the refrigerator for up to 5 days or in the freezer for up to 2 months.

Texas Black Bean Soup

2	cans (19 ounces each) black beans
2	large carrots
2	cloves garlic
1	large Spanish (yellow) onion
2	tablespoons olive oil
1	cup canned tomato puree
1	tablespoon low-sodium chicken bouillon granules
2	tablespoons dry sherry
6	cups water
1	teaspoon chili powder
$\frac{1}{4}$–$\frac{1}{2}$	teaspoon ground red pepper
1	teaspoon dried oregano
1	teaspoon liquid smoke

Makes 8 servings

Per serving: 136 calories, 6 g protein, 19 g carbohydrates, 4 g total fat, 0.5 g saturated fat, 0 mg cholesterol, 6 g dietary fiber, 416 mg sodium

1. Drain the beans. Rinse well and drain again. Set aside.

2. Peel the carrots and cut into ¼" to ½" pieces. Set aside.

3. Peel the garlic and chop finely. Peel the onion and cut into rough ½" to 1" pieces. Warm the oil in a 6- to 8-quart pot over medium heat. Add the garlic and onion and cook, stirring often, for about 15 minutes, or until the onion turns light brown. Add water, 1 tablespoon at a time, as necessary to prevent burning.

4. Add the beans, carrots, tomato puree, bouillon, sherry, water, chili powder, red pepper, and oregano. Cook over medium heat for 50 to 55 minutes, or until the soup is medium-thick. Stir in the liquid smoke. Add more spices to taste. Add more water if you prefer a thinner soup. Serve hot or warm.

Roasted Acorn Squash Soup

1	large acorn squash
3	large carrots
1	large Spanish (yellow) onion
1	clove garlic
1	tablespoon olive oil
1	bay leaf
½	teaspoon salt or 1 tablespoon liquid aminos
2	teaspoons dried rosemary
1	teaspoon dried sage
¼	cup chicken bouillon granules
8	cups water

Makes 8 servings

Per serving: 65 calories, 1 g protein, 11 g carbohydrates, 2 g total fat, 0.5 g saturated fat, 0 mg cholesterol, 2 g dietary fiber, 162 mg sodium

1. Preheat the oven to 400°F. Cut the squash in half and remove the seeds. Place the squash on a baking sheet, cut side up. Bake for 45 minutes to 1 hour, or until soft. Set aside to cool. When cool enough to handle, scoop out the insides and set aside in a bowl.

2. Meanwhile, peel the carrots and chop into 1" to 2" chunks. Set aside.

3. Peel the onion and garlic. Cut the onion into rough ½" to 1" pieces. Chop the garlic finely. Warm the oil in a 6- to 8-quart pot over medium heat. Add the onion and garlic and cook, stirring often, for about 15 minutes, or until the onion turns light brown. Add water, 1 tablespoon at a time, as necessary to prevent burning.

4. Add the carrots, bay leaf, salt or aminos, rosemary, sage, bouillon, and water. Cook over low heat for 30 minutes, or until the carrots have softened. Remove and discard the bay leaf. Stir in the cooked squash.

5. Puree in a blender or food processor fitted with the chopping blade, or use an immersion blender directly in the pot. Blend or process until creamy and medium-thick. Return to the pot and simmer for 15 minutes longer. Serve hot or warm. Transfer cooled leftovers into covered containers and store in the refrigerator or freezer.

Chunky Mixed Vegetable Soup

1	large zucchini
2	ribs celery
1	medium red bell pepper
1	medium turnip
1	medium parsnip
1	medium Idaho potato
2	cloves garlic
1	large Spanish (yellow) onion
1	tablespoon olive oil
1	bag (1 pound) baby carrots
1	can (15 ounces) chopped or whole tomatoes
½	teaspoon salt or 2 tablespoons liquid aminos
8–10	cups water or canned vegetable broth
1	cup fresh basil leaves, chopped
	Ground black pepper

This is a filling and yummy soup. Feel free to use any vegetables you like.

Makes 8 servings

Per serving: 108 calories, 3 g protein, 21 g carbohydrates, 2 g total fat, 0.5 g saturated fat, 0 mg cholesterol, 5 g dietary fiber, 275 mg sodium

1. Chop the zucchini and celery into 1" pieces. Remove seeds from the bell pepper and cut into 1" pieces. Set aside.

2. Peel the turnip, parsnip, and potato. Chop each into ½" to 1" pieces. Set aside.

3. Peel the garlic and onion. Chop the garlic roughly. Cut the onion into ⅛" to ¼" pieces. Warm the oil in a 6- to 8-quart pot over medium heat. Add the onion and garlic and cook, stirring often, for about 10 minutes, or until the onion just starts to brown. Add water, 1 tablespoon at a time, as necessary to prevent burning.

4. Add the zucchini, celery, bell pepper, turnip, parsnip, potato, baby carrots, tomatoes (with juice), salt or aminos, water or broth, basil, and black pepper to taste. Simmer over low heat for 45 to 60 minutes, stirring occasionally to break up the whole tomatoes (if using). Add more water if the soup seems too thick. Serve hot or warm. Transfer cooled leftovers into covered containers and store in the refrigerator or freezer.

Wild Mushroom Soup

2	cloves garlic
1	large Spanish (yellow) onion
1	tablespoon olive oil
12	ounces white mushrooms
8	ounces shiitake mushrooms (and/or other mushrooms such as oyster or maitake)
½	teaspoon salt or 2 tablespoons liquid aminos
1	bay leaf
½	teaspoon dried oregano
½	teaspoon dried basil
6	cups water

If you want a creamy version of this soup, add a 14-ounce can of evaporated skim milk at the end.

Makes 8 servings

Per serving: 49 calories, 2 g protein, 8 g carbohydrates, 2 g total fat, 0.5 g saturated fat, 0 mg cholesterol, 1 g dietary fiber, 276 mg sodium

1. Peel the garlic and onion. Chop the garlic roughly. Cut the onion into ⅛" to ¼" pieces. Warm the oil in a 6- to 8-quart pot over medium heat. Add the garlic and onion and cook, stirring often, until the onion is soft, about 10 minutes. Add water, 1 tablespoon at a time, as necessary to prevent burning.

2. Gently wash the mushrooms. Slice the mushrooms. Add to the pot and cook over medium-low heat for 20 minutes, or until the mushrooms are golden brown.

3. Add the salt or aminos, bay leaf, oregano, basil, and water. Simmer over low heat for 25 minutes.

4. Remove and discard the bay leaf. Puree half of the soup in a blender or food processor fitted with the chopping blade, or use an immersion blender until the mixture is medium-thick. Return to the pot. Serve hot or warm. Transfer cooled leftovers into covered containers and store in the refrigerator.

Roasted Garlic and White Bean Spread

1 bulb garlic (whole head)
1 can (15 ounces) cannellini beans, rinsed and drained
½ cup low-fat mayonnaise
½ teaspoon ground cumin
¼ teaspoon salt or ½ teaspoon liquid aminos
2–3 tablespoons lemon juice
Ground black pepper
3 tablespoons chopped parsley

Makes 1½ cups

Per 2 tablespoons: 65 calories, 2 g protein, 8 g carbohydrates, 3 g total fat, 0 g saturated fat, 3 mg cholesterol, 0 g dietary fiber, 134 mg sodium

1. Preheat the oven to 350°F. Place the unpeeled whole garlic bulb in a shallow baking dish or on a baking sheet and bake for about 1 hour, or until soft. (It is acceptable for the skin to char.) Remove from the oven and let cool.

2. Squeeze out at least 2 or 3 cloves of roasted garlic, removing the peel, or as many as you like. Place in the bowl of a food processor fitted with the chopping blade. Add the beans, mayonnaise, and cumin. Process for about 20 seconds, or until light and creamy. Transfer to a medium bowl, and mix in the salt or aminos, lemon juice, and pepper to taste. Stir in the parsley.

3. Serve as a dip or in lightly toasted whole wheat pitas or on whole wheat crackers.

Lemony Hummus

1 clove garlic
1 can (15 ounces) chickpeas
  Grated peel and juice of 1 lemon
3 tablespoons olive or canola oil
2 teaspoons tahini sauce (optional)
¼ teaspoon salt or ½ tablespoon liquid aminos
¼ teaspoon ground black pepper
2 tablespoons chopped parsley

Makes 1½ cups

Per 2 tablespoons: 64 calories, 1 g protein, 5 g carbohydrates, 4 g total fat, 1 g saturated fat, 0 mg cholesterol, 1 g dietary fiber, 105 mg sodium

1. Peel the garlic and place in the bowl of a food processor fitted with the chopping blade. Process for 5 seconds, or until the garlic is chopped. Drain the chickpeas well, rinse, and drain again. Add to the food processor, along with the lemon peel, lemon juice, oil, tahini (if using), salt or aminos, pepper, and parsley. Process for about 20 seconds, or until smooth.

2. Serve as a dip or in lightly toasted whole wheat pitas or on whole wheat crackers.

Lentil Salad with Lemon and Feta

1¾ cups dried lentils
1 large beefsteak tomato or 3 or 4 plum tomatoes
1 scallion (green onion)
1 cup fresh cilantro leaves
4 ounces feta cheese
2 tablespoons extra-virgin olive oil
  Grated peel of 1 lemon
  Juice of 2 lemons (about ¼ cup)
¼ teaspoon ground black pepper

Makes 8 servings

Per serving: 168 calories, 12 g protein, 28 g carbohydrates, 6 g total fat, 3 g saturated fat, 12 mg cholesterol, 12 g dietary fiber, 166 mg sodium

1. In a 2-quart saucepan, bring 3 cups of water to a boil. Add the lentils and return the heat to boiling. Simmer over medium-low heat for about 25 minutes, or until the lentils are tender but still hold their shape. Drain the lentils and rinse under cold water. Drain again and set aside.

2. Chop the tomato(es) into ¼" pieces and place in a medium bowl. Chop the scallion and cilantro finely and add to the bowl. Crumble the cheese into the bowl and add the lentils.

3. In a small bowl, whisk the oil, lemon peel, lemon juice, and pepper. Add to the lentil mixture and toss well. Refrigerate for at least 1 hour or overnight and serve.

Bean and Barley Salad

Dressing

Juice of ½ lemon
¼ teaspoon salt or ½ tablespoon liquid aminos
1 clove garlic
2½ tablespoons extra-virgin olive oil
2 tablespoons water
2 teaspoons Dijon mustard
2 teaspoons fresh basil or ¾ teaspoon dried
2 teaspoons fresh oregano or ¾ teaspoon dried
Ground black pepper

Makes 8 servings

Per serving: 159 calories, 5 g protein, 22 g carbohydrates, 7 g total fat, 1 g saturated fat, 0 mg cholesterol, 5 g dietary fiber, 196 mg sodium

Salad

2 cups water or low-sodium chicken broth
1 cup quick-cooking barley
1 small zucchini
1 small carrot
1 tablespoon olive oil
1 cup broccoli florets
1 cup cauliflower florets
1 cup canned black beans, rinsed and drained

1. *To prepare the dressing:* In a small bowl, combine the lemon juice and salt or aminos, stirring until the salt dissolves. Peel the garlic and chop finely. Add the garlic, oil, water, mustard, basil, oregano, and pepper to taste. Mix well with a fork.

2. *To prepare the salad:* Bring water and barley to a boil in a 2-quart heavy saucepan, then reduce heat and simmer, covered, until barley is tender, about 10 minutes. Remove from heat and let stand, covered, 5 minutes. Drain barley in a colander, then rinse under cold water and let cool to room temperature.

3. Meanwhile, cut the zucchini and carrot into ¼" slices. Warm the oil in a large nonstick skillet over medium heat. Add the carrot and cook for about 4 minutes. Add the broccoli and cauliflower, and cook for 3 minutes longer, or until they just start to cook. Add the zucchini and cook for 1 or 2 minutes longer, or until the vegetables are just cooked but still a little crisp.

4. In a large bowl, combine the barley, vegetable mixture, and beans. Add the dressing and toss well. Serve the salad immediately or refrigerate until ready to serve. (The salad can be made up to 4 days in advance.)

Mexican Rice and Beans

³/₄ cup brown rice
2¼ cups water
2 cans (15 ounces each) low-sodium red kidney beans
1 clove garlic
1 medium Spanish (yellow) onion
1 tablespoon olive oil
1 scallion (green onion), roughly chopped
2 tablespoons chopped fresh cilantro
1 teaspoon ground cumin
¼ teaspoon salt or 1 teaspoon liquid aminos
Ground black pepper

1. In a medium saucepan, combine the brown rice and water. Cook, covered, over medium heat for 45 minutes to 1 hour, or until the water is absorbed and the rice is tender. Drain the beans, rinse well, and drain again. Set aside.

2. Meanwhile, peel the garlic and chop roughly. Peel the onion, halve it, and slice. Warm the oil in a 3-quart saucepan over medium heat. Add the garlic and onion and cook, stirring often, for about 7 minutes, or until the onion starts to brown. Add the beans and cook for 4 minutes, or until the beans are heated through.

3. In a large bowl, combine the bean mixture with the rice, scallion, cilantro, cumin, salt or aminos, and pepper to taste. Serve immediately.

While I've suggested using red kidney beans, you may use any beans you like. By using canned beans, you'll save a lot of time. You can also use rice left over from another meal, which will turn this into a super-fast dish. If using precooked rice, place it in a dish covered with plastic wrap and microwave on high power for 2 minutes.

Makes 4 servings

Per serving: 296 calories, 13 g protein, 52 g carbohydrates, 5 g total fat, 1 g saturated fat, 0 mg cholesterol, 15 g dietary fiber, 160 mg sodium

Brown Rice Pilaf

2½	cups water
1	cup brown rice
1	medium Spanish (yellow) onion
1	clove garlic
1	tablespoon olive oil
¼	teaspoon salt or 2 teaspoons liquid aminos
2	tablespoons pine nuts (optional)

1. In a 2-quart saucepan, combine the water and rice and cook over medium heat for 45 minutes to 1 hour, or until the water is absorbed and the rice is tender. Be sure not to overcook. Rice grains should separate easily. Set aside to cool.

2. Peel the onion and cut into ⅛" slices. Peel the garlic and chop finely.

3. Warm the oil in a large nonstick skillet over medium heat. Add the onion, garlic, and salt or aminos. Cook, stirring often, for about 7 minutes, or until the onion starts to brown. Add water, 1 tablespoon at a time, as necessary to prevent burning. Cool.

4. Combine the cooled rice with the onion mixture. If using pine nuts, toast them in a nonstick skillet over medium heat for about 3 minutes, or until they start to brown. Then toss the toasted nuts with the rice mixture. Serve immediately or refrigerate.

*B*ecause it's made with brown rice, this dish is an excellent way to incorporate more fiber into your diet. It's delicious without the pine nuts, but adding them takes the flavor to the next level.

Makes 4 servings

Per serving: 241 calories, 4 g protein, 40 g carbohydrates, 7 g total fat, 1 g saturated fat, 0 mg cholesterol, 3 g dietary fiber, 142 mg sodium

Italian Risotto with Wild Mushrooms

4	cups low-sodium vegetable broth
½	cup dried porcini mushrooms
½	cup boiling water
1	large Spanish (yellow) onion
2	tablespoons olive oil
1	cup Arborio rice
½	cup dry white wine
½	cup sliced shiitake mushrooms
¼	teaspoon salt
1	tablespoon chopped parsley
¼	cup (1 ounce) grated Parmesan cheese

Makes 4 servings

Per serving: 331 calories, 8 g protein, 50 g carbohydrates, 9 g total fat, 2 g saturated fat, 5 mg cholesterol, 1 g dietary fiber, 543 mg sodium

1. Pour the broth into a 3-quart saucepan and warm over low heat. Soak the porcini mushrooms in the water for about 10 minutes, or until soft. Strain the soaking liquid and set both the mushrooms and liquid aside.

2. Meanwhile, peel the onion and chop into ⅛" pieces. Warm the oil in a 2-quart pot over medium heat. Add the onion and cook over medium-low heat for 7 to 10 minutes, or until the onion is soft and transparent. Add broth, 1 tablespoon at a time, as necessary to prevent the onion from browning.

3. Add the rice to the pot and continue cooking over low heat for 3 to 5 minutes, or until the rice turns opaque. Add the wine and cook until it is absorbed. Then add 1 cup of the broth. Cook, stirring frequently, until the rice has absorbed the broth, about 15 minutes.

4. Add the reserved mushroom soaking liquid and ½ cup of broth. Continue to simmer, stirring frequently, until all the liquid has been absorbed. Add the reserved porcini mushrooms, shiitake mushrooms, and 1/2 cup of broth. Stir frequently until the rice has absorbed all the broth.

5. If the rice is still too firm, continue adding the remaining broth, ½ cup at a time, and stir until the broth is absorbed and the rice becomes tender. The rice should be a little chewy and creamy. Stir in the salt, parsley, and cheese. Serve immediately as a side dish.

Jasmine Rice Pilaf

1   cup jasmine rice
1½ cups water
1   small leek
1   medium onion
1   rib celery
1   tablespoon olive oil
    Ground black pepper

Makes 4 servings

Per serving: 232 calories, 4 g protein, 45 g carbohydrates, 4 g total fat, 1 g saturated fat, 0 mg cholesterol, 2 g dietary fiber, 21 mg sodium

1. Rinse the rice under running water until the water turns clear. In a 1-quart saucepan, combine the rice and water. Bring to a boil and cover. Reduce the heat to very low and cook for 20 minutes. Turn off the heat and leave undisturbed for 10 minutes. Let cool.

2. Cut off the green leafy part of the leek and discard. Halve the white part lengthwise and rinse thoroughly. Cut into ⅛" to ¼" slices. Peel the onion and cut into ⅛" to ¼" slices. Cut the celery into ⅛" to ¼" slices. Warm the oil in a large nonstick skillet over medium-low heat. Add the leek, onion, and celery. Cook for about 10 minutes, or until the onion turns soft and lightly brown. Add water, 1 tablespoon at a time, as necessary to prevent burning. Let cool.

3. Combine the onion mixture, cooled rice, and pepper to taste.

Quinoa with Fried Onions

½ cup quinoa
1 cup water
2 medium onions
2 tablespoons olive oil
2 tablespoons chopped parsley
¼ cup (1 ounce) grated Parmesan cheese
Ground black pepper

1. Rinse the quinoa under cold running water until the water turns clear.

2. In a 2-quart saucepan, combine the quinoa and water. Simmer over medium-low heat for about 15 minutes, or until the quinoa begins to soften. Remove from the heat and drain.

3. Meanwhile, peel the onions and cut into ⅛" to ¼" slices. Warm the oil in a large skillet over medium-low heat. Add the onions and cook for about 10 minutes, or until they soften and brown. Add water, 1 tablespoon at a time, as necessary to prevent burning.

4. In a medium bowl, combine the quinoa, onions, parsley, cheese, and pepper to taste. Toss well. Serve as a side dish.

*P*ronounced "keen-wah," this grain, native to South America, has been cultivated for more than 5,000 years. In fact, it is not a true grain at all, but a relative of spinach and Swiss chard. Over the past 20 years, it has enjoyed a resurgence on plates across America. This might have to do with its nutty flavor or maybe the fact that it has more iron than any other grain around and is a great source of vitamins, minerals, and protein.

Makes 4 servings

Per serving: 199 calories, 6 g protein, 22 g carbohydrates, 10 g total fat, 2 g saturated fat, 5 mg cholesterol, 2 g dietary fiber, 126 mg sodium

Middle Eastern Tabbouleh Salad

Juice of 1 lemon
½ cup bulgur
2 large ripe plum tomatoes
2 medium cucumbers
2 tablespoons extra-virgin olive oil
¼ teaspoon salt or 2 teaspoons liquid aminos
Ground black pepper
¼ cup chopped parsley
2 tablespoons chopped fresh mint

1. Place the lemon juice in a 1-cup measure and add enough cold water to make 1 cup. Place the bulgur in a small bowl and add the lemon-water mixture. Stir, then allow to sit for 30 minutes, or until soft.

2. Chop the tomatoes into ¼" pieces and place in a medium bowl. Peel and seed the cucumbers. (To seed a cucumber, halve it lengthwise and scoop out the seeds with a spoon.) Slice the cucumber halves into ¼" pieces and add to the bowl.

3. Add the bulgur, olive oil, salt or aminos, pepper to taste, parsley, and mint. Mix well. Stir in additional parsley and mint to taste. Serve the salad immediately or refrigerate until ready to serve (can be made up to 2 days in advance).

*B*ulgur—also known as cracked wheat—has a slightly nutty flavor and comes from wheat berries. The coolest thing about this refreshing salad? No cooking. Simply soaking the grains for about a half hour "cooks" them.

Makes 4 servings

Per serving: 152 calories, 3 g protein, 21 g carbohydrates, 7 g total fat, 1 g saturated fat, 0 mg cholesterol, 6 g dietary fiber, 144 mg sodium

Roasted Vegetable Lasagna

1	large Spanish (yellow) onion
1	clove garlic
2	tablespoons olive oil
2¾	cups canned low-sodium tomato puree
1	tablespoon tomato paste
1	teaspoon dried oregano
1	teaspoon dried basil
3–4	cups Roasted Vegetables (page 267), with beets omitted
6	oven-ready lasagna noodles or 6 semicooked regular lasagna noodles
1	cup (4 ounces) grated low-fat mozzarella cheese
2	tablespoons (½ ounce) grated Parmesan cheese

Makes 6 servings

Per serving: 421 calories, 17 g protein, 67 g carbohydrates, 12 g total fat, 3 g saturated fat, 12 mg cholesterol, 7 g dietary fiber, 276 mg sodium

1. Preheat the oven to 350°F.

2. Peel the onion and chop into ⅛" to ¼" pieces. Peel the garlic and chop finely. Warm the oil in a 2-quart saucepan over medium heat. Add the onion and garlic and cook, stirring often, for about 10 minutes, or until the onion just starts to brown. Add water, 1 tablespoon at a time, as necessary to prevent burning. Add the tomato puree, tomato paste, oregano, and basil and cook for about 20 minutes, or until the sauce thickens.

3. While the sauce is cooking, cut the roasted vegetables into ½" to 1" pieces.

4. Coat a 9" x 5" baking pan with cooking spray. Spread ½ cup of the tomato sauce on the bottom of the pan.

5. Place 2 noodles, overlapping, on top of the sauce. Spread about 1 cup of the roasted vegetables over the noodles, then sprinkle with about 3 tablespoons mozzarella. Top with ½ cup of tomato sauce, then place another layer of noodles on top.

6. Keep layering—vegetables, mozzarella, sauce, noodles—until all the noodles are used and the roasted vegetables with cheese are on top. There should be 3 layers.

7. Top with the remaining sauce. Sprinkle the Parmesan and remaining mozzarella on top and cover the pan with aluminum foil. Bake for about 45 minutes to 1 hour, or until bubbling and heated completely through.

8. Remove from the oven and let rest for 10 minutes before serving.

Sesame Noodles

8	ounces linguini
1	large carrot
2	scallions (green onions)
2	cloves garlic
2	tablespoons all-natural peanut butter
2	teaspoons sesame oil
2	tablespoons low-sodium soy sauce
1	tablespoon honey
½	teaspoon chili powder
4	teaspoons rice wine or apple cider vinegar

Makes 4 servings

Per serving: 310 calories, 10 g protein, 52 g carbohydrates, 7 g total fat, 1 g saturated fat, 0 mg cholesterol, 1 g dietary fiber, 331 mg sodium

1. Cook the pasta according to package directions. Drain and set aside.

2. While the pasta cooks, peel the carrot and grate on the wide-holes side of a box grater. Chop the scallions roughly. Peel the garlic and crush with the side of a knife.

3. In a blender or food processor fitted with the chopping blade, combine the carrot, scallions, garlic, peanut butter, oil, soy sauce, honey, chili powder, and vinegar. Blend or process for 15 to 30 seconds, or until smooth.

4. In a bowl, combine the pasta and sauce and mix well. Serve immediately or refrigerate for up to 3 days.

Mac and Cheese

12	ounces elbow macaroni
2½	cups fat-free milk
3	tablespoons unbleached all-purpose flour
3	teaspoons dry mustard
	Ground black pepper
1	cup (4 ounces) shredded fat-free Cheddar cheese
2½	cups (10 ounces) shredded reduced-fat Cheddar cheese

Makes 8 servings

Per serving: 344 calories, 22 g protein, 39 g carbohydrates, 9 g total fat, 5 g saturated fat, 26 mg cholesterol, 1 g dietary fiber, 430 mg sodium

1. Preheat the oven to 350°F. Coat a 2-quart baking dish with cooking spray. Set aside.

2. Prepare the macaroni according to package directions. Drain.

3. In a large bowl, combine 1 cup of the milk with the flour, mustard, and pepper, to taste. Whisk until smooth.

4. Pour the remaining 1½ cups milk into a 2- to 4-quart pot and bring to a simmer over medium heat, stirring constantly. Add the milk-and-flour mixture and keep stirring for 3 to 5 minutes, or until thick and bubbling. Reduce the heat. Add the fat-free and reduced-fat cheese. Mix until the cheese melts.

5. Remove the pot from the stove and add the macaroni. Transfer the macaroni mixture to the prepared baking dish. Bake for 35 to 40 minutes, or until hot and bubbling around the edges. Serve hot.

Pasta Primavera

2 cups fusilli (corkscrew) pasta
1 medium zucchini
1 red bell pepper
1 large or 2 medium cloves garlic
1 large onion
2 tablespoons extra-virgin olive oil
1 cup broccoli florets
2 cups canned low-sodium tomato puree
1 tablespoon tomato paste
½ teaspoon salt or 2 teaspoons liquid aminos
Ground black pepper
1 teaspoon dried oregano
1 teaspoon dried basil
3 tablespoons chopped fresh basil
1 cup fresh or frozen peas

Makes 8 servings

Per serving: 190 calories, 7 g protein, 33 g carbohydrates, 4 g total fat, 1 g saturated fat, 0 mg cholesterol, 4 g dietary fiber, 186 mg sodium

1. Cook the pasta according to package directions. Drain and set aside.

2. Cut the zucchini into ¼" x 3" strips and set aside. Remove the ribs and seeds from the bell pepper and cut into ¼"-wide strips and set aside. Peel the garlic and chop roughly. Peel the onion and cut into ⅛" to ¼" slices.

3. Heat 1 tablespoon of the oil in a large skillet over medium heat. Add the garlic and onion and cook, stirring often, for about 10 minutes, or until the onion starts to brown. Add water, 1 tablespoon at a time, as necessary to prevent burning.

4. Add the zucchini, bell pepper, broccoli, tomato puree, tomato paste, salt or aminos, black pepper to taste, oregano, dried basil, and the remaining 1 tablespoon oil. Cook for 10 minutes on medium-low heat. Add the fresh basil and fresh peas (if using) and cook for 15 minutes longer. If using frozen peas, stir them in the last 2 minutes.

5. In a large bowl, combine the pasta and sauce and toss well. Serve immediately or refrigerate for up to 3 days.

Salmon or Tuna Burgers

2   small yellow onions
1   tablespoon olive oil
1   can (14 ounces) salmon or 3 cans (6 ounces each) water-packed solid-white tuna, drained and flaked with a fork
1   egg white
3   tablespoons dried bread crumbs
1   teaspoon dried basil
1   teaspoon dried oregano
1   tablespoon toasted wheat germ
¼   teaspoon salt or 1 tablespoon liquid aminos
    Ground black pepper

Makes 6

Per serving: 125 calories, 12 g protein, 6 g carbohydrates, 6 g total fat, 1 g saturated fat, 29 mg cholesterol, 1 g dietary fiber, 415 mg sodium

1. Preheat the oven to 375°F. Coat a baking sheet with nonstick spray. Set aside.

2. Peel the onions and cut into ⅛" to ¼" pieces. Warm the oil in a large skillet over medium heat. Add the onions and cook, stirring often, for about 10 minutes, or until they start to brown. Remove from the heat, transfer to a large bowl, and let cool for 10 minutes.

3. To the same bowl, add the salmon or tuna, egg white, bread crumbs, basil, oregano, wheat germ, salt or aminos, and pepper to taste. Mix well. Shape the mixture into 6 burgers and place on the baking sheet.

4. Bake for 15 minutes. Turn each burger. Bake for 10 to 20 minutes longer, or until heated all the way through and browned. Serve immediately.

Turkey Burgers

3	medium yellow onions
1	clove garlic
2	tablespoons olive oil
1⅓	pounds ground turkey breast
3	tablespoons dried bread crumbs
2	tablespoons barbecue sauce
3	tablespoons quick-cooking oats (not instant)
1	teaspoon dried basil
1	teaspoon dried oregano
1	tablespoon toasted wheat germ
¼	teaspoon salt or 1 tablespoon liquid aminos
	Ground black pepper

Makes 9

Per serving: 146 calories, 17 g protein, 8 g carbohydrates, 5 g total fat, 1 g saturated fat, 39 mg cholesterol, 1 g dietary fiber, 145 mg sodium

1. Peel the onions and cut into ⅛" to ¼" pieces. Peel the garlic and chop finely. Warm the oil in a large skillet over medium heat. Add the onions and garlic and cook over medium heat, stirring often, for about 10 minutes, or until the onions start to brown. Add water, 1 tablespoon at a time, as necessary to prevent burning. Remove from the heat, transfer to a large bowl, and let cool for 10 minutes.

2. To the same bowl, add the turkey, bread crumbs, barbecue sauce, oats, basil, oregano, wheat germ, salt or aminos, and pepper to taste. Mix well. Shape the mixture into 9 burgers.

3. Coat a large nonstick skillet with cooking spray. Cook the burgers over medium heat for about 5 minutes, or until browned and crispy. Flip the burgers carefully and cook for 5 minutes longer, or until golden brown and a thermometer inserted in the center registers 165° and the meat is no longer pink. Serve the burgers hot.

Deli Sandwiches with Russian Yogurt Dressing

Russian Yogurt Dressing

1/3	cup fat-free plain yogurt
1	tablespoon low-fat mayonnaise
2	teaspoons ketchup
1/4	teaspoon dried oregano
1/4	teaspoon dried basil
	Ground black pepper

Sandwiches

4	leaves romaine lettuce
8	slices whole grain or whole wheat bread, 4 whole wheat pitas (halved and split to form a pocket), or 4 split oat bran English muffins, toasted
1	pound thinly sliced roast beef or turkey breast
2	ripe tomatoes, sliced thinly

*W*hether you make it at home or get it from the deli counter, roast beef is surprisingly lean. Add some vegetables and a lower-fat Russian dressing, and you've got a sandwich to crow about. Feel free to use sliced turkey breast instead of the roast beef, if you prefer.

Makes 4

Per serving: 354 calories, 32 g protein, 32 g carbohydrates, 11 g total fat, 3 g saturated fat, 79 mg cholesterol, 4 g dietary fiber, 346 mg sodium

1. *To make the dressing:* In a small bowl, combine the yogurt, mayonnaise, ketchup, oregano, basil, and pepper to taste. Whisk until well-blended.

2. *To make the sandwiches:* Cut or tear the lettuce into 1" strips.

3. For each sandwich, spread 2 tablespoons of the dressing on 2 slices of bread, inside 2 pita halves, or on 2 English muffin halves. Place 1/4 each of the meat, lettuce, and tomatoes on or in the prepared breads.

Vegetarian Asian Tofu Sandwiches

Dressing

- 4 ounces soft tofu, drained
- 1 teaspoon peanut butter or tahini
- 1 tablespoon low-fat mayonnaise
- 1 teaspoon miso (fermented soy paste)
- 1 tablespoon lemon juice
  Ground black pepper

Makes 4

Per serving: 285 calories, 11 g protein, 37 g carbohydrates, 12 g total fat, 1 g saturated fat, 0 mg cholesterol, 8 g dietary fiber, 415 mg sodium

Sandwiches

- 4 pieces romaine, red leaf, or green leaf lettuce or 2 cups mixed baby greens
- 2 ripe tomatoes
- 1 cucumber
- 1 ripe avocado
- 4 whole wheat pitas (halved and split to form a pocket) or 8 slices whole grain or whole wheat bread

1. *To make the dressing:* In a blender or food processor fitted with the chopping blade, combine the tofu, peanut butter or tahini, mayonnaise, miso, lemon juice, and pepper to taste. Blend or process for 15 seconds, or until well-mixed.

2. *To make the sandwiches:* If using large lettuce, cut or tear into bite-size pieces. Slice the tomatoes. Peel the cucumber, halve, and scoop out the seeds. Cut into ¼" slices. Peel the avocado, remove the pit, and cut into ¼" slices. In a large bowl, combine the lettuce, tomatoes, cucumber, and avocado.

3. Add the dressing and toss lightly until coated. Divide among the pitas or bread. Serve immediately.

South of the Border Fajitas

1	pound chicken breast tenders or boneless, skinless breast halves
2	cloves garlic
3–4	tablespoons lime juice
2	teaspoons ground cumin
1/4	teaspoon red-pepper flakes
1/4	teaspoon salt or 1 tablespoon liquid aminos
1	red bell pepper
1	yellow bell pepper
2	medium red onions
3	tablespoons olive oil
1 1/2	cups chopped fresh cilantro
8	low-fat wheat tortillas (10" diameter)
4	ounces fat-free sour cream
1	cup salsa

Makes 8

Per serving: 236 calories, 18 g protein, 28 g carbohydrates, 8 g total fat, 1 g saturated fat, 33 mg cholesterol, 5 g dietary fiber, 410 mg sodium

1. Rinse the chicken and blot dry with paper towels. If using the breast halves, slice across the grain into 1/4"-wide strips. Peel the garlic and chop finely. In a large bowl or resealable plastic bag, place the chicken, garlic, lime juice, cumin, red-pepper flakes, and salt or aminos. Stir. Cover the bowl if using. Refrigerate for 1 to 24 hours.

2. Remove and discard the seeds and ribs from the bell peppers and slice into 1/4"-wide strips. Set aside. Peel the onions and cut into 1/4" slices. Set aside.

3. Heat 1 1/2 tablespoons oil in a large skillet over medium-high heat. Add the peppers and cook for about 5 minutes, or until the peppers begin to soften slightly. Add the onions and continue cooking until the onions are browned. Remove from the heat. Transfer the cooked vegetables to a medium bowl and set aside. Drain the chicken from the marinade. Discard the marinade.

4. In the same skillet, add the remaining 1 1/2 tablespoons oil and chicken. Cook on medium heat, stirring occasionally, for about 10 minutes, or until the chicken is no longer pink when tested with a knife. Add the reserved cooked vegetables and cilantro and cook for about 1 minute longer.

5. Divide the chicken and vegetable mixture evenly among the tortillas and place 2 tablespoons of sour cream in each fajita. Roll up or fold in half. Serve the fajitas with the salsa on the side.

Bean Enchiladas

1	green bell pepper
2	medium carrots
1	medium-large zucchini
1	clove garlic
1½	tablespoons olive oil
3½	cups black beans, red kidney beans, or pinto beans
2	cups canned tomato puree
1	teaspoon ground red pepper
¼	teaspoon salt or 1 tablespoon liquid aminos
3	teaspoons chili powder
	Ground black pepper
6	corn or wheat tortillas (10" diameter)
2	scallions (green onions)
1	lime

Makes 6

Per serving: 295 calories, 14 g protein, 52 g carbohydrates, 6 g total fat, 1 g saturated fat, 0 mg cholesterol, 10 g dietary fiber, 499 mg sodium

1. Preheat the oven to 300°F. Remove and discard the seeds and ribs from the pepper and cut into ¼"-wide strips. Peel the carrots and cut into ¼" pieces. Cut the zucchini into ¼" pieces. Peel the garlic and chop roughly.

2. Warm the oil in a large nonstick skillet over medium-high heat. When the pan is hot, add the garlic and cook for 30 seconds. Then add the bell pepper, carrots, and zucchini and cook, stirring frequently, for 12 minutes, or until the vegetables are cooked through. Remove from the heat and set aside.

3. Drain the beans and rinse well. Drain again. In a large bowl, combine the cooked vegetables, beans, 1½ cups tomato puree, red pepper, salt or aminos, chili powder, and black pepper to taste. Mix well.

4. Wrap each tortilla in a damp paper towel and microwave on high power for 15 seconds, or until the tortillas are warm and soft.

5. Coat a 13" x 9" baking pan with cooking spray. Spoon ¼ cup tomato puree into the bottom of the pan and set aside.

6. Lay 1 tortilla on a plate or work surface and place ⅓ cup bean-vegetable mixture on the lower third of the tortilla and roll up. Place the rolled tortilla in the baking pan. Repeat the procedure until all the tortillas are filled and placed in the baking pan.

7. Top with the remaining bean mixture and tomato puree. Cover the pan with aluminum foil and bake for 10 minutes. Remove the foil and bake for 10 minutes longer. Meanwhile, cut the scallions into ¼" pieces. Cut the lime into ¼" slices.

8. Remove the pan from the oven and let cool for a few minutes. Place 1 tortilla on each plate and garnish with a lime slice and a sprinkle of chopped scallions.

Grilled Chicken-Veggie Wrap

Sauce

¼–½	red bell pepper
2	tablespoons fat-free mayonnaise
2	ounces low-fat plain yogurt
1	clove garlic, peeled

Wrap

1	medium yellow onion (optional)
1	tablespoon olive oil (optional)
1	grilled chicken breast half (about 6 ounces)
4	whole wheat tortillas (10" diameter) or 4 flat-breads (10")
1	cup Roasted Vegetables (see page 267), cut into bite-size pieces

*T*hese sandwiches are a terrific use for leftover chicken and Roasted Vegetables. You can also customize them to your tastes or whatever you happen to have on hand. For instance, you can exclude the chicken and use grilled portobello mushrooms, or just use leftover roasted vegetables.

Makes 4

Per serving: 203 calories, 17 g protein, 24 g carbohydrates, 7 g total fat, 1 g saturated fat, 37 mg cholesterol, 4 g dietary fiber, 312 mg sodium

1. *To make the sauce:* Preheat the broiler. Place the pepper on a broiler pan and broil about 2" from the heat. Cook, turning with the tongs, for 15 to 20 minutes, or until the skin is evenly blackened.

2. Transfer the pepper to a small bowl. Cover and let sit for about 10 minutes. Peel, seed, and cut the pepper into chunks. In a blender or food processor fitted with the chopping blade, combine the pepper, mayonnaise, yogurt, and garlic. Blend for about 30 seconds, or until smooth and well-blended. Refrigerate the sauce until ready to use (it will last for 5 days, covered).

3. *To make the wrap:* If using the onion, peel it and cut into ¼" slices. Warm the oil in a medium nonstick skillet over medium heat. Add the onion and cook, stirring often, for about 8 minutes, or until the onion starts to brown. Add water, 1 tablespoon at a time, as necessary to prevent burning. Set aside to cool.

4. Slice the chicken into ¼"-thick strips. Spread each tortilla or flatbread with 2 tablespoons of the sauce. Lay ¼ of the chicken, ¼ of the onions (if using), and ¼ cup of the Roasted Vegetables on the bottom third of the tortilla or flatbread. Roll up and serve.

Eggplant Parmesan

3 medium eggplants
2 cloves garlic
1 large Spanish (yellow) onion
2 tablespoons olive oil
3 cups canned low-sodium tomato puree
3 ounces tomato paste
2 teaspoons dried oregano
2 teaspoons dried basil
2 cups (8 ounces) shredded low-fat mozzarella cheese
¼ cup (1 ounce) grated Parmesan cheese

Makes 6 servings

Per serving: 293 calories, 17 g protein, 33 g carbohydrates, 12 g total fat, 5 g saturated fat, 25 mg cholesterol, 4 g dietary fiber, 413 mg sodium

1. Preheat the oven to 350°F. Peel the eggplants and cut into ½"-thick rounds (you should have about 30 slices). Coat a large nonstick skillet with cooking spray. Warm the skillet over medium heat, and add 3 or 4 slices of eggplant. Fry the eggplant for about 10 minutes, or until each side is brown and soft in the middle. Remove the eggplant to a plate. Coat the skillet again, and continue frying the eggplant in batches until it is all cooked.

2. Peel the garlic and chop roughly. Peel the onion and chop it into ¼" pieces. Warm the oil in a 2-quart pot over medium heat. Add the garlic and onion and cook, stirring often, for about 10 minutes, or until the onion starts to become transparent. Add the tomato puree, tomato paste, oregano, and basil. Cook on medium heat for 15 to 20 minutes, or until the sauce thickens slightly.

3. Coat a 13" x 9" baking pan with cooking spray. Spread ¼ cup of the tomato sauce over the bottom. Place a layer of cooked eggplant slices on top of the sauce to cover the bottom of the pan. On top of the eggplant, spread 3 to 4 tablespoons of tomato sauce and a thin layer (about 3 tablespoons) of mozzarella.

4. Repeat the layers until all the eggplant and mozzarella are used and the sauce finishes on top. Sprinkle the Parmesan over the top. Cover the pan with aluminum foil and bake for 30 minutes.

5. Remove the foil and continue baking for 10 minutes longer, or until the top is lightly browned.

Spaghetti Squash Marinara

1   medium spaghetti squash
1   large Spanish (yellow) onion
1   clove garlic
1   small zucchini
1   small yellow squash
1   medium red bell pepper
2   tablespoons olive oil
2   cups canned tomato puree
1   cup loosely packed fresh basil leaves
½   teaspoon salt
    Ground black pepper

Spaghetti squash is a very interesting vegetable. Although it is a squash, when cooked, the flesh turns stringy like strands of spaghetti. This is a filling and lower-calorie version of traditional spaghetti with tomato sauce.

Makes 8 servings

Per serving: 97 calories, 3 g protein, 16 g carbohydrates, 4 g total fat, 1 g saturated fat, 0 mg cholesterol, 4 g dietary fiber, 386 mg sodium

1. Prick the spaghetti squash all over with a fork. Place the squash in a microwave-safe dish and microwave on high power for 15 to 20 minutes, or until the squash gets soft. Remove from the microwave and let cool. (Be careful because it gets very hot.)

2. When the squash is cool enough to handle, halve it lengthwise and scrape out the seeds and some fibrous strings. Set aside.

3. Meanwhile, peel the onion and halve it. Cut each half into long, thin strips and set aside. Peel the garlic and chop very finely. Cut the zucchini and yellow squash into ¼" by 4" strips. Set aside. Remove the seeds from the bell pepper and cut into ¼" by 4" strips. Set aside.

4. Warm 1 tablespoon oil in a 4- to 6-quart pot over medium heat. Add the onion and garlic and cook, stirring often, for about 10 minutes, or until the onion starts to brown. Add water, 1 tablespoon at a time, as necessary to prevent burning. Add the remaining 1 tablespoon oil, zucchini, yellow squash, and bell pepper to the skillet and cook for about 10 minutes, or until the vegetables soften slightly.

5. Add the tomato puree and basil and simmer over low heat for about 15 minutes.

6. While the sauce is simmering, gently remove the squash strands with 2 forks and place in a medium bowl. Stir in the salt and black pepper to taste. Add the spaghetti squash to the sauce and cook for 1 or 2 minutes longer, or until the squash is heated through. Serve.

Spinach and Cheese Pie

2	packages (10 ounces each) frozen chopped spinach, thawed
2	scallions (green onions)
1	tablespoon olive oil
¼	cup chopped parsley
2	tablespoons chopped fresh dill
	Ground black pepper
1	egg, lightly beaten
	Grated peel of 1 lemon
1	cup (4 ounces) shredded low-fat mozzarella cheese
½	cup (2 ounces) crumbled feta cheese
12	sheets phyllo dough
2	tablespoons (½ ounce) grated Parmesan cheese

Makes 4 servings

Per serving: 388 calories, 21 g protein, 40 g carbohydrates, 17 g total fat, 6 g saturated fat, 84 mg cholesterol, 3 g dietary fiber, 488 mg sodium

1. Preheat the oven to 350°F. Squeeze out as much moisture as you can from the thawed spinach. Chop the spinach roughly and place in a medium bowl. Set aside. Slice the scallions thinly.

2. Warm the oil in a large skillet over medium heat. Add the scallions and cook for 2 minutes. Add the spinach, parsley, dill, and pepper to taste. Cook for 2 minutes longer. Transfer to a medium bowl and set aside to cool.

3. When the spinach mixture is cooled, add the egg, lemon peel, mozzarella, and feta. Mix well. Set aside.

4. Coat a 9" x 9" baking pan with cooking spray. Place 1 sheet of phyllo dough in the bottom of the pan and trim the sides to fit. Coat with cooking spray. Repeat this procedure until there are 6 sheets of phyllo dough in the bottom of the pan. Spread the spinach mixture evenly over the dough.

5. Top the spinach with the remaining 6 sheets of phyllo dough, coating each sheet with cooking spray. Top the pie with the Parmesan.

6. Bake for 40 to 50 minutes, or until brown. Let sit for about 10 minutes before cutting. Serve hot or at room temperature. Refrigerate leftovers for up to 1 day.

Salmon, Chicken, or Tofu Teriyaki

2   scallions (green onions)
1   clove garlic
4   teaspoons grated fresh ginger
½   cup low-sodium soy sauce
3   tablespoons sweet rice wine (mirin) or apple juice
3   tablespoons honey
5   tablespoons lemon juice
4   salmon fillets or chicken cutlets (5 ounces each) or 1 pound firm or extra-firm tofu, drained

1. Cut the scallions into ⅛" to ¼" pieces. Peel and crush the garlic. In a gallon-size, resealable plastic bag, combine the scallions, garlic, ginger, soy sauce, rice wine or apple juice, honey, and lemon juice.

2. If using salmon or chicken, rinse under running water and blot dry with paper towels. If using tofu, drain and then cut the block into 4 equal pieces. Add the salmon, chicken, or tofu to the plastic bag and seal. Shake the bag well and refrigerate for 1 to 24 hours, turning occasionally.

3. Coat a broiler pan with cooking spray. Preheat the broiler. Transfer the salmon, chicken, or tofu to the broiler pan and place in the oven about 4" from the heat. Discard the leftover marinade. Broil the salmon for 10 to 12 minutes, or until the fish is opaque. Broil the chicken for 10 to 15 minutes, turning after 8 minutes. The chicken is done when a thermometer inserted in the thickest portion registers 160°F and the juices run clear. Broil the tofu for 6 to 8 minutes, turning after 4 minutes. The tofu is cooked when heated through and browned on both sides.

*W*hether you prefer to use salmon, chicken, or tofu, this teriyaki marinade works beautifully. When you serve this with steamed vegetables, such as broccoli and carrots, and brown rice, you've got a delicious, wholesome, and filling dinner.

Makes 4 servings

Per serving for salmon teriyaki: 245 calories, 30 g protein, 9 g carbohydrates, 9 g total fat, 1 g saturated fat, 78 mg cholesterol, 0 g dietary fiber, 619 mg sodium

Per serving for chicken teriyaki: 199 calories, 34 g protein, 9 g carbohydrates, 2 g total fat, 0.5 g saturated fat, 82 mg cholesterol, 0 g dietary fiber, 649 mg sodium

Per serving for tofu teriyaki: 207 calories, 19 g protein, 14 g carbohydrates, 10 g total fat, 1 g saturated fat, 0 mg cholesterol, 1 g dietary fiber, 573 mg sodium

Simple Poached Salmon

2   salmon steaks (6 ounces each)
1   large lemon

1. Rinse the salmon steaks and blot dry with paper towels. Place the salmon in a microwaveable dish. Squeeze the lemon over the salmon, using as much as you like. Cover the dish with a microwaveable cover or use microwaveable plastic wrap.

2. Microwave the salmon on high power for 3 to 4 minutes (longer if the salmon is thick). Remove the salmon and let it rest for 5 minutes so that it can continue to cook. The salmon should be opaque and light pink. If you prefer it cooked more, microwave it for 30 seconds to 1 minute longer.

Makes 2 servings

Per serving: 190 calories, 26 g protein, 3 g carbohydrates, 8 g total fat, 1 g saturated fat, 71 mg cholesterol, 0.5 g dietary fiber, 56 mg sodium

Oven-Baked Crispy Sole

½   cup dried bread crumbs
4   sole fillets (7 ounces each)

1. Preheat the oven to 400°F. Coat a baking sheet with olive oil cooking spray. Place the bread crumbs on a plate or in a shallow bowl.

2. Rinse the sole. While it's still damp, place 1 fillet in the bread crumbs to cover both sides well. Place the sole on the baking sheet. Repeat with each piece of fish.

3. Coat the top of each fillet with cooking spray. Bake for about 10 minutes, then check to see that it's not overcooking. If it is underdone, bake for 2 minutes longer, or until the fish flakes easily. Serve hot with lemon slices for garnish.

This recipe couldn't be easier. If you like, you can add your favorite dried herbs or spices to the bread crumbs for a flavor boost.

Makes 4 servings

Per serving: 231 calories, 39 g protein, 9 g carbohydrates, 3 g total fat, 1 g saturated fat, 96 mg cholesterol, 0.5 g dietary fiber, 253 mg sodium

Tuna with Green-Herb Pesto

1   bunch fresh parsley (about 1½ cups loosely packed)

1   bunch fresh basil and/or cilantro (about 1½ cups loosely packed leaves)

2   medium cloves garlic, peeled

2   teaspoons pine nuts

    Grated peel and juice of 1 lemon

2   tablespoons extra-virigin olive oil

¼   teaspoon salt

    Ground black pepper

4   tuna steaks (4–5 ounces each)

Brown rice, jasmine rice, or boiled baby potatoes go very well with this dish.

Makes 4 servings

Per serving: 208 calories, 28 g protein, 4 g carbohydrates, 9 g total fat, 1 g saturated fat, 51 mg cholesterol, 1 g dietary fiber, 186 mg sodium

1. Cut off most of the stems from the parsley, basil, and/or cilantro. Place the leaves in the bowl of a food processor fitted with the chopping blade. Add the garlic and process for about 15 seconds, or until the herbs and garlic are well cut up. Add the pine nuts, lemon peel, half of the lemon juice, 1 tablespoon oil, salt, and pepper to taste. Process for 30 seconds, or until the mixture comes together to form a sauce. Place in a bowl and cover with plastic wrap.

2. Rinse the tuna and blot dry with paper towels. Sprinkle each side with salt and pepper to taste.

3. Warm the remaining 1 tablespoon of oil in a large nonstick skillet over medium-high heat. Add the fish and cook for 5 minutes. Turn the tuna over and cook for 3 to 5 minutes longer, or until the fish is just opaque.

4. Serve with 1 tablespoon of the pesto spooned on top of each tuna steak and drizzle with remaining lemon juice.

Mama's Meat Loaf

1	medium carrot
½	medium yellow onion
1	pound ground turkey breast
2	tablespoons Italian-style bread crumbs
2	tablespoons toasted wheat germ
½	cup canned tomato puree
2	egg whites
1	teaspoon garlic powder
1	teaspoon dried basil
1	teaspoon dried oregano
8	tablespoons ketchup
1	tablespoon honey

Makes 6 servings

Per serving: 162 calories, 21 g protein, 16 g carbohydrates, 2 g total fat, 0.5 g saturated fat, 44 mg cholesterol, 1 g dietary fiber, 375 mg sodium

1. Preheat the oven to 350°F. Grate the carrot finely using the small holes on a box grater. Peel the onion and grate finely.

2. In a large bowl, combine the carrot, onion, turkey, bread crumbs, wheat germ, tomato puree, egg whites, garlic powder, basil, oregano, and 6 tablespoons ketchup. Mix well. Transfer the mixture into a 9" x 5" loaf pan. Bake for about 55 minutes, or until the meat loaf is firm and browned. A thermometer inserted in the center should register 165°F.

3. Spread the remaining 2 tablespoons of ketchup and the honey on top of the loaf and bake for 5 minutes longer. Remove from the oven, let sit for 5 minutes, and serve.

Shepherd's Pie

Topping

3	medium red potatoes (1 pound)
6	ounces fat-free sour cream
¼	teaspoon salt or 2 teaspoons liquid aminos

Pie

3	medium yellow onions
2	tablespoons olive oil
1	pound ground turkey breast
1	cup canned tomato sauce
3	teaspoons dried oregano
2	teaspoons chili powder
1	package (12 ounces) frozen mixed vegetables, thawed
¼	cup (1 ounce) grated Parmesan cheese

Makes 8 servings

Per serving: 229 calories, 19 g protein, 26 g carbohydrates, 6 g total fat, 1 g saturated fat, 35 mg cholesterol, 2 g dietary fiber, 271 mg sodium

1. *To make the topping:* Quarter the potatoes, then cut each quarter in half. Place the potatoes in a 2-quart pot filled with water. Boil for about 12 minutes, or until the potatoes are soft and can be pierced easily with a fork or knife. Drain the potatoes and let cool slightly.

2. Place the potatoes in a medium bowl. Add the sour cream and salt or aminos. Mash with a fork until smooth. Add more sour cream if the mixture is too stiff. Set aside.

3. *To make the pie:* Preheat the oven to 350°F. Coat a 9" x 5" loaf pan with cooking spray. Set aside.

4. Peel the onions and cut into ⅛" slices. Warm the oil in a large skillet over medium heat. Add the onions and cook, stirring often, for about 10 minutes, or until the onions start to brown. Add water, 1 tablespoon at a time, as necessary to prevent burning. Transfer to a bowl to cool slightly.

5. Cook the turkey over medium heat in the same skillet used for the onions. Stir to crumble the meat. Cook until the meat is no longer pink. Add the tomato sauce, oregano, chili powder, and onions. Cook until the mixture is heated through.

6. Spoon the turkey mixture into the prepared pan. Arrange the mixed vegetables in a layer over the top. Then spread the mashed potatoes over the vegetables and top with the Parmesan.

7. Bake, uncovered, for about 35 minutes, or until the top is light brown. Cool for 10 minutes before serving.

Unfried Chicken Breasts

4 boneless, skinless chicken breast halves (about 6 ounces each)
³/₄ cup Italian-style bread crumbs
1 clove garlic
½ teaspoon ground black pepper

1. Preheat the oven to 450°F. Rinse the chicken and blot dry with paper towels.

2. Place the bread crumbs in a pie plate. Peel the garlic and chop very finely. Add to the bread crumbs along with the pepper. Toss the bread crumb mixture with a fork.

3. Coat each chicken breast with cooking spray and coat each side well with the bread crumbs.

4. Place the chicken breasts on an ungreased baking sheet and bake for 15 minutes. Turn the chicken over and cook for about 10 minutes longer on the other side, or until a thermometer inserted in the thickest portion registers 160° and the juices run clear. Serve hot.

If you want a variation on this easy, crunchy chicken dish, add a teaspoon or two of your favorite spices and/or dried herbs to the bread crumbs. I personally like to add paprika, ground red pepper, or even Cajun spice mix.

Makes 4 servings

Per serving: 263 calories, 42 g protein, 14 g carbohydrates, 3 g total fat, 1 g saturated fat, 99 mg cholesterol, 1 g dietary fiber, 249 mg sodium

Tender Chicken Salad

4	small boneless, skinless chicken breast halves (about 4 ounces each)
1	rib celery
1	large carrot
1	small apple
½	small red onion
½	cup raisins
½	cup low-fat mayonnaise
¼	cup chopped cilantro or parsley (optional)
	Ground black pepper
4	large lettuce leaves

If you like, adding a teaspoon or two of curry powder to this chicken salad brings it to a whole new level.

Makes 4 servings

Per serving: 298 calories, 28 g protein, 26 g carbohydrates, 10 g total fat, 0.5 g saturated fat, 76 mg cholesterol, 3 g dietary fiber, 94 mg sodium

1. Preheat the oven to 350°F. Rinse the chicken breasts and blot dry with paper towels. Place the chicken on a baking sheet coated with cooking spray. Bake for 25 to 35 minutes (depending on the thickness), or until a thermometer inserted in the thickest portion registers 160°F. Let cool.

2. Remove and discard the celery leaves and cut the celery rib into ⅛" to ¼" pieces. Peel the carrot, apple, and onion. Cut each into ⅛" to ¼" pieces. Place in a large bowl.

3. With your fingers, shred the cooked chicken into small pieces and add to the bowl. Add the raisins, mayonnaise, cilantro or parsley (if using), and pepper to taste. Mix well.

4. Line each of 4 plates with a lettuce leaf. Scoop the salad onto each leaf and serve.

Chicken and Root Vegetable Stew

4 large carrots
1 medium turnip
1 large parsnip
1 large Spanish (yellow) onion
1 clove garlic
2 boneless, skinless chicken breast halves (about 5 ounces each)
½ cup cauliflower florets
½ cup chopped fresh cilantro
1 teaspoon dried oregano
1 teaspoon dried basil
1 teaspoon dried rosemary
½ cup white wine
2 cups canned low-sodium tomato puree
2 tablespoons tomato paste

Makes 2 servings

Per serving: 459 calories, 42 g protein, 62 g carbohydrates, 3 g total fat, 1 g saturated fat, 82 mg cholesterol, 15 g dietary fiber, 236 mg sodium

1. Preheat the oven to 350°F. Peel the carrots, turnip, and parsnip and cut into 1" to 2" pieces. Peel the onion and garlic. Cut the onion into 1" pieces. Chop the garlic finely. Wash the chicken and blot dry with paper towels. Cut the chicken into 1" pieces.

2. In a 3- or 4-quart baking dish, combine the carrots, turnip, parsnip, onion, garlic, chicken, cauliflower, cilantro, oregano, basil, rosemary, wine, tomato puree, and tomato paste. Mix well.

3. Cover the baking dish and bake for 45 minutes to 1 hour, or until the vegetables are soft and the chicken is no longer pink and the juices run clear. Serve hot.

Stir-Fried Chicken and Vegetables

1   large Spanish (yellow) onion
2   cloves garlic
1   large red or yellow bell pepper
1   large zucchini
1   large carrot
2   scallions (green onions)
2   boneless, skinless chicken breast halves (about 5 ounces each)
2   tablespoons canola oil
2   tablespoons toasted (dark) sesame oil
2   tablespoons low-sodium soy sauce
1   tablespoon minced fresh ginger
1   cup broccoli florets
1   cup cauliflower florets
1   cup snow peas

*S*erve this dish with a helping of brown rice and you've got a tasty, and complete, meal.

Makes 4 servings

Per serving: 275 calories, 21 g protein, 16 g carbohydrates, 15 g total fat, 2 g saturated fat, 41 mg cholesterol, 5 g dietary fiber, 346 mg sodium

1. Peel the onion and garlic. Cut the onion into ¼" to ½" pieces. Set aside. Chop the garlic very finely and set aside.

2. Remove the seeds and ribs from the pepper. Cut the pepper into thin strips and set aside. Cut the zucchini into thin strips and set aside. Grate the carrot on the wide-holes side of a box grater and set aside. Slice the scallions into ⅛" to ¼" pieces and set aside.

3. Wash the chicken and blot dry with paper towels. Cut the chicken into 1" pieces. Set aside.

4. Warm 1 tablespoon each of the canola and sesame oils in a large nonstick skillet over medium heat. Add 1 tablespoon soy sauce, ½ tablespoon ginger, and half of the chopped garlic. Cook for 30 seconds to 1 minute. Add the onion, pepper, zucchini, carrot, broccoli, cauliflower, and snow peas. Cook over medium-high heat for about 10 to 15 minutes, or until the vegetables soften slightly but are cooked through. Transfer to a large bowl.

5. In the same skillet, heat the remaining 1 tablespoon each of the canola and sesame oils. Add the remaining 1 tablespoon soy sauce, the remaining half of the garlic, and the remaining ½ tablespoon ginger. Add the chicken and cook on medium-high heat for 8 minutes, or until the chicken is no longer pink and the juices run clear. Add the scallions and cook for 30 seconds longer.

6. Combine the chicken with the cooked vegetables. Toss together and serve. Refrigerate leftovers for up to 3 days.

Chicken Spring Rolls

Spring Rolls

2	large carrots
1	scallion (green onion)
¼	head napa cabbage
1	tablespoon olive oil
1	tablespoon low-sodium soy sauce
1	tablespoon minced fresh cilantro
¼	teaspoon ground black pepper
3	ounces dried bean thread noodles
1	pound grilled boneless chicken breasts
16	8" rice-paper spring-roll wrappers
2	teaspoons slivered fresh basil

Dipping Sauce

¼	cup low-sodium soy sauce
1	tablespoon honey
1½	teaspoons toasted (dark) sesame oil
½	clove garlic, chopped finely
1	teaspoon minced fresh ginger
1	tablespoon finely chopped fresh cilantro

This is an exotic and full-flavored recipe. The next time you stoke up your barbecue, grill some chicken breasts to use for this dish later. You can also substitute firm tofu for the chicken or just have plain veggie spring rolls. You can find dried bean thread noodles and spring-roll wrappers at Asian grocery stores.

Makes 16

Per roll: 164 calories, 12 g protein, 20 g carbohydrates, 3 g total fat, 1 g saturated fat, 28 mg cholesterol, 1 g dietary fiber, 378 mg sodium

1. *To make the spring rolls:* Peel the carrots and cut into ⅛" x 3" strips. Cut the scallion into ¼" slices. Thinly slice the cabbage to make ⅓ cup.

2. In a large bowl, combine the carrots, scallion, cabbage, olive oil, soy sauce, cilantro, and pepper. Mix well. Let sit at room temperature for 10 minutes, stirring occasionally.

3. Meanwhile, place the noodles in a medium bowl. Cover with boiling water and soak for about 30 minutes, or until softened. Drain well and chop into 2" pieces. Set aside. Slice the chicken breasts thinly.

4. Pour hot water into a large bowl. Using tongs, dip 1 rice-paper wrapper into the water for 5 seconds. Remove from the water and place on a wet towel. Let stand for 30 seconds. (It should be soft and pliable. If still stiff, sprinkle with more water.) Be careful not to oversoak the wrapper or it will fall apart. Repeat until all the wrappers are moistened.

5. Place a scant 2 tablespoons of the noodles, a scant 2 tablespoons of the vegetable mixture, and 1 ounce of chicken breast 1" from the lower edge of each wrapper. Sprinkle each portion with the basil. Fold the bottom edge over the filling, fold in both sides, and roll up tightly. Press to seal.

6. *To make the dipping sauce:* In a small bowl, combine the soy sauce, honey, sesame oil, garlic, ginger, and cilantro. Mix well. Serve the dipping sauce with the spring rolls.

Filet Mignon with Mushrooms

2	filet mignon steaks (4–5 ounces each)
¼	teaspoon salt
	Ground black pepper
1	clove garlic
2	large or 3 medium shallots
½	pound mushrooms
6	teaspoons olive oil
¼	cup dry red or white table wine
3	tablespoons chopped parsley

1. Season the steaks well with the salt and pepper to taste. Set aside for 15 minutes to 1 hour, or until the steaks reach room temperature.

2. Peel the garlic and shallots. Chop the garlic finely and the shallots roughly. Set aside.

3. Wash or brush the mushrooms well and dry. Cut off the bottoms of the mushroom stems. Cut the mushrooms and trimmed stems into rough ¼" to ½" chunks and set aside. Preheat the oven to 200°F.

4. Warm a cast-iron skillet over high heat until very hot. Swirl 2 teaspoons oil around the skillet for about 30 seconds. Add the steaks and let cook, undisturbed, for 5 minutes. Turn the steaks over with tongs and cook for 4 minutes longer. Transfer the steaks to an ovenproof plate and place in the oven to keep warm.

5. Reduce the heat on the stove top to medium-low. Add the remaining 4 teaspoons oil to the skillet. Add the shallots and cook for about 2 minutes, or until they start to soften. Add the mushrooms. Cook, stirring occasionally, for about 5 minutes. Add the garlic and continue cooking for 5 minutes longer. Add the wine and continue cooking, stirring and scraping the bottom of the skillet with a wooden spoon, until the wine is evaporated. Stir in the parsley and add salt and pepper to taste. Serve the mushrooms on top of the steaks.

This is a special-occasion dish because filet mignon is expensive, and while it is meltingly tender and leaner than most cuts of beef, filet mignon (especially with a nice mushroom sauce) is not exactly low-fat. To bring out the most flavor, it's best to cook filet mignon to no more than medium-rare. The main secret of cooking a great steak at home is to use a well-heated cast-iron skillet and to turn the steak only once (or twice at most) during the cooking process. A variety of wild mushrooms, including shiitake, cremini, and oyster, make the sauce a little more complex, but regular white button mushrooms work just fine, too.

Makes 2 servings

Per serving: 506 calories, 23 g protein, 8 g carbohydrates, 41 g total fat, 13 g saturated fat, 80 mg cholesterol, 2 g dietary fiber, 331 mg sodium

Oatmeal Raisin Cookies

6	tablespoons light butter or margarine
¾	cup packed light brown sugar
3	tablespoons fat-free liquid egg substitute or 2 tablespoons egg whites mixed with 1 tablespoon fat-free plain yogurt
1½	teaspoons vanilla extract
1	cup unbleached all-purpose flour
1	cup quick-cooking oats (not instant)
½	teaspoon baking soda
¾	cup raisins
1	teaspoon ground cinnamon

Makes 42

Per cookie: 48 calories, 1 g protein, 9 g carbohydrates, 1 g total fat, 1 g saturated fat, 3 mg cholesterol, 0.5 g dietary fiber, 23 mg sodium

1. Preheat the oven to 325°F. Line two baking sheets with parchment paper. Set aside.

2. In the bowl of a food processor or with an electric mixer, combine the butter or margarine, brown sugar, egg substitute or egg white mixture, and vanilla extract. Process or mix until smooth. In a large bowl, combine the flour, oats, and baking soda. Add the flour mixture to the butter or margarine mixture, and process or mix well. Stir in the raisins and cinnamon.

3. Drop rounded teaspoonfuls of dough onto the lined baking sheets, spacing them 1½" apart. Flatten each cookie slightly with the tip of a spoon or fingers dampened with water.

4. Bake for 15 to 18 minutes, or until lightly browned and crisp. Cool on the sheets on racks for 1 minute. Remove to the racks and cool completely.

Scones

1½ cups unbleached all-purpose flour
½ cup quick-cooking oats (not instant)
2 tablespoons sugar
2 teaspoons baking powder
½ teaspoon baking soda
1 teaspoon ground cinnamon (optional)
⅓ cup light butter or margarine, cold, cut into small pieces
1 egg white
6–8 ounces fat-free plain yogurt
½ cup raisins
2 tablespoons fat-free milk or 1 lightly beaten egg white

Makes 12

Per scone: 124 calories, 4 g protein, 21 g carbohydrates, 3 g total fat, 2 g saturated fat, 9 mg cholesterol, 1 g dietary fiber, 138 mg sodium

1. Preheat the oven to 375°F. Combine the flour, oats, sugar, baking powder, baking soda, and cinnamon (if using). Using 2 knives or a pastry cutter or fork, blend the butter or margarine into the flour mixture until it looks like fine crumbs. Add the egg white and enough of the yogurt to form a stiff dough (start with ¾ cup of yogurt and then add more if needed). Mix well. Stir in the raisins.

2. Form the dough into a ball and place on a lightly floured surface. With floured hands, pat the dough into a 7" circle (about 1" thick).

3. Using a 1" round cookie cutter, cut out 12 circles. (As needed, form the scraps into a new ball and flatten.) Place the cut dough on a nonstick baking sheet and brush the tops with the milk or lightly beaten egg white.

4. Bake for 10 to 15 minutes, or until light brown. Remove from the oven and let cool at least 10 minutes before eating.

Muffins Galore

1 cup quick-cooking oats (not instant)
1 tablespoon baking powder
½ cup sugar
2 cups unbleached all-purpose flour
2 egg whites
1 cup fat-free milk
⅓ cup melted light butter or margarine
2 ounces fat-free plain yogurt
1 teaspoon vanilla extract

As you'll see at the end of this recipe, this is a very adaptable muffin. Mix up the muffin base, then add your choice of flavoring to the muffin cups before baking. By adding the flavoring to the individual muffin cups instead of the whole batter, you can make a batch of 12 muffins in 12 different flavors (not that you'd want to go that crazy, but you could).

1. Preheat the oven to 350°F. Coat a 12-cup nonstick muffin pan with cooking spray or line with paper baking cups.

2. In a medium bowl, combine the oats, baking powder, sugar, and flour. Mix well. In a large bowl, combine the egg whites, milk, butter or margarine, yogurt, and vanilla extract. Mix well. Add the dry ingredients to the wet ingredients, carefully mixing them all. Do not overmix. It is acceptable if the batter is lumpy.

3. Use any of the following flavor boosters mixed inside the individual muffin cups. Bake for about 20 minutes, or until the muffins turn light brown on top.

Makes 12

Per muffin: 163 calories, 5 g protein, 29 g carbohydrates, 3 g total fat, 2 g saturated fat, 9 mg cholesterol,1 g dietary fiber, 137 mg sodium

---

Cranberry-Orange Muffin: 2 heaping tablespoons muffin base, 10 fresh or dried cranberries, and ¼ teaspoon orange juice concentrate. Or add 1 cup cranberries and 1 tablespoon orange juice concentrate to the whole recipe.

Banana-Raspberry Muffin: 2 heaping tablespoons muffin base, 2 tablespoons chopped bananas, and 5 fresh or frozen (unthawed) raspberries. Or add 1 chopped banana and ¾ cup fresh or frozen raspberries to the whole recipe.

Apple-Cinnamon Muffin: 2 heaping tablespoons muffin base, 1 tablespoon stewed apples (or 2 tablespoons peeled and chopped fresh apple), and ⅛ teaspoon ground cinnamon. Or add 1 medium apple, peeled and chopped, and ½ tablespoon ground cinnamon to the whole recipe.

Corn Muffin: 2 heaping tablespoons muffin base, 1 tablespoon cornmeal, and 2 tablespoons corn kernels. Or add ½ cup cornmeal and ¾ cup corn kernels to the whole recipe.

Blueberry Muffin: 2 heaping tablespoons muffin base and 10 fresh or frozen (unthawed) blueberries. Or add 1 cup fresh or frozen blueberries to the whole recipe.

Apple-Berry-Raisin Crumble

6–8	medium Granny Smith apples, peeled and thinly sliced (about 8 cups)
1	tablespoon cornstarch
2	cups any variety of mixed fresh or frozen berries
½	cup raisins
¼	cup + 3 tablespoons frozen apple juice concentrate, thawed
2	tablespoons honey
4	tablespoons wheat germ
3	cups quick-cooking oats (not instant)
¼	cup packed light brown sugar
1	teaspoon ground cinnamon

A nice addition to this crumble is ginger. For Apple-Ginger Crumble, add 1 teaspoon ground ginger to the filling.

Makes 10 servings

Per serving: 249 calories, 5 g protein, 55 g carbohydrates, 2 g total fat, 0.5 g saturated fat, 0 mg cholesterol, 4 g dietary fiber, 9 mg sodium

1. Preheat the oven to 375°F. In a large bowl, toss the apples with the cornstarch. Add the berries, raisins, ¼ cup juice concentrate, and honey, and toss to mix. Place the mixture in a 9" deep-dish pie pan, or use an 8" x 8" or 9" x 9" baking pan. Combine the wheat germ, oats, brown sugar, cinnamon, and the remaining 3 tablespoons juice concentrate. Mix until moist and crumbly. Sprinkle the topping over the fruit.

2. Bake for 45 minutes, or until the filling is bubbly and the topping is golden brown. Serve warm.

Baked Apples

2   large Granny Smith or other baking apples
2   tablespoons raisins
2   tablespoons honey
2   teaspoons vanilla extract
1   teaspoon ground cinnamon
2   tablespoons maple syrup

Makes 2 servings

Per serving: 245 calories, 1 g protein, 62 g carbohydrates, 1 g total fat, 0.5 g saturated fat, 0 mg cholesterol, 4 g dietary fiber, 24 mg sodium

1. Preheat the oven to 350°F. Core the apples to within ½" of the bottom. Alternatively, core the apples with an apple corer. Cut ½" of the bottom of the core and "plug" the bottoms of the apples. Peel a 1" strip of skin around the middle of each apple, or peel the upper half of the apples to prevent splitting.

2. Coat a 9" pie pan with cooking spray, and add ¼" of water to the bottom. Place the apples in the pan. Put 1 tablespoon of raisins, 1 teaspoon of honey, and 1 teaspoon of vanilla extract in each apple. Sprinkle the apples with the cinnamon. Add the remaining honey and the maple syrup to the water in the pan.

3. Cover with foil and bake for 40 minutes, basting (spooning the pan liquids over the apples) every 20 minutes. Remove the foil and bake uncovered for 10 minutes longer. Let cool for at least 10 minutes before serving. (These get very hot, so be careful.)

Blueberry Angel Food Cake

1	cup cake flour
1¼	cups sugar
1	cup fresh or frozen and unthawed blueberries
10	egg whites, at room temperature
2	teaspoons vanilla extract
¼	teaspoon almond extract (optional)

1. Preheat the oven to 350°F. Sift the flour and ½ cup of the sugar 3 times and set aside. Toss the blueberries with 2 tablespoons of the flour-sugar mixture. Set aside.

2. Using the whisk attachment of an electric hand or stand mixer, beat the egg whites until foamy. Gradually add the remaining ¾ cup sugar, 2 tablespoons at a time, while beating the egg whites. Add the vanilla extract and almond extract (if using) with the last addition of sugar. Continue to beat the egg whites until soft peaks form. Do not overbeat.

3. With a spatula, gently fold the flour-sugar mixture into the beaten egg whites, being careful not to deflate the egg whites. Very gently fold in the blueberries. Gently spoon the batter into an ungreased 10" x 4" tube pan.

4. Bake for 40 to 45 minutes, or until the cake is golden brown and springs back to the touch. Remove from the oven and immediately invert the cake onto a funnel or bottle to cool. Serve at room temperature.

*A*ngel food cake hangs upside down to cool so that its delicate structure won't collapse in on itself. In most tube pans, either the rim has feet on it or the funnel in the center is slightly higher than the rim, so the pan can balance itself as it cools. Otherwise, you can hang your pan on a heatproof funnel or bottle to cool.

Makes 12 servings

Per serving: 131 calories, 4 g protein, 29 g carbohydrates, 0.5 g total fat, 0.5 g saturated fat, 0 mg cholesterol, 0.5 g dietary fiber, 47 mg sodium

Banana-Date Cake

2	cups whole wheat flour
2¼	teaspoons baking soda
1	teaspoon cream of tartar
1	teaspoon ground cinnamon
¼	teaspoon ground nutmeg
¾	cup honey
¼	cup maple syrup
2	teaspoons vanilla extract
2	egg whites
2	very ripe bananas, pureed
1	large ripe banana, chopped
½	cup boiled water
¾	cup chopped dried dates
2	egg whites, lightly beaten

Makes 12 servings

Per serving: 219 calories, 4 g protein, 52 g carbohydrates, 1 g total fat, 0.5 g saturated fat, 0 mg cholesterol, 4 g dietary fiber, 91 mg sodium

1. Preheat the oven to 325°F. Coat a 9" Bundt pan with cooking spray. Set aside.

2. In a large bowl, combine the flour, ¾ teaspoon of the baking soda, cream of tartar, cinnamon, and nutmeg.

3. In a medium bowl, combine the honey, maple syrup, vanilla extract, 2 egg whites, and the pureed and chopped bananas. Stir in the flour mixture until just blended.

4. In a blender or food processor, combine the water, dates, and the remaining 1½ teaspoons baking soda. Blend or process on high speed until the dates are pureed. Stir into the flour-banana mixture. Gently stir the lightly beaten egg whites into the batter. Do not overmix. Spoon the batter into the Bundt pan. Bake for 1 hour, or until a toothpick inserted in the center comes out clean. Let cool.

Cinnamon Apple Crumb Cake

Cake

$2/3$	cup unbleached all-purpose flour
$2/3$	cup whole wheat flour
$1/2$	cup sugar
$1\frac{1}{2}$	teaspoons baking powder
$1/4$	teaspoon ground nutmeg
$1/2$	cup fat-free milk
$1/2$	cup unsweetened applesauce
1	egg white
3–4	peeled and sliced Granny Smith apples (2 cups)

Crumb Topping

$3/4$	cup quick-cooking oats (not instant)
1	tablespoon packed brown sugar
1	tablespoon maple syrup
$1\frac{1}{2}$	teaspoons ground cinnamon
$1\frac{1}{2}$	teaspoons toasted wheat germ

Makes 9 servings

Per serving: 179 calories, 4 g protein, 40 g carbohydrates, 1 g total fat, 0.5 g saturated fat, 0.5 mg cholesterol, 3 g dietary fiber, 72 mg sodium

1. Preheat the oven to 350°F. Coat a 9" x 9" baking pan with cooking spray. Set aside.

2. *To make the cake:* In a large bowl, combine the all-purpose flour, whole wheat flour, sugar, baking powder, and nutmeg. Add the milk, applesauce, and egg white. Mix well. Pour the batter into the baking pan, and arrange the apples on top.

3. *To make the topping:* In a medium bowl, combine the oats, brown sugar, maple syrup, cinnamon, and wheat germ. Sprinkle the topping over the apples.

4. Bake for about 40 minutes, or until a toothpick inserted into the center comes out clean. Cool and serve.

Very Creamy Cheesecake

½ cup graham cracker crumbs (from 5–6 crushed large graham crackers)
1 tablespoon + ½ cup sugar
1 package (8 ounces) reduced-fat cream cheese (Neufchâtel)
1 package (8 ounces) fat-free cream cheese
14 ounces low-fat ricotta cheese
2 eggs
2 egg whites
¼ cup + 2 tablespoons unbleached all-purpose flour
2 teaspoons vanilla extract

Makes 12 servings

Per serving: 177 calories, 11 g protein, 18 g carbohydrates, 7 g total fat, 4 g saturated fat, 59 mg cholesterol, 1 g dietary fiber, 328 mg sodium

1. Preheat the oven to 325°F. Coat a 9" springform pan with cooking spray.

2. Combine the graham cracker crumbs and 1 tablespoon sugar. Press into the pan.

3. In a blender or food processor fitted with the chopping blade, combine the reduced-fat cream cheese, fat-free cream cheese, ricotta cheese, eggs, egg whites, flour, the remaining ½ cup sugar, and vanilla extract. Blend or process until smooth. Spread over the crust. Bake for 1 hour, or until the center is set.

4. Let cool in the oven with the door ajar for 45 minutes. Chill for 8 hours or overnight.

INDEX

Underscored page references indicate boxed text. **Boldface** references indicate illustrations.

G

Conversion Chart

These equivalents have been slightly rounded to make measuring easier.

VOLUME MEASUREMENTS

U.S.	Imperial	Metric
¼ tsp	–	1 ml
½ tsp	–	2 ml
1 tsp	–	5 ml
1 Tbsp	–	15 ml
2 Tbsp (1 oz)	1 fl oz	30 ml
¼ cup (2 oz)	2 fl oz	60 ml
⅓ cup (3 oz)	3 fl oz	80 ml
½ cup (4 oz)	4 fl oz	120 ml
⅔ cup (5 oz)	5 fl oz	160 ml
¾ cup (6 oz)	6 fl oz	180 ml
1 cup (8 oz)	8 fl oz	240 ml

WEIGHT MEASUREMENTS

U.S.	Metric
1 oz	30 g
2 oz	60 g
4 oz (¼ lb)	115 g
5 oz (⅓ lb)	145 g
6 oz	170 g
7 oz	200 g
8 oz (½ lb)	230 g
10 oz	285 g
12 oz (¾ lb)	340 g
14 oz	400 g
16 oz (1 lb)	455 g
2.2 lb	1 kg

LENGTH MEASUREMENTS

U.S.	Metric
¼"	0.6 cm
½"	1.25 cm
1"	2.5 cm
2"	5 cm
4"	11 cm
6"	15 cm
8"	20 cm
10"	25 cm
12" (1')	30 cm

PAN SIZES

U.S.	Metric
8" cake pan	20 × 4 cm sandwich or cake tin
9" cake pan	23 × 3.5 cm sandwich or cake tin
11" × 7" baking pan	28 × 18 cm baking tin
13" × 9" baking pan	32.5 × 23 cm baking tin
15" × 10" baking pan	38 × 25.5 cm baking tin (Swiss roll tin)
1½ qt baking dish	1.5 liter baking dish
2 qt baking dish	2 liter baking dish
2 qt rectangular baking dish	30 × 19 cm baking dish
9" pie plate	22 × 4 or 23 × 4 cm pie plate
7" or 8" springform pan	18 or 20 cm springform or loose-bottom cake tin
9" × 5" loaf pan	23 × 13 cm or 2 lb narrow loaf tin or pâté tin

TEMPERATURES

Fahrenheit	Centigrade	Gas
140°	60°	–
160°	70°	–
180°	80°	–
225°	105°	¼
250°	120°	½
275°	135°	1
300°	150°	2
325°	160°	3
350°	180°	4
375°	190°	5
400°	200°	6
425°	220°	7
450°	230°	8
475°	245°	9
500°	260°	–